A Beginner's Guide to Targeted Cancer Treatments

A Beginner's Guide to Targeted Cancer Treatments

Elaine Vickers, PhD

Science Communicated Ltd

WILEY Blackwell

Registered Office(s)
John Wiley & Sons, Inc., 111 River Street, Hoboken, NJ 07030, USA
John Wiley & Sons Ltd, The Atrium, Southern Gate, Chichester, West Sussex, PO19 8SQ, UK

Editorial Office
9600 Garsington Road, Oxford, OX4 2DQ, UK

For details of our global editorial offices, customer services, and more information about Wiley products visit us at www.wiley.com.

Wiley also publishes its books in a variety of electronic formats and by print-on-demand. Some content that appears in standard print versions of this book may not be available in other formats.

Library of Congress Cataloging-in-Publication Data

Names: Vickers, Elaine (Elaine Ruth), author.
Title: A beginner's guide to targeted cancer treatments / by Elaine Vickers.
Description: Hoboken, NJ : Wiley, 2018. | Includes bibliographical references
    and index. |
Identifiers: LCCN 2018000469 (print) | LCCN 2018000728 (ebook) |
    ISBN 9781119126836 (pdf) | ISBN 9781119126829 (epub) | ISBN 9781119126799 (pbk.)
Subjects: | MESH: Neoplasms–drug therapy | Molecular Targeted
    Therapy–methods
Classification: LCC RC271.C5 (ebook) | LCC RC271.C5 (print) | NLM QZ 267 |
    DDC 616.99/4061–dc23
LC record available at https://lccn.loc.gov/2018000469

Cover Design: Wiley
Cover Images: (Sphere bacteria cells) © neyro2008/Gettyimages;
(Antibodies attacking cancer cells) © Eraxion/Gettyimages

Set in 9.5/13pt Palatino by SPi Global, Pondicherry, India
Printed and bound in Singapore by Markono Print Media Pte Ltd
10 9 8 7 6 5 4 3

Contents

Acknowledgments

I would like to thank Heather Phillips, Sue Bailey, and Carrie Weller for their generous support and encouragement over many years, and for providing advice and feedback on the contents of this book.

Thanks also go to the people (nurses, doctors, pharmacists, trials coordinators, and others) who read through various chapters and provided valuable comments and suggestions. They are Maggie Uzzell, Anne Croudass, Dan Collins, Ben Hood, Kate Searle, Nikki Hayward, Richard Berks, Sandra Gutcher, Sue Brook, Tom Taylor, Jo Bird, Zahid Bashir, Kate Montague-Hellen, Alasdair Rankin, and Jean Tremlett.

A special thanks goes to Ruth McLaren, who first suggested I should teach nurses and who made it possible. I would also like to thank her for inspiring me to make cancer education my full-time occupation.

Finally, I would like to thank my parents for their unending love, and my husband Rowan, for always listening and for being hugely enthusiastic about everything I do.

About the Author

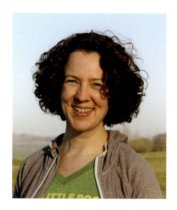

Elaine Vickers has worked as a science educator and writer for over fifteen years. Since setting up her company, Science Communicated Ltd. (www.sciencecommunicated.co.uk), she has created numerous study days and modules that explain the science behind targeted cancer treatments. Each year, she teaches hundreds of cancer nurses, doctors, and clinical research staff in hospitals and research centers throughout the United Kingdom. She is also the author and presenter of "Demystifying Targeted Cancer Treatments," an online course commissioned by Cancer Research UK. Elaine has a degree in Medical Science from the University of Birmingham and a PhD in Molecular Biology from the University of Manchester. Her goal is to unravel the complexities of cancer biology and new cancer treatments, and to make these topics interesting and accessible to non-scientists. She loves hiking and going to the ballet, and considers herself incredibly lucky to live in Manchester with her husband Rowan.

How to Use This Book

I have written *A Beginner's Guide to Targeted Cancer Treatments* because I couldn't find a resource that described how new cancer treatments worked without relying on vague generalizations or that didn't overwhelm the reader with scientific detail.

Every year, I teach hundreds of nurses, trials coordinators, pharmacists, and others involved in the delivery of cancer clinical trials and treatments. I felt I owed it to the people I teach to provide a resource that would avoid unnecessary jargon and be written in the same everyday language that I use to teach. I also wanted to give readers access to some of the illustrations I have developed during my years of teaching.

As you'll quickly realize, although I have called this book "A beginner's guide …" I do include a lot of science. I also don't try to hide the complexity of the subject I am attempting to describe. However, I hope that by including a general overview of cancer biology in Chapter 1, and an overview of monoclonal antibodies and kinase inhibitors in Chapter 2, you'll feel prepared for the later chapters.

You'll also notice that I don't describe any advances in radiotherapy or surgery. These omissions are because I'm a molecular biologist and don't feel qualified to stray into other disciplines. I have also not covered any advances made in the design or use of chemotherapy. This is partly because chemotherapies are relatively untargeted, and also because I presumed that my readers would already have a reasonable idea as to how they work. If you're looking for information on hormone therapies, you'll find it in Chapter 6, when I discuss treatments for breast cancer and prostate cancer. Also, what I can't do in this book is to pass on any medical or practical knowledge of the treatments I write about, because I have none. So if you're looking for information about the best course of treatment for a patient, or for practical advice, that information will need to come from elsewhere.

One problem I had when writing this book is the rapid pace of cancer research and drug development. For example, when I first started writing back in January 2015, just one checkpoint inhibitor (ipilimumab) was licensed in the United States and Europe to treat one type of cancer, malignant melanoma. But now, in December 2017, four checkpoint inhibitors are licensed in Europe, five in the United States, and they're used to treat people with a wide range of solid tumors and Hodgkin lymphoma. Thus, although I have done my best to make this book up to date, this up-to-dateness will be quickly eroded by the creation of new treatments and new approvals in the months and years to come. Despite this, I hope that because I have focused on the mechanisms of action of new treatments, rather than their stage of development, you will find this book relevant to you.

When writing, I have presumed that you will be coming at this subject area from one of four angles:

1. Because you've heard about **a particular treatment** and want to learn more about it – in which case you might want to start with the index and go from there.

2. Because you're involved in the care of people affected by **a particular type of cancer**, and you want to know about the treatments that are relevant to them – in which case you might be best off navigating to the section about that cancer in Chapter 6 or 7.

3. Because you've heard about **a group of treatments**, such as CDK inhibitors or checkpoint inhibitors, and you want to know how they work – in which case Chapter 3, 4, or 5 might be your starting point.

4. Because you're working in clinical trials or on wards in which you come into contact with **various new treatments**, and you want to know more about how all these treatments work – in which case you might want to start at the beginning!

Whatever your reason for reading this book, my sincere hope is that you will find it useful.

CHAPTER 1

An Introduction to Cancer Cell Biology and Genetics

IN BRIEF

It is impossible to describe targeted cancer treatments without mentioning what it is they target. And when I try to explain what it is they target, I find myself going back to the beginning and explaining where cancers come from, what faults they contain, and why they behave as they do. And in order to explain that, I need explain concepts such as different types of DNA damage, oncogenes and tumor suppressor genes, and the hallmarks of cancer cells.

Hence, in this chapter, I provide an overview of the causes and consequences of DNA mutations in cells. And I describe how even just a handful of key mutations can force a healthy cell to become a cancer cell.

I also describe the cancer microenvironment – the cells and structures that cancer cells live among. Cancer cells have the ability to exploit their microenvironment and in many instances manipulate it. I explain what impact this has when doctors come to treat people with the disease.

In addition, I tackle topics such as genomic instability and intratumoral heterogeneity. Perhaps these are topics that right now don't mean anything to you, and you're unsure of why you need to know about them. But it's only through understanding these concepts that you can appreciate the limitations of targeted (and standard) cancer treatments and the promise of immunotherapy. It is also important to understand why cancer spreads and how cancers evolve and change over time.

Finally, I wrap up the chapter with a brief overview of why cancer is so difficult to treat successfully and why so many people currently cannot be cured.

1.1 INTRODUCTION

This book is all about the science behind targeted cancer treatments. And, almost without exception, **all targeted cancer treatments work by targeting proteins** that are either inside or on the surface of cancer cells or the cells around them. So in order to explain how targeted cancer treatments work, I need to describe the proteins found in cancer cells and how they differ from those in healthy cells. In order to do this, I need to explain the different types of DNA damage that cancer cells contain, **because a cell's DNA is its instruction**

A Beginner's Guide to Targeted Cancer Treatments, First Edition. Elaine Vickers.
© 2018 John Wiley & Sons Ltd. Published 2018 by John Wiley & Sons Ltd.

manual telling it how to make proteins. If we know what DNA damage a cell contains, this will tell us what faulty proteins it's making. And if we know what faulty proteins it's making, we will know which targeted treatments might work against it.

A general understanding of the DNA damage that cancer cells contain, and what impact this has on cancer cells, should help you make sense of why some treatments are applicable to some cancer patients and not others. It should also help you understand why it can be helpful to test a patient's cancer cells for the presence or absence of various DNA mutations.

So this chapter is all about cancer cells, DNA, and proteins. And, along with the chapter that follows (which is all about the two main groups of targeted cancer treatments: monoclonal antibodies and kinase inhibitors), this chapter will hopefully provide you with all the background information you need to make sense of the rest of the book.

However, even in this chapter, I've made some assumptions about what you do and don't know. For example, I've assumed that you have a rough idea of what DNA is and how cells use their DNA to make proteins. I'm also assuming that you know what proteins are and a bit about what some of them do. If you're not familiar with these concepts, I would recommend first of all taking a look at the Appendix, which contains a list of reading material about cells, DNA, chromosomes, genes, and proteins. When you've had a look at that, you'll be ready to read further.

1.2 DNA DAMAGE IS THE CAUSE OF EVERY CANCER

Our cells' DNA is essentially a huge instruction manual telling our cells what proteins to make, how to make them, when to make

them, what to do with them, and when to destroy them. In turn, the proteins our cells make dictate their behavior. For this reason, if you damage a cell's DNA, you also end up with damaged proteins, leading to abnormal behavior.

A cancer starts to develop when a single cell accumulates DNA damage that causes it to make various faulty proteins that force it to behave abnormally. This normally doesn't happen. A cell that finds its DNA is damaged usually either tries to repair the damage, or it self-destructs through a process called apoptosis.[1] But, if a cell doesn't notice the damage and survives and later accumulates more damage, it might ultimately become a cancer cell.

Over the past 40 years or so, scientists have been gradually discovering what DNA damage cancer cells contain and how this affects their proteins. The scientists' primary focus has been to study the DNA that contains the instructions to make proteins – our cells' genes. This protein-coding DNA only takes up about 1% or so of our cells' total DNA [1]. (What exactly the other 99% of our cells' DNA is for is a matter of continued debate among scientists.)

Through initiatives such as The Cancer Genome Atlas [2] and the International Cancer Genome Consortium [3], hundreds of scientists have amassed an incredible catalog of information about the thousands of different DNA mutations cancer cells contain [4]. They've also discovered that different types of cancer differ from one another in terms of the mutations they contain and the treatments they respond to. And as well as the differences, we know that important similarities can exist between cancers that arise in different organs. For example, some breast cancer patients may have tumors that overproduce[2] a protein called HER2, as do the tumors of some patients with stomach cancer [5].

---

[1] Apoptosis is also referred to as "programmed cell death."
[2] Scientists generally talk about proteins being "over-expressed" rather than "overproduced," but they essentially mean the same thing.

Box 1.1   The names of genes and their proteins

As you read this book you might notice that protein names are written normally but that gene names are written in *italics*. For example, the *HER2* gene contains the instructions for making HER2 protein. You might also notice that sometimes the gene and protein have different names. An example of this is the *TP53* gene, which contains the instructions for making a protein called p53. It's also possible for a gene to contain the instructions for making more than one protein. For instance, the *CDKN2A* gene (sometimes referred to as the *CDKN2A* locus) contains the instructions for making several proteins, two of which are called p16^{INK4a} and p14^{ARF}.

To add to the confusion, some genes and proteins have more than one name. For example, the HER2 gene is also called *ErbB2* and *NEU*. The reasons behind the various names often have a lot to do with what organism or group of cells the gene/protein was discovered in; if it's similar to another gene/protein that has already been discovered; what role the gene/protein is thought to play in the cells or organism it was found in; and whether or not abnormalities in the gene/protein cause disease. For example, HER2 stands for human epidermal growth factor receptor-2, because it's similar in structure to HER1 (although we usually refer to HER1 as the EGF-Receptor). *HER2* is also called *ErbB2* because a very similar gene, called *Erb-b*, was discovered in a disease-causing virus called the avian erythroblastosis virus. And *HER2* is also called *NEU* because a faulty version of it can cause a cancer called neuroblastoma in rodents.

A final point to note is that gene names are often written in capital letters, whereas protein names aren't. But this convention isn't always adhered to.

Because there is lots to say about the DNA mutations in cancer cells, I'm going to split it up into different topics. First, I'll talk about what causes the DNA mutations found in cancer cells (Section 1.2.1). Then I'll describe what types of mutation occur (see Section 1.2.2), how the number of mutations in cancer cells varies (see Section 1.2.3), and which mutations have the greatest effect on cell behavior (see Section 1.2.4). Then I'll talk about some of the most common gene mutations in cancer cells and what impact they have (Section 1.2.5).

Later in the chapter, we will look at the defining characteristics of cancer cells (Section 1.3), how cancer cells in a tumor can be genetically different from one another (Section 1.4); how they interact with and influence the non-cancer cells that live alongside them (Section 1.5), and how they invade and spread (Section 1.6).

All of this information is gradually helping scientists create new, more targeted cancer treatments, which are the subject of the rest of this book.

1.2.1 Causes of DNA Mutations

There are many different reasons why our cells' DNA gets damaged. Some of this damage is natural and unavoidable, whereas some of it is down to our lifestyle, behaviors, exposures, geographical location, and even local customs.[3] We can also inherit DNA damage from our parents. Depending on

---

[3] For example, in countries like Iran, people are used to drinking much hotter tea than people do in the United Kingdom, and this has been linked to a higher incidence of esophageal cancer.

what sort of data scientists look at (e.g., whether they examine individual cells or whole organs or tissues, or look at populations of people in different countries), they end up drawing very different conclusions about what proportion of cancers could be avoided [6]. So although I've listed some of the causes of DNA damage below, I haven't tried to pin down exactly how many cancers are caused by each one.[4]

Where DNA Damage Comes from – Lifestyle and Exposures

Cells that are exposed to high levels of **carcinogens** (anything that causes cancer is called a carcinogen) are particularly vulnerable to becoming cancer cells. This includes cells that line our lungs, skin, bowel, and stomach. Carcinogens include various constituents of cigarette smoke, alcohol, sunlight, radiation from X-rays, some viruses, asbestos, and food toxins [7, 8].

Our cancer risk is also linked to our **diet** (including our consumption of fruit and vegetables, red and processed meat, high salt intake, and low fiber), our level of **physical activity**, and our **weight**. This is a huge topic. If you would like to read more, I suggest looking at the Cancer Research UK [9, 10] and American Cancer Society [11] websites.

Where DNA Damage Comes from – Inherited Mutations

Some people are **born with DNA faults** that put them at higher risk of cancer than the people around them. Sometimes the fault has been passed down from generation to generation, with many family members affected. For example, actress and film director Angelina Jolie has inherited a fault in one copy of her

BRCA1 gene. Because this fault is shared by many of her relatives, she lost her mother, grandmother, and aunt to cancer [12]. Faults in high-risk genes such as BRCA genes are generally rare, but they can have an enormous impact on a person's cancer risk. More commonly, subtle variations in many genes will combine to affect our risk.

Faults can also arise in a mother's egg or a father's sperm. If the faulty egg or sperm goes on to create an embryo, this fault will be present in every cell. Or, the fault might occur later, as the growing embryo is developing. For example, faults that occur in an embryo's white blood cells as its immune system forms can cause infant or childhood leukemia [13].

Where DNA Damage Comes from – Chemical Reactions

Unfortunately for us, **our cells' DNA gets damaged every second of every day** – it is estimated that even without the influence of external factors like diet, smoking, or sunlight, each of our cells sustains damage to its DNA roughly 20,000 times each day [14].

Much of this damage is caused by the products of chemical reactions that are essential to keep us alive. For example, many of our cells' important chemical reactions produce oxygen free radicals[5] – high-energy oxygen atoms that essentially bash into and break DNA [15]. Our cells contain well over 100 different DNA repair proteins to fix this damage [16]. But sometimes they fail to spot all the damage, or they simply can't keep up.

Where DNA Damage Comes from – DNA Polymerase

Tissues that need to renew and replenish their cells often (such as the lining of our bowel, our

---

[4] If you do want to learn more about what you can do to reduce your risk, I would recommend looking at the Cancer Research UK website: http://www.cancerresearchuk.org/about-cancer/causes-of-cancer/can-cancer-be-prevented.
[5] These are also called reactive oxygen species – ROS.

skin, and immune system) are the most at risk of cancer [17–19].[6] This is because for a cell to multiply, it has to make a complete copy of all of its DNA – all 3,000 million base pairs of it [20]. The enzyme that copies DNA, called DNA polymerase, although spectacularly fast and accurate, does occasionally make mistakes [21]. Therefore, cells that have to multiply often are at a greater risk of becoming cancer cells than cells that rarely, if ever, multiply.

Where DNA Damage Comes from – APOBEC Enzymes

APOBEC[7] enzymes are a family of proteins that our cells use to help protect them from virus infections. APOBEC enzymes attack viruses by introducing mutations into their DNA. However, if an uninfected cell accidentally makes APOBEC enzymes, the enzymes will attack the cell's own DNA and introduce lots of mutations that could cause cancer [22]. Also, even when the cell has become a cancer cell, APOBEC enzymes continue to add more and more damage to the cell's genes [23].

Where DNA Damage Comes from – Cancer Treatments

Most chemotherapies and radiotherapy work by causing so much DNA damage that cancer cells die. However, not every cell is killed. Cells that sustain damage to their DNA and yet survive may later become cancer cells. Because of this, people treated for cancer sometimes develop second cancers months or even many years later.

The Influence of Sex Hormones

When discussing the causes of cancer, we shouldn't ignore the influence of sex hormones such as estrogen, progesterone, and testosterone. These tiny, fat-soluble chemicals encourage cells that contain receptors for them to survive, grow, and multiply (estrogen can also cause DNA damage [24]). Cancers that develop from hormone-sensitive tissues in the breast and prostate often retain their sensitivity to hormones. These cancers respond to treatments that block the production of hormones in the body or that block the impact of hormones on cancer cells.

In women, the risk of various cancers, including breast, ovarian, and endometrial cancer, is linked to their body's exposure to sex hormones such as estrogen. Reproductive factors (such as age of menarche[8] and menopause, along with the number of pregnancies and length of time they breast-fed) and bodyweight affect their lifetime exposure to estrogen and thus also influence their cancer risk.

The Influence of Inflammation

For many people, their cancer diagnosis was preceded by years of inflammation, infection, or irritation [25]. For example, people with chronic hepatitis B or hepatitis C are at high risk of liver cancer, whereas people with inflammatory bowel disease are at an increased risk of bowel cancer [25]. It seems that the presence of white blood cells in a tissue can increase the DNA mutation rate in the tissues' cells and encourage the cells to multiply, raising the risk of cancer [26].

---

[6] If this seems like a simple and straightforward association, don't be fooled. There is huge controversy around the exact relationship between cancer risk and tissue renewal, number of stem cells, and DNA damage by environmental versus natural mechanisms. I've supplied a handful of references if you want to explore further.
[7] In case you're curious, APOBEC stands for apolipoprotein B mRNA editing enzyme, catalytic polypeptide-like.
[8] The age at which a girl has her first period.

The Influence of Epigenetics

Epigenetics refers to chemical changes to the DNA double helix and to histone proteins that DNA wraps around [27, 28]. Epigenetic changes don't alter the sequence of the four bases in DNA. But epigenetic changes do affect how compact and tightly coiled DNA is. This in turn affects whether the information in genes is accessible to the cell's transcription factors and whether the genes can be used to make proteins. For example, if a stretch of DNA in a chromosome is very compact, it won't be transcribed. But if it's relaxed, it's available for transcription. The pattern of epigenetic changes in our DNA appears to be partly inherited from our parents, but it may also be affected by inflammation, exposure to some chemicals, nutrition, and our own and possibly even our parents' lifestyles. Epigenetics is also affected by many of the gene mutations found in cancer cells [29].

Causes of DNA Mutations – Summary

Our risk of cancer in any particular place in our body is therefore a combination of:

- Our age
- The natural rate that the cells multiply in that tissue
- The extent to which DNA polymerase, oxygen free radicals, and APOBEC enzymes have caused mutations in the tissue's cells (the amount of damage will gradually increase as we age)
- Our sex, our lifestyle, and behaviors (which will be hugely impacted by our cultural background, physical location, and personal choices and opportunities)
- Our cells' exposure to carcinogens, hormones, and factors that cause inflammation
- Our inherited genetic and epigenetic makeup

Cancer Research UK estimates that around 42% of cancers are potentially preventable through changes to lifestyle, behaviors, exposures, and weight [30, 31]. However, we cannot influence factors such as the activity of APOBEC enzymes or the accuracy of DNA polymerase. As I said before, estimating what proportion of cancers can be prevented is an incredibly contentious topic, and estimates vary widely depending on how the research was done.

1.2.2 Types of DNA Mutations

As we've seen, DNA damage is caused by a wide variety of different factors. Some causes of damage are natural and unavoidable, and others are potentially avoidable.

DNA mutations also come in many forms. For the sake of simplicity, I'm going to split them into two groups: (1) mutations affecting long stretches of DNA and whole chromosomes and (2) mutations affecting just a few DNA base pairs.

Mutations Affecting Long Stretches of DNA and Whole Chromosomes

For a start, many cancers are aneuploid – that is, the cells contain the wrong number (i.e., not the normal 23 pairs) of chromosomes [32]. However, although this is no doubt important, it's not always clear what impact this is having on the cell. Because the detection of extra chromosomes in cancer cells doesn't generally help doctors decide what treatment to use, I'm not going to talk about this further.

What can be more helpful is detecting chromosome faults such as translocations, inversions, insertions, deletions, and amplifications.

Chromosome Translocations and Rearrangements

A chromosome translocation is when two chromosomes break, and the cell accidentally sticks them back together incorrectly (see Figure 1.1). Chromosomal rearrangements are similar, but both breaks occur in a single chromosome. More often than not, the

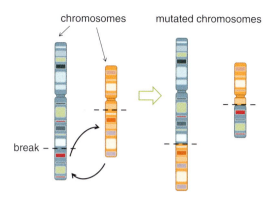

chromosomes   mutated chromosomes

break

Figure 1.1 A chromosome translocation. Two chromosomes (colored turquoise and orange) break. The cell accidentally sticks them back together incorrectly. If the chromosomes have broken where genes are located, this may result in the creation of a gene fusion.

chromosomes break in regions that don't contain any genes (remember that the information to make proteins only takes up 1% or so of our chromosomes). However, **sometimes translocations and rearrangements do affect genes**, and this can have dire consequences. For example, the cancer cells of chronic myeloid leukemia (CML) almost always contain a translocation in which chromosome 9 and chromosome 22 have broken and been stitched back together incorrectly. This causes the *BCR* gene on chromosome 22 to become fused together with the *ABL* gene on chromosome 9 [33]. The fusion of these two genes forces the cell to make a Bcr-Abl **fusion protein** (a protein made from the information in the fusion gene), which forces the cells to grow and multiply.

In other cancers, you find translocations and rearrangements in which a control region from one gene (a promoter or enhancer[9]) has become fused to the protein-coding region[10] of

a second gene. This has often happened during the development of prostate cancer and some forms of blood cancer such as non-Hodgkin lymphomas and multiple myeloma. In prostate cancer, the rearrangement often involves the *ERG* and *TMPRSS2* genes on chromosome 21. The rearrangement places the promoter from the *TMPRSS2* gene (a gene which is always active in prostate cells) next to the protein-coding region from a powerful, pro-growth protein called *ERG* [34] (see Figure 1.2). The consequence of this rearrangement is the massive overproduction of ERG protein, which forces the prostate cell to multiply.

Chromosome Insertions
This occurs when **part of one chromosome is inserted into another chromosome** (Figure 1.3). It can also occurs when part of a chromosome is re-inserted back into the chromosome it came from, but in the wrong place. An example is the "internal tandem duplications" affecting the *FLT3* gene that are found in the cancer cells of around a third of people with acute myeloid leukemia (AML) [35]. The insertion involves part of the FLT3 gene, which is copied and re-inserted back into the gene. This causes the cell to make an extra-large, overactive version of FLT3 protein. FLT3 inhibitors are in clinical trials. (See Chapter 7, Section 7.10.1 and Figure 7.21 for more about FLT3 mutations in AML.)

Chromosome Deletions
Not surprisingly, a chromosome deletion is when **part of a chromosome gets deleted** (Figure 1.4a). Examples include deletion of the part of chromosome 17 that contains the *TP53* gene, and deletion of the part of chromosome 9 containing the *CDKN2A* gene. Both *TP53*

---

[9] The Khan Academy website has a nice description of gene regulation: https://www.khanacademy.org/science/biology/gene-regulation/gene-regulation-in-eukaryotes/a/overview-of-eukaryotic-gene-regulation.
[10] That is, the part of the gene that contains the instructions to make a protein.

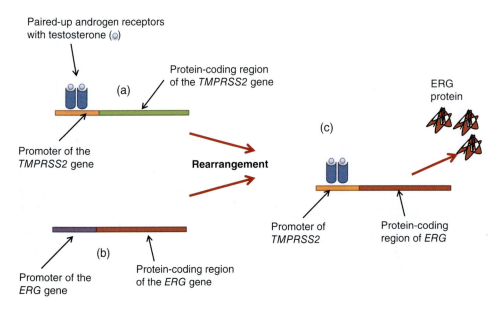

Figure 1.2 **The TMPRSS2-ERG gene fusion found in prostate cancer cells**. **(a)** In healthy prostate cells, androgen receptors pair up due to the presence of testosterone. Paired-up receptors then attach to the TMPRSS2 gene promoter and cause the cell to produce TMPRSS2 protein. **(b)** In contrast, prostate cells only rarely produce ERG, because the ERG gene does not contain attachment sites for androgen receptors. **(c)** 50% of prostate cancers contain a chromosome rearrangement which puts the protein-coding region of the ERG gene under the control of the promoter from the TMPRSS2 gene. This mutation causes the cell to produce ERG, which in turn forces the cell to multiply.

and *CDKN2A* are vital tumor suppressor genes that prevent our cells from becoming cancer cells (there is more about *TP53* and *CDKN2A* in Section 1.2.5). Their loss means that part of the cell's protection against cancer has gone.

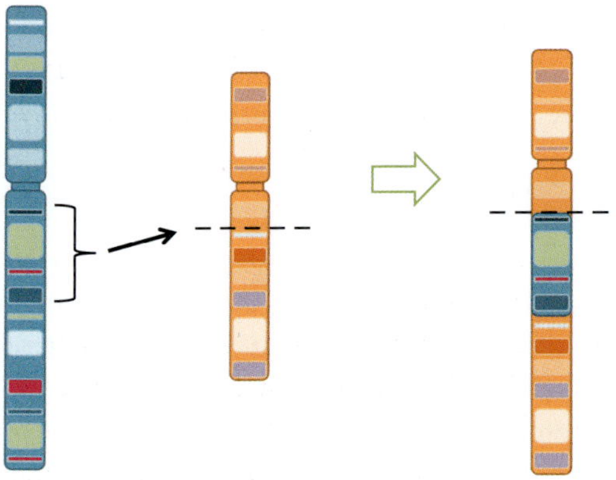

Chromosome Inversions

Inversions (Figure 1.4b), in which part **of a chromosome is cut out, flipped over, and then re-inserted**, can also disrupt genes. For example, an inversion of part of chromosome 2 is found in about 4% of non-small cell lung cancers (this is the most common type of lung cancer). The inversion joins together the *ALK* gene with part of the *EML4* gene, creating an uncontrollable fusion protein that forces the cells to multiply [36]. Three ALK inhibitors are now licensed treatments for ALK-mutated lung cancers; they are crizotinib (Xalkori), alectinib (Alacensa), and ceritinib (Zykadia). (For more about ALK mutation in lung cancer, and ALK inhibitors, see Chapter 4, Section 4.2.4 and Chapter 6, Section 6.4.4.)

Figure 1.3 **A chromosome insertion** – part of one chromosome is inserted into another chromosome (as shown) or back into the same chromosome but in the wrong location.

(a)　　　　　　　(b)

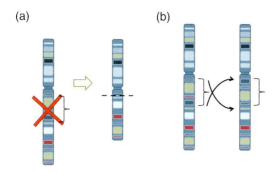

Figure 1.4 Chromosome deletions and inversions. (a) In a chromosome deletion, part of a chromosome is (not surprisingly) deleted. An example is the deletion of part of chromosome 17 containing the *TP53* gene in chronic lymphocytic leukemia, bowel cancer, and other cancers. **(b) Chromosome inversion** – a segment of the chromosome is cut out, flipped over, and inserted back into the chromosome; for example, inversions involving the *ALK* gene on chromosome 2 in lung cancer.

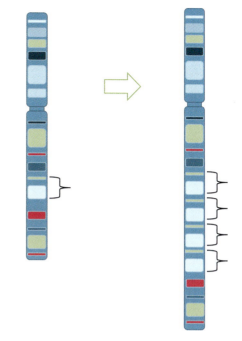

Figure 1.5 Gene amplification. The cell accidently makes extra copies of part of a chromosome. The duplicate segments are inserted into other chromosomes or back into the same chromosome; for example, amplification of a segment of chromosome 17 containing the *HER2* gene in breast cancer.

Gene Amplification

Lastly, one of the most commonly looked for types of chromosome damage is gene amplifications. Gene amplifications occur when a cell's DNA replication machinery **accidentally makes extra copies of a region of a chromosome** that contains one or more genes (see Figure 1.5). As a consequence, the cell overproduces (over-expresses) the proteins made from the amplified genes. A common amplification is that of the *HER2* gene (the HER2 gene is also commonly called *Neu* or *ErbB*), which is amplified in about 18%–20% of breast cancers [37].

Point Mutations

A point mutation is when **one DNA base is accidentally added, deleted, or swapped** for a different one. Most point mutations have no impact on the cell as they occur outside of genes. However, if a point mutation (such as

a base substitution, addition, or deletion) occurs within a gene, it can have various consequences (see Figure 1.6).[11] Point mutations are classed as missense, nonsense, or silent, depending on what consequence the mutation has on protein production. They are also classified as "in-frame" or "frameshift" mutations.

Missense Mutations

If one DNA base is substituted for a different one, this might mean that the **protein made from that gene differs by one amino acid** from the normal protein (three DNA bases in a gene equate to one amino acid in the resulting

---

[11] If you need a refresher on gene transcription and translation at this point, I suggest taking a look at some of the resources suggested in the Appendix.

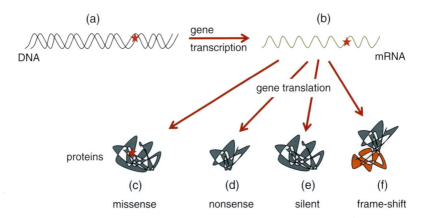

Figure 1.6 **Point mutations.** A point mutation (shown by a red star) is when one DNA base is added, deleted, or swapped for a different one in the cell's DNA **(a)**. If the mutation is in a gene, the mutation will be copied into the mRNA **(b)** and it may alter the resulting protein. The consequence might be that **(c)** due to a **missense mutation,** the protein made by the cell differs from the normal (the so-called "wild-type") version of the protein by one amino acid, **(d) a nonsense mutation in** the DNA introduces a stop signal into the mRNA, and the cell makes an extra-short (truncated) protein, **(e)** a **silent mutation** has no impact on the protein produced, **(f)** a **frameshift** mutation causes the cell to make a very different protein compared to the normal protein, one which is only partly the same as the original.

protein) (Figure 1.6c) [38]. Two examples are the faulty version of the B-Raf protein (called V600E), which is often found in the cancer cells of people with malignant melanoma, and some of the faulty versions of EGFR (epidermal growth factor receptor), which are found in the cancer cells of some people with lung cancer. In both cases, the faulty proteins (both of which contain hundreds of amino acids) are just one amino acid different from the healthy version of the protein. However, even changing that one amino acid is sufficient to create a massively overactive version of B-Raf or EGFR.

Nonsense Mutations

Nonsense mutations are those that cause the cell to make a shortened (truncated) version of the protein (Figure 1.6d). This happens because the change to the DNA sequence creates a "stop codon" in the resulting mRNA strand. As you might already know, proteins are made from 20 different amino acids, and

each set of three bases (called a codon) in the mRNA strand tells the ribosome what amino acid to add next to the protein it's making.[12] But there are three codons (UAA, UAG, and UGA) which tell the ribosome to stop adding any more amino acids. If a DNA point mutation creates one of these stop codons part way through the mRNA from a gene, then the ribosome will stop part way through making the protein. For example, some of the inherited *BRCA* gene mutations that increase a woman's risk of breast and ovarian cancer cause her cells to produce a shortened version of a BRCA protein [39].

Silent Mutations

These point mutations don't have any impact on the protein the cell makes even if they occur within a gene (Figure 1.6e). For example, if a ribosome comes across the mRNA sequence CCC, this tells it to add a proline amino acid to the protein it's making. If a point mutation

---

[12] If you're struggling to make sense of this, I would suggest looking at the Appendix and learning a bit about gene transcription and translocation.

changes the mRNA from CCC to CCA, this has no impact because the sequence CCA also tells the ribosome to add a proline.

In-Frame and Frameshift Mutations

If one or two DNA bases are added or deleted to a gene's sequence, this can create a frameshift mutation that has an enormous impact on what protein is produced (Figure 1.6f). An example is if one DNA base is added to a gene that changes the mRNA from ....CGACGACGA.... to ...CCGACGACGA.... Now, instead of reading the sequence as …CGA CGA CGA… adding three arginine amino acids to the protein, the ribosome reads …CCG ACG ACG A… and adds a proline followed by two threonines. The ribosome carries on going from there, adding a completely different selection of amino acids from the normal selection. As a result, **the protein the cell makes may bear very little resemblance to the normal protein**. Frameshift mutations also commonly introduce stop codons that create truncated proteins.

An "in-frame" mutation is opposite to a frameshift mutation – that is, it is a mutation that either swaps one base for a different one, or one in which bases are added in multiples of three, so they don't alter the rest of the protein made. For example, if three bases are added to ....CGACGACGA.... so that it becomes ....CGA**CCC**CGACGA…, the ribosome will insert an extra proline in between the arginines, but it has no further impact on the rest of the protein.

1.2.3 Numbers and Patterns of DNA Mutations in Cancer Cells

In recent years, technologies have been developed that allow scientists to pinpoint the location of thousands of DNA mutations inside cancer cells. They have discovered that **different cancers contain different numbers, types, and patterns of mutations that arise due to different mutational processes**. For example, lung cancers from smokers contain lots of point mutations in which a C has been changed to an A. A different pattern of mutations – where there are lots of insertions and deletions of more than three DNA bases at a time – is common in people with cancers associated with inherited *BRCA* gene mutations. Other patterns are linked to overactive APOBEC enzymes. In all, scientists have so far discovered 30 different patterns of mutations, which they call "mutation signatures" [40]. And, of course, it's possible for one cancer cell to contain multiple patterns of mutations because the cancer has arisen due to a combination of causes.

The amount of damage in cancer cells' DNA varies greatly from cancer type to cancer type [41]. For example, cancers that have come about because of the effects of powerful carcinogens often contain a vast amount of DNA damage. Therefore, lung cancers in people who smoke or have smoked in the past contain ten times the number of mutations as lung cancers in people who have never smoked. Malignant melanoma skin cancers, which are almost always caused by UV light from the sun, also contain a vast number of mutations [41]. In general, cancers in older people contain more mutations than those in children and young adults. Older peoples' cells have simply had many more years in which to accumulate mutations.

Although cancer cells often contain hundreds or even thousands of mutations, the majority of these mutations have no discernible impact on the cell's behavior. They have occurred because the cancer cell is damaged and unstable and is picking up new mutations all the time. The mutations that are important in driving the cancer cells' abnormal behavior are referred to by scientists as **driver mutations**. Mutations that add little or nothing to the cells' behavior are called **passenger mutations**.

Perhaps not surprisingly, scientists are much more interested in finding a cancer's driver mutations than its passenger mutations. They want to know what's driving the cells' behavior so that they can do something about it.

1.2.4 Driver Mutations – Those That Affect Cancer Cell Behavior

In order for DNA damage to cause cancer, some of it must occur in genes that control the cell's behavior. These "driver mutations" affect cell processes and behaviors such as:

- How fast the cell grows
- How frequently it multiplies
- The way it communicates with neighboring cells
- How often and how well it checks its own health
- Its ability to survive in adverse conditions such as low oxygen levels
- Its ability to move through the body's tissues
- Whether it goes through all the normal checks and balances during the cell cycle[13]
- Whether it still has the ability to self-destruct
- The way it produces energy
- Whether it can hide from or suppress the person's immune system

The genes that have caused these changes in behavior are classed as oncogenes, tumor suppressor genes, and DNA repair genes.

Oncogenes

Many of the proteins made from these genes encourage our cells **to survive, grow, and multiply**. Others can make cells more **mobile and invasive** or help them to **hide from the immune system**. All these genes need to be tightly controlled to avoid cancer. In cancer cells, they're damaged in a way that they're overproduced and/or overactive. Examples of oncogenes include *EGFR, RAS, B-RAF, MYC, HER2,* and *SRC.*

Tumor Suppressor Genes

The proteins made from these genes **slow down or stop cell growth and proliferation and trigger cell death (apoptosis)**. In cancer cells, they're damaged in a way that causes their protection to be lost. Examples include *TP53, PTEN, RB1,* and *APC.*

DNA Repair Genes

The proteins made from these genes **sense and repair DNA damage**. In cancer cells, they're damaged in such a way that they can no longer do their job properly. Because of this, cancer cells pick up more and more DNA damage as time goes on. Examples of DNA repair genes include *BRCA1, BRCA2, ATM, ATR, RAD51,* and *ERCC1.*

In healthy cells, the proteins made from DNA repair genes keep the cell's DNA free from faults. There is also a balancing act between the oncogenes and the tumor suppressor genes. For example, a protein called Bcl-2 protects cells from death, whereas a protein called p53 triggers death. The gene for making Bcl-2 (called *BCL2*) is an oncogene; the gene for making p53 (called *TP53*) is a tumor suppressor gene. Healthy cells contain strict amounts of both proteins that balance each other out. But cancer cells often contain too much Bcl-2 and too little, or faulty, p53.

Multiple Driver Mutations Are Necessary for a Cell to Become a Cancer Cell

The sequence of events that leads to bowel cancer is often given as an example of how the gradual accumulation of mutations in several oncogenes, tumor suppressor genes, and DNA repair genes can ultimately cause someone to develop cancer.

---

[13] The cell cycle is the normal, step-by-step process our cells go through when they multiply.

Our bowel is lined by orderly layers of cells known as epithelial cells. Because bowel cells are constantly getting scraped off by food passing through, our bowel cells have to multiply pretty often in order to keep the number of cells constant. Cells that multiply are prone to picking up mutations. So our bowel cells tend to contain more and more mutations as we get older. If a mutation affects a gene called *APC*, this is bad news as *APC* is an important tumor suppressor gene. But the situation isn't desperate as it's only one mutation, which isn't enough to cause cancer. However, if it's followed by a mutation in *KRAS*, then the situation becomes worse; *KRAS* is a powerful growth-promoting oncogene that forces the cell to multiply more rapidly. As the cells multiply, they pick up yet more mutations. The cell still isn't a cancer cell because other protective proteins are still doing their job. But if genes such as *PIK3CA* (an oncogene), *SMAD4* (a tumor suppressor gene), and *TP53* (a tumor suppressor gene) become faulty, then the cell will become a full-blown cancer cell [41] (see Figure 1.7 for an illustration of this process).

In other cancers, a similar **combination of mutations in a handful of important genes** is thought to drive their behavior [42].

1.2.5 The "Usual Suspects" – Genes Commonly Mutated in Many Cancers

Some gene mutations are common only in one or two types of cancer. These include the *VHL* mutations that are very common in kidney cancer and some of the translocations that are very common in hematological cancers (such as leukemias, lymphomas, and multiple myeloma). But **other gene mutations crop up time and time again** in many different cancer types. I'll be mentioning some of these gene mutations again and again in this book, so I've listed a handful of them in Table 1.1 to give you a rough idea of what they do.

One thing that might (or might not!) jump out at you from the table is that that many of the most commonly mutated genes in cancer cells are involved in **cell communication pathways**. These pathways are used by all our

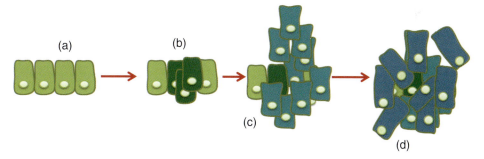

(a)   (b)   (c)   (d)

Figure 1.7 The series of mutations leading to many bowel cancers. (a) Orderly, well-connected cells line the bowel. **(b)** A random mutation in a bowel cell lead to loss of APC activity; this cell starts to multiply slightly faster than its neighbors, forming a little lump – an adenoma. The faulty cells are not yet cancer cells, but because they are multiplying more quickly than normal, they are prone to collecting more mutations. **(c)** Weeks, months, or years later, a mutation in the *KRAS* gene causes the K-Ras protein to become overactive; the cells now multiply rapidly and in a disorderly fashion. **(d)** Finally, genes like *TP53*, *PIK3CA*, and *SMAD4* are mutated. The faulty cells are now full-blown cancer cells, able to invade through local tissues and spread to other parts of the body.
Abbreviations: *APC* – adenomatous polyposis coli; *TP53* – tumor protein 53; *PIK3CA* -phosphatidylinositol-4,5-bisphosphate 3-kinase catalytic subunit alpha; *SMAD4* – SMAD family member 4

Table 1.1   A selection of some of the most commonly mutated oncogenes, tumor suppressor genes, and DNA repair genes in human cancers.

Gene name (protein name)	What protein is made from this gene?	What is the consequence for the cell if the gene is mutated?
Oncogenes		
RAS (Ras)	The three Ras proteins (K-Ras, N-Ras, and H-Ras) are enzymes involved in cell communication. There are three versions of the gene (*KRAS, NRAS,* and *HRAS*), which contain the instructions for making the three proteins [43].	All the proteins made from these genes are involved in cell communication pathways – the sequences of events triggered inside a cell when it receives a signal to grow and multiply from its neighbors. Therefore, all these proteins cause cells to grow and multiply. Overactive communication pathways also force cells to survive (even when damaged) and to become more mobile and invasive.
PIK3CA (p110-alpha)	The PI3K protein is an enzyme involved in cell communication. It comes in many different forms and is made up of two component parts: an enzyme part and a regulatory part. The *PIK3CA* gene encodes an enzyme part called p110alpha (p110α) [44].	
HER2/NEU/ ERBB2 (HER2)	A receptor found on the cell surface; it activates cell communication pathways inside the cell [45].	For more on cell communication pathways and how they work, see Chapter 3, Section 3.2.
MYC (MYC)	A transcription factor – it attaches to various gene promoters and triggers gene transcription. Many of the genes it controls are involved in cell growth and proliferation [46].	
BRAF (B-Raf)	An enzyme involved in cell communication and activated by Ras proteins [47].	
EGFR (EGFR)	A receptor found on the cell surface; it activates cell communication pathways inside the cell [45].	
Tumor suppressor genes		
TP53 (p53)	A transcription factor activated by DNA damage and other triggers – it attaches to various gene promoters and triggers gene transcription. The proteins produced as a result of p53 block cell proliferation and cause cell death [48].	If p53 is not working properly or is missing from a cell, the cell loses the ability to stop multiplying or die in response to DNA damage.
PTEN (PTEN)	An enzyme involved in cell communication that blocks the activity of PI3K. PTEN also helps cells avoid DNA damage [49].	If PTEN is not working properly or is missing from a cell, the PI3K-controlled communication pathway becomes overactive.
RB (RB)	It has a pocket in it that fits E2F proteins, which control entry into the cell cycle[a]. RB holds onto and blocks E2F proteins, and this prevents the cell from entering the cell cycle [50].	If RB is not working properly or is missing from a cell, E2F can force the cell into the cell cycle (for more about RB and E2F, see Chapter 4, Section 4.5).
CDKN2A (p16 INK4a)	p16[INK4a] is a protein that blocks a set of enzymes called the CDKs. The CDKs force RB to let go of E2F proteins (see the description of RB above). Hence, p16 prevents cells from entering the cell cycle (see Chapter 4, Figures 4.18 and 4.19) [50].	If p16 [INK4a] is not working properly or is missing from a cell, E2F can force the cell into the cell cycle.
NF1 (neuro-fibromin)	A large protein that inactivates Ras proteins (see the description of Ras earlier in this table) [51].	If neurofibromin is not working properly or is missing from a cell, Ras proteins become overactive.
APC	The surface of the APC protein has various different regions through which it interacts with many different proteins involved in cell communication, mobility, adhesion to neighboring cells, and other processes [52].	If APC is not working properly or is missing from a cell, then levels of another protein, beta-catenin (β-catenin), rise. Beta-catenin causes cells to multiply.

Table 1.1   (Continued)

DNA repair genes

***BRCA1* (BRCA1) & BRCA2 (BRCA2)**	BRCA1 and BRCA2 are both necessary for a DNA repair process called homologous recombination (HR). Our cells use HR to accurately repair double-strand breaks in their DNA (see Chapter 4, Section 4.3. for more information on BRCA proteins).	If either BRCA1 or BRCA2 is not working properly or is missing from a cell, the cell can no longer perform HR. It is therefore liable to pick up lots of DNA mutations.
ATM & ATR	These are enzymes whose activity is triggered when a cell detects that its DNA is damaged. They coordinate the cell's response to the damage [53].	If either ATM or ATR is damaged or missing from a cell, its ability to respond to DNA damage is compromised.

Abbreviations: *PIK3CA* – phosphatidylinositol-4,5-bisphosphate 3-kinase catalytic subunit alpha; HER2 – human epidermal growth factor receptor-2; EGFR – epidermal growth factor receptor; TP53 – tumor protein p53; PTEN – phosphatase and tensin homologue; RB – retinoblastoma protein; NF1 – neurofibromatosis type 1; APC – Adenomatous polyposis coli; BRCA – Breast cancer susceptibility gene; ATM – ataxia-telangiectasia mutated; ATR – ATM- and Rad3-Related
[a] The cell cycle is the very orderly and precise sequence of events that a cell goes through in order to multiply.
Source: Kandoth C et al. (2013). Mutational landscape and significance across 12 major cancer types. *Nature* **502**: 333–339.

body's cells to sense and respond to: changes in their environment, signals sent out by neighboring cells, the presence or absence of hormones, and signals sent out by white blood cells. A wide variety of communication pathways exist in our cells. And there are some proteins like Ras and PI3K that are involved in many different signaling pathways. These pathways are often the target of new cancer drugs, and the whole of Chapter 3 is dedicated to explaining them and the cancer drugs that block them.

1.3 THE DEFINING FEATURES (HALLMARKS) OF CANCER CELLS

All cancers are presumed to begin with a single cell that has sustained damage to its DNA and has multiplied out of control. As an adult, it's probably true that every cell in our body contains some sort of damage to its DNA.

However, what sets a cancer cell apart from a non-cancer cell is:

- The **amount** and **type** of DNA damage the cells contain
- The **location** of this damage in oncogenes, tumor suppressor genes, and DNA repair genes
- The **changes in behavior** that the damage causes

The behavioral changes that set a cancer cell apart from a healthy cell are collectively known as "the hallmarks of cancer." Six hallmarks were listed and described by two scientists called Douglas Hanahan and Robert Weinberg back in 2000 [54], and they added two more in 2011 [55]. I've described all eight below.

1.3.1 The Eight Hallmarks of Cancer

1. They can tell themselves to multiply. A normal cell only multiplies when it receives an instruction[14] to do so. A cancer cell can generate those instructions itself.

---

[14] This instruction is usually in the form of small proteins known as "growth factors" released by the cells' near neighbors – see Chapter 3, Section 3.2.1 for more on this.

2. **They are insensitive to negative feedback**, because proteins that would normally tell them to stop multiplying and die (like p53) have been lost or don't work properly.

3. **They resist death**. Every day, millions of cells in our body self-destruct because they have worn out or become damaged. Cancer cells have defects that make it almost impossible for them to do this.

4. **Cancer cells can multiply forever** because they contain a protein called telomerase. Healthy cells lack this protein and eventually stop multiplying.

5. **They gain a blood supply**. Cancer cells release a tiny protein called VEGF that tells nearby blood vessels to sprout and grow (a process called **angiogenesis**). New blood vessels supply the growing cancer with oxygen and nutrients.

6. **They can invade and spread**. Most of our body's cells are connected to each other in orderly arrangements. Cancer cells have lost connective proteins from their surface, and they are independent and mobile.

7. **They have changed the way they produce energy**. Healthy cells use sugars from our food to make energy using a highly efficient, oxygen-dependent process. Cancer cells use an inefficient process that requires less oxygen but helps them multiply more quickly.

8. **They can avoid destruction by the immune system**. White blood cells constantly patrol our body looking for defective cells. Cancer cells hide from white blood cells; suppress cancer-fighting white blood cells; co-opt white blood cells for their own purposes (there is lots more about this in Chapter 5 on immunotherapy).

1.4 GENETIC VARIATION AMONG CANCER CELLS IN A SINGLE TUMOR

A major reason why many tumors fail to respond to treatment or become resistant later is **intratumoral heterogeneity** – the fact that inside a tumor there are various populations of cancer cells that are genetically different from one another (see Figure 1.8).

In fact, scientists analyzing multiple biopsies from a single tumor have found huge variations in the number, type, and chromosome location of genetic mutations in the cancer cells. One of the first and most

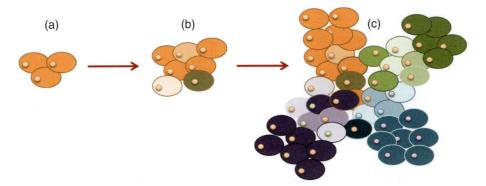

Figure 1.8 Genome instability drives intratumoral heterogeneity. (a) In a microscopic cluster of cancer cells, all the cells are likely to contain the same genetic faults. However, the cells are genomically unstable and likely to pick up more mutations. **(b)** The cells start to evolve and become different from one another. **(c)** As time goes on, the cells diverge from each other more and more, creating distinct populations of cells driven by different sets of mutations.

comprehensive analyses of this phenomenon was conducted by a group of British scientists who studied tumor biopsy samples from people with kidney cancer [56]. When investigating 12 samples from one patient, they found that only a third of the 128 DNA mutations they discovered were present in all 12 samples. A similar study investigating tumor samples from eight people with esophageal cancer has revealed a similar story [57, 58].

It seems that as a cancer grows, the cells within it evolve and change. This is because cancer cells are **genomically unstable** – they accumulate DNA damage at a faster rate than healthy cells. There are various reasons for this instability, some of the most important of which are the following [59, 60]:

- Cancer cells contain faults in DNA repair genes that compromise their ability to detect and repair DNA damage.
- Cancer cells' apoptosis machinery is faulty, which means they stay alive despite containing lots of DNA damage.
- The normal mechanisms that ensure the cell has the correct number of chromosomes and help to avoid chromosome breakages and fusions are lost.
- The cells' ability to replicate their DNA accurately is compromised.
- Some cancer cells are continually exposed to mutagens such as cigarette smoke or UV light from the sun.
- The cancer cells contain mutations in powerful oncogenes that destabilize the cell and lead to further mutations.

Because of genomic instability, over the weeks, months, and years that go by before a cancer is diagnosed (and in the weeks, months, and years afterward), cancer cells emerge that have different combinations of mutations compared to their predecessors. And, as time goes on, the cancer cells within a tumor become more and more diverse.

1.5 THE CANCER MICROENVIRONMENT

Tumors are not lumps of tissue made from millions of identical cancer cells. Instead, they **contain a variety of non-cancer cells** (collectively known as stromal cells) such as fibroblasts (these are common, structural cells found in many locations around the body), white blood cells, cells that make up the blood vessels (endothelial cells and pericytes), fat cells (adipoctyes), nerve cells, and other cell types (see Figure 1.9) [61]. In fact, in some tumors there are more non-cancer cells than there are cancer cells [61].

The cells in a tumor are also embedded in a network of proteins and complicated sugar molecules known as the ECM – the extracellular matrix[15]. This intricate web surrounds the cells in all our tissues and organs, and its makeup and role differs from place to place around the body. When a cancer develops, cancer cells and non-cancer cells (which are now under the cancer cells' influence) cause the makeup and density of the ECM to change. For example, in breast cancer, the ECM becomes stiffer, and this seems to help cancer cells to move and escape into the lymph vessels and bloodstream [62].

1.5.1 The Role of White Blood Cells

The number, type, and actions of white blood cells in a cancer can vary enormously. Solid tumors are often **host to millions of white**

---

[15] Examples of ECM proteins include collagen, fibronectin, laminin, and elastin. The complex sugar molecules (called glycoseaminoglycans) are generally chemically linked to proteins to form protein-sugar hybrids called proteoglycans. These proteoglycans form a jelly-like substance in which the fibrous proteins are embedded.

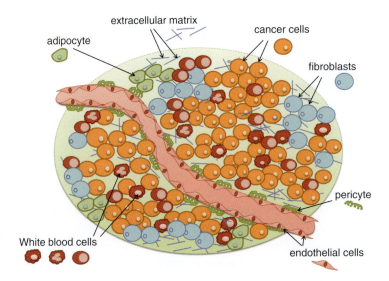

Figure 1.9 The cancer microenvironment contains many different types of cells. Tumors contain cancer cells, many different types of white blood cells, fibroblasts, fat cells (adipocytes) and other cell types (not shown). Winding their way through them are blood vessels, which are made up of endothelial cells and pericytes. Lymph vessels might also be present (not shown). All of these proteins are embedded in a protein scaffold called the extracellular matrix (ECM).

blood cells such as macrophages, mast cells, lymphocytes (B and T cells), and neutrophils. These cells can supply [63]:

- Small proteins known as growth factors that sustain the cancer cells' proliferation[16]
- Small proteins and chemicals collectively called "survival factors" that help cancer cells stay alive despite being in a hostile and toxic environment[17]
- Small proteins and chemicals that promote cancer cell migration, invasion, and metastasis
- Pro-angiogenic growth factors (see Section 1.5.3 below) and enzymes that destroy the extracellular matrix (ECM), providing an escape route for cancer cells

- Toxic molecules that cause cancer cells to mutate further

Each person's tumor will have a different collection of white blood cells inside it and at its outer fringes. The type of cells present, their number, and their behavior have a huge impact on how quickly or slowly the tumor grows and whether the person can be cured [64]. As yet, we're not in a position to use information about the number and type of white blood cells in a cancer before deciding what treatment to give someone. But it's likely that this will happen in the next few years [65].

There's more about the interactions between white blood cells and cancer cells in Chapter 5 on immunotherapy.

---

[16] We return to the topic of growth factors in Chapter 3 as many cancer treatments work by blocking growth factor receptors.

[17] This might not seem obvious, but because cancer cells grow in a haphazard manner and there aren't enough decent blood vessels around to supply them with everything they want and to take toxins away, their environment is toxic.

1.5.2 The Role of Other Cell Types

Fibroblasts sit in our tissues, and they normally produce structural proteins (such as collagen, elastin, fibronectin, and laminin) that form the ECM [66]. In tumors, the fibroblasts change in response to chemicals and signals sent out by cancer cells. They become perpetually activated and behave as though they are in a damaged tissue. For example, they release vast quantities of ECM proteins – much more than normal – and they produce growth factors and chemicals that encourage cancer cells to multiply [61].

Also found in some tumors are fat-storing cells called adipocytes. Again, the adipocytes found within tumors aren't normal; they've been altered by signals sent out by cancer cells. And, like the fibroblasts in tumors, the adipocytes also encourage and help cancer cells to grow and multiply [61].

1.5.3 Angiogenesis

Angiogenesis (the sprouting and growth of blood vessels) is almost always necessary for a cancer to become life-threatening. A tumor can grow to around $1\,mm^3$ without angiogenesis,[18] but to get beyond this it must have a blood supply [67]. (A $1\,mm^3$ tumor will typically have around 1 million cells, and it could have taken several years for it to get to this size.) By the time a cancer has reached $1\,mm^3$, the cells will be experiencing a drop in oxygen levels (hypoxia). To gain a blood supply and the necessary supplies of oxygen and nutrients, the cancer cells trigger angiogenesis.

The most important trigger for angiogenesis is a tiny protein called VEGF (vascular endothelial growth factor), which is released by cancer cells (and other cells) when oxygen levels drop. VEGF attaches to receptor proteins on the surface of endothelial cells – the cells that line our small blood vessels. Once VEGF has attached to its receptors, the endothelial cells multiply and move into place to form a new blood vessel.

When properly controlled, angiogenesis is an important and entirely healthy process. It happens normally: during the healing of cuts and wounds, during a woman's menstrual cycle, during the formation of the placenta in pregnancy, and in a growing embryo. However, when angiogenesis happens in cancer, it helps the cancer to grow and spread by supplying the cells with oxygen and nutrients and providing access to the bloodstream (see Figure 1.10).

1.6 CANCER SPREAD/METASTASIS

As soon as a cancer spreads (metastasizes) to another part of the body, treatment becomes more complicated, and the person's likelihood of being cured of their disease drops dramatically [68, 69]. Scientists estimate that metastasis is responsible for around 90% of cancer deaths [70]. Sadly, once a cancer has metastasized, the various new cancer growths quickly become resistant to treatment and eventually disrupt and destroy vital tissues and organs.

And, even when a cancer doesn't *appear* to have spread, there can be individual cancer cells, or microscopic clumps of cells that are circulating in the person's blood or lodged in distant organs or tissues [69]. These initially dormant cells can later cause metastasis and relapse.

---

[18] This is roughly equivalent to the size of a pin head or a grain of Demerara sugar.

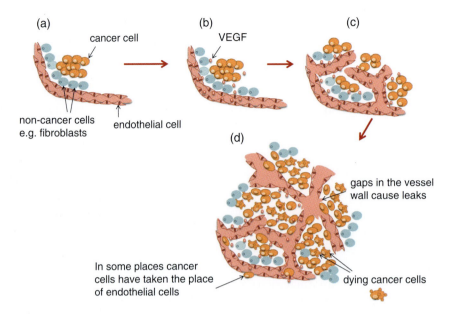

Figure 1.10 Cancer angiogenesis. (a) A cluster of cancer cells is too far away from the nearest blood vessel to receive an adequate blood supply. **(b)** The drop in oxygen levels triggers the cancer cells to release VEGF into their surroundings. **(c)** VEGF attaches to VEGF receptors on the surface endothelial cells, causing the blood vessel to sprout and grow. **(d)** The tumor contains a convoluted, lumpy, leaky network of blood vessels; many cancer cells now have sufficient blood supply, but many others do not. **Abbreviations:** VEGF – vascular endothelial growth factor

There are numerous reasons why cancers metastasize. For example:

- DNA mutations that some cancer cells contain might force them into behaviors that cause metastasis.
- Cancer cells that are on the move might enter a blood or lymph vessel and get carried along by the blood/lymph to distant sites.
- The cells, proteins, and structures in the cancer cells' environment, and the cancer cells' limited access to oxygen, can encourage cancer cells to become more mobile or to move in specific directions.

One important thing to realize is that cancer cells that metastasize might contain lots of mutations and display behaviors that aren't present in cancer cells that stay put. As a result, a patient's metastases might behave differently and respond to different treatments than the primary tumor.

1.6.1 Routes through Which Cancers Spread

There are five main routes through which a cancer can spread [71]:

- Local invasion
- Lymph vessels
- Blood vessels
- Nerves
- Fluid in the abdomen

Routes of Cancer Spread – via Local Invasion

"Local invasion" describes the process whereby cancer cells digest the ECM proteins that surround them and gradually move into, infiltrate, and destroy nearby tissues. Local invasion is often the first step toward metastasis to distant organs.

Routes of Cancer Spread – via Lymph Vessels (Lymphatic)

The fluid around our cells drains into lymphatic vessels and from there into lymph nodes (also called lymph glands) and finally back into the bloodstream.[19] Cancer cells that have become detached from the cells around them are often caught up in this flow and carried to nearby lymph nodes.

Routes of Cancer Spread – via Blood Vessels (Vascular)

Individual cancer cells (and small clusters) are sometimes able to squeeze their way into small blood vessels. The red and white blood cells in the vessel then sweep the cancer cells along until they get stuck somewhere else. Cancer cells that have found their way into the bloodstream are called circulating cancer cells or circulating tumor cells (CTCs).

Routes of Cancer Spread – via Nerves (Perineural)

This is a relatively rare but dangerous route of cancer spread in which cancer cells spread along the course of nerve bundles. This type of spread is often very painful because cancer cells produce chemicals that trigger nerve activity.

Via Fluid in the Abdomen or (Transcoelomic)

Cancers that arise in the abdomen, particularly ovarian cancers, are liable to spread via the fluid that circulates within the abdomen. Cancer cells on the surface of the tumor break away and float in the abdominal fluid (this fluid bathes our internal organs). Cancer cells are carried along in the fluid and then adhere to tissues and organs in the abdomen such as the omentum[20] or bowel.

Once a cancer cell has reached a new location in the body, it won't necessarily cause a new cancer to grow. In fact, the vast majority of breakaway cancer cells die in the lymph or blood, are killed by white blood cells, or simply remain dormant (see Figure 1.11). In order for the cell to cause metastasis, it must survive and thrive in its new environment. And only a tiny proportion of breakaway cancer cells are ultimately able to go through this process.

1.6.2 Locations to Which Cancers Spread

Some cancers have particular routes of spread that are more likely than others (e.g., breast cancer commonly spreads via the lymph system). And each type of cancer is also more likely to spread to some locations than others [72]. For example:

- Breast cancers often spread to the bones, brain, liver, and lungs.
- Prostate cancers often spread to bones.
- Bowel cancers often spread to the liver, lungs, and the lining of the abdominal cavity (peritoneum).
- Lung cancers often spread to the adrenal glands, bone, brain, liver, and/or into the other lung.
- Melanoma skin cancers often spread to the lungs, brain, skin, and liver.

The preference that cancers have to spread to some locations rather than others is often due to the anatomical layout of lymph and blood vessels. For example, the blood supply to the bowel goes from there to the liver, hence the liver is where bowel cancers often spread to first [73].

---

[19] For a colorful illustration of the lymph system, see the Cancer Research UK website: http://www.cancerresearchuk.org/what-is-cancer/body-systems-and-cancer/the-lymphatic-system-and-cancer [accessed April 4, 2017].
[20] The omentum is a fold of fatty tissue that hangs down from the stomach and covers our intestines and other organs.

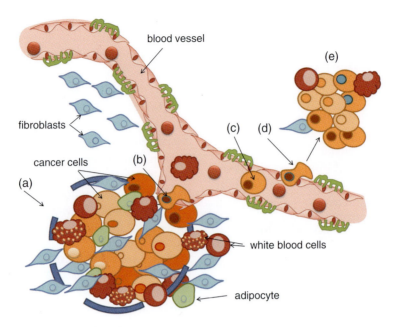

Figure 1.11 **The path to metastasis. (a)** A primary tumor containing many different cell types. **(b)** A cancer cell that is particularly mobile might invade locally and squeeze its way into blood vessels. **(c)** A cancer cell circulating in the blood. **(d)** The cancer cell squeezes out of the blood vessel into a new environment. **(e)** In its new location, the cancer cell may die or remain dormant for weeks or even years, kept in check by its new environment. However, eventually a change in its environment or the gain of new mutations might enable it to multiply and create a metastasis.

1.6.3 Reasons Why Cancers Spread

Many of the cells in a cancer seem to be relatively inert and dormant, perhaps because of low oxygen levels or in response to signals sent out by their cancer and non-cancer neighbors. However, other cancer cells can be highly mobile and likely to cause metastasis. Scientists believe that these mobile cells have gone through a change in appearance and behavior called **the epithelial-to-mesenchymal transition (EMT)** [74] (see Figure 1.12).

The EMT is a change that some healthy cells undergo in a developing embryo or in an adult when a tissue is damaged. It's when a stationary, well-connected epithelial cell becomes more like a mobile, independent mesenchymal cell. During the EMT, the cell produces more ECM proteins, becomes more resilient, and changes shape [74].

The EMT is thus a natural process that is hijacked and reactivated by cancer cells [74]. Understandably, if a cancer cell goes through this change, it's more likely to cause metastasis than other cancer cells.

Triggers that encourage cancer cells to go through the EMT include growth factors and other chemicals released by neighboring cells, low oxygen levels, and contact with various ECM proteins [75].

The EMT appears to be very important and poses huge problems for doctors. For example, cancers that contain a high proportion

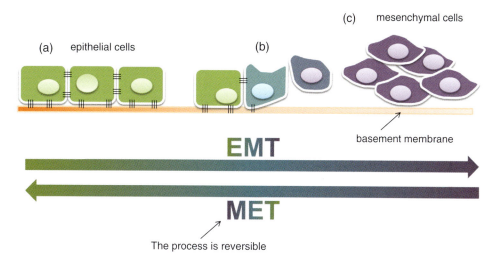

Figure 1.12 **The epithelial-to-mesenchymal transition (EMT). (a)** All our body's organs and tissues are lined with epithelial cells. Epithelial cells tend to be lined-up and well connected to one another. They are also physically attached to the basement membrane. **(b)** During the EMT, cells gradually lose epithelial proteins and gain mesenchymal proteins. **(c)** Mesenchymal cells are mobile and resilient and less well connected to one another and the basement membrane.
Abbreviations: EMT – epithelial-to-mesenchymal transition; MET – mesenchymal to epithelial transition

of mesenchymal cells are more likely to resist treatment and spread quickly [76]. Also, some treatments seem to cause cancer cells to go through the EMT, helping them survive the effects of treatment and causing metastasis [77].

1.7 CANCER STEM CELLS

Over the past 20 years or so, scientists have increasingly become convinced that a proportion of cancer cells behave somewhat like our body's stem cells[21] and can be classed as cancer stem cells. That is, they not only have the ability to multiply to generate further cancer stem cells, but they can

also produce cancer cells with other properties. Therefore, if you kill all the other cells in a tumor but leave the stem cells behind, they will cause the cancer to return. Evidence suggests that cancer stem cells are relatively rare, slow-growing, drug-resistant cancer cells that can survive many cancer treatments [78]. The strength of evidence for their existence varies from cancer type to cancer type [78].

The precise properties of cancer stem cells and where they come from are hotly debated by scientists. Some scientists suggest that they could start out life as healthy adult stem cells that, due to DNA mutations, start behaving like cancer cells. Other scientists point to the

---

[21] Adult stem cells are slow growing, versatile cells found in small numbers in our organs and tissues. When they multiply they create mature, specialized cells that replenish, repair, and renew the tissue and keep it healthy. The number of stem cells differs from organ to organ and tissue to tissue around the body, depending on the turnover of cells in that tissue. For example, there are many stem cells in the lining of the bowel because cells are continually being scraped off as food passes through, and the scraped-off cells need to be replaced.

similarities between cancer stem cells and cancer cells that have gone through the EMT. And they suggest that cancer stem cells are derived from cancer cells that have gone through the EMT and that have later undergone further changes [79].

Two of the problems scientists face when trying to study cancer stem cells are that (1) they are highly changeable and adaptable cells and that (2) what constitutes a cancer stem cell varies from cancer to cancer and even from patient to patient [80]. So it's best not to get too worked up about the label "cancer stem cell." Instead, we will simply acknowledge that there are often cells in a cancer that are not easily destroyed by treatments and that can cause a cancer to return weeks, months, or years later.

1.8 OBSTACLES THAT PREVENT US FROM CURING CANCER

In this chapter, I've explained some of what we now know about how cancers come about and why cancer cells behave as they do. I've also described some of the behaviors that cancer cells exhibit. And I've described the diversity that often exists within tumors in terms of the types of cells found in them and the genetic diversity among cancer cells. Armed with all this knowledge about cancer, it's tempting to believe that we might know enough to cure everyone affected by the disease. However, as I'm sure you know, this isn't the case.

So what is it that still thwarts us? What features of cancer cells and cancer behavior are responsible for our inability to cure it, particularly when it has metastasized?

As a conclusion to this introductory chapter, I'm going to go through some of the chief obstacles to curing more cancer patients:

- The similarities between cancer cells and healthy cells

- The great dissimilarities between different types of cancer
- The fact that cancer spreads
- Genomic instability and intratumoral heterogeneity
- The tumor microenvironment

There are, of course, other obstacles to successfully curing a patient of cancer. Not least are the issues of late diagnosis, the difficulty of eliminating every single microscopic cancer cell, and the fact that many cancer patients are relatively elderly and frail and have other medical complaints that often preclude the use of aggressive treatments. However, these issues are beyond the scope of this book, so I'll stick to describing the five obstacles I've listed above.

1.8.1 The Similarity between Healthy Cells and Cancer Cells

All our cells **have the same repertoire of roughly 21,000 genes** that contain the instructions for making all the proteins our cells will ever need. And as you might have already gathered from the rest of this chapter, cancer cells never do anything completely new. Instead, they overproduce or produce faulty, overactive versions of proteins that help them grow, multiply, and stay alive. And they underproduce or produce dysfunctional versions of proteins that would normally limit their growth or encourage them to die.

So, although we might think that a cancer is an unnatural aberration that needs destroying, a patient's body doesn't necessarily think the same. And although it's true that our immune system is powerful enough to rid the body of cancer, it often doesn't do so (although it's impossible to say exactly how many of us have avoided cancer thanks to the vigilance of our immune system).

Because **cancer cells are very similar to healthy cells**, it's very difficult to create drugs that can kill one without the other. Newspapers and web pages are often littered with stories about chemicals from many different sources that can kill cancer cells grown in a lab. But that isn't difficult. The difficulty is finding chemicals that can the kill cancer cells in a person while leaving their healthy cells alone. And this is virtually impossible. So every treatment, no matter how targeted we might think it is, will kill some healthy cells alongside killing cancer cells. And that means that every cancer treatment causes side effects. The severity of a treatment's side effects often limits how much of the treatment can be given to a patient safely, and that ultimately compromises the treatment's ability to cure them.

1.8.2 Differences between Different Cancer Types

I'm often asked whether there will ever be "a cure for cancer." And if all cancers shared the same DNA mutations and behaviors, my answer might perhaps be "yes." But as it is, there are many, many different types of cancer. And each cancer has its own unique vulnerability to different treatments. And not only is it possible to develop liver cancer, stomach cancer, bowel cancer, skin cancer, and so on, but there are also many different types of cancer that can occur in each location. For example, there are adenocarcinoma and squamous cell carcinoma versions of non-small cell lung cancer, estrogen receptor positive and estrogen receptor negative breast cancer, and various different types of skin cancer.

In recent years, scientists have uncovered more and more information about the various forms of cancer, what drives them, and what impacts their behavior. And this knowledge is gradually improving our ability to treat people more effectively. However, the complexity is mind-blowing. And even when two cancers appear to be driven by the same mutations, it's not necessarily the case that they will respond to the same treatments. It depends on precisely how the cells' internal proteins

interact with one another, and how the cancer cells interact with the cells around them. For example, in 50% of people with melanoma skin cancer, the cancer cells contain a mutation in a gene called *BRAF*. Treatment with a B-Raf inhibitor shrinks 50%–80% of these cancers [81]. The same *BRAF* mutation is also found in the cancer cells of 8%–10% of people with bowel cancer. But in bowel cancer, a B-Raf inhibitor does not work, at least not unless it's combined with at least two other treatments [82, 83].

So, for every cancer, and for every subset of every cancer, we have to discover exactly how the cells are wired up – what's driving them and what's protecting them – before we can uncover how best to treat them. As a result, there will never be "one cure" for all cancers.

1.8.3 Cancer Spread

Cancer metastasis has important implications for treatment. For example, cancer cells in distant organs might contain different mutations compared to those in the original (primary) tumor. Consequently, they wouldn't be destroyed by a cancer treatment chosen by a doctor for its ability to target the primary tumor [69].

Also, there is often a lag between the cancer cells' arrival in a new location and their growth into a metastasis. During the lag period, the cancer cells are dormant and unlikely to be killed by chemotherapy or other cancer treatments [84]. The length of time the cancer cells remain dormant, and the likelihood that they will cause metastasis, varies from cancer to cancer. For example, relapses several years after surgery are common in people with breast, prostate, kidney, and melanoma skin cancer [84].

In addition, cancer cells that have traveled to locations like the brain or bone marrow will receive protection and support from their new environment. The brain, in particular, is difficult for drugs to penetrate, has a large nutrient supply, and is relatively protected from the immune system [85]. Also, the bone marrow is full of white blood cells and other cells that churn out survival-promoting chemicals that can help cancer cells survive and multiply [86].

Lastly, scientists have made lots of progress in identifying the gene mutations that cause cancer and that drive its growth. They've also created many treatments that target the consequences of these mutations. However, a lot less progress has been made in identifying the mutations that drive metastasis. And they've developed very few treatments that specifically target metastatic cancer cells [69]. So once a cancer has metastasized and become resistant to treatments, doctors currently have very little to offer their patients.

1.8.4 Genomic Instability and Intratumoral Heterogeneity

Genomic instability and intratumoral heterogeneity[22] are huge obstacles for scientists and doctors.

One problem that intratumoral heterogeneity causes is that a biopsy sample taken from a patient's cancer might not be representative of their cancer as a whole. So if you analyze a biopsy sample for the presence of a particular protein or a particular mutation and then treat the patient accordingly, you may end up killing only a minority of the cancer cells [87, 88] (see Figure 1.13a). For example, it might have seemed from a biopsy that a cancer is driven by the high numbers of EGFR proteins on the cells' surface. However, in reality, these cells were in the minority, and the majority of cancer cells were driven by a different protein. Because of this, giving the patient an EGFR-targeted treatment would have little impact.

In addition, if you use a treatment that targets one particular protein (as is the case with many of the treatments mentioned in this book), it is inevitable that there will be cells in the tumor that have mutations that make them impervious to your treatment (see Figure 1.13b & c) [89, 90].

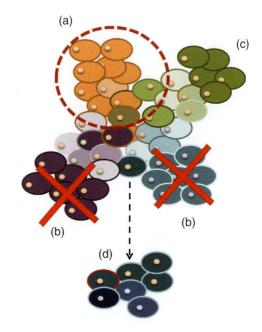

Figure 1.13 Intratumoral heterogeneity is an obstacle to effective cancer treatment. Due to the genomic instability of cancer cells, cancers often contain multiple populations of cancer cells driven by different combinations of mutations (represented by the different colors). **(a)** A biopsy sample (illustrated by the dotted red circle) does not contain representative cells from the whole cancer and may give scientists a skewed view of what mutations are driving the cells' behavior. **(b)** Some cancer cells are killed by a treatment (red crosses). **(c)** However, many other cells contain mutations that make them resistant and able to survive. **(d)** A cancer cell that leaves the original tumor and creates a metastasis elsewhere in the body may have very different properties from the original tumor.

---

[22] As you might remember from Section 1.4, intratumoral heterogeneity is the phrase scientists use to describe the fact that most cancers contain multiple populations of cancer cells driven by different combinations of gene mutations.

In fact, often there are multiple treatment-resistant cancer cells, each with a different resistance-causing mutation. And when the cancer returns, each new cancer growth may be driven by a different set of mutations [91].

In general, cancers that contain the most mutations (e.g., melanoma skin cancer and lung cancers in smokers) are also those that evolve most quickly and contain the highest degree of intratumoral heterogeneity [92, 93]. These cancers also have the shortest durations of response to treatment, and the patient's cancer quickly starts growing again [89].

A final problem caused by intratumoral heterogeneity is the way it enables cancers to change over time. Therefore, the cancer cells that drive recurrence and metastasis often contain different gene mutations and have different survival mechanisms than the cancer cells that were first present (Figure 1.13d) [88]. So when a cancer starts growing again, it's likely to be impervious to the treatments used previously (any cancer cell that was vulnerable to that treatment is already dead), hence the cancer gets harder and harder to treat. And referring back to an archived tumor sample might not tell you what is driving the cancer now, nor give you accurate information about what treatment to use [88].

Thus, intratumoral heterogeneity is a huge barrier to the successful treatment of cancer patients. Efforts to overcome this problem center on:

- Using logical combinations of drugs that target different faulty proteins and pathways and that synergize with one another to kill a more diverse range of cancer cells than any individual treatment used on its own
- Innovations in the analysis of cancer cells circulating in a patient's bloodstream, and using these cells to track the cancer cells' evolution and predict drug resistance-causing mechanisms
- Taking multiple biopsies from a tumor and its metastases to gain a fuller picture of the mutations driving the cancer
- Developing treatments such as immunotherapies that are less selective and may be able to kill a broad range of cancer cells driven by different mutations (see Chapter 5)

A final note: in the past, intratumoral heterogeneity was uniformly considered to be a bad thing because it causes rapid drug resistance. However, the creation of new immunotherapies (like checkpoint inhibitors – Chapter 5, Section 5.3) has led some scientists to think differently, as it seems that patients with cancers with the most mutations are also the most likely to benefit from immunotherapy (although it's not always that black and white) [94]. As a result the frustration of rapid resistance to targeted treatments is now balanced by optimism about the possibilities of immunotherapy.

1.8.5 The Cancer Microenvironment

The environment in which cancer cells live can have an enormous impact on whether a treatment given to a patient is effective. Even if a drug is highly targeted and (in theory) highly effective against a patient's cancer, it still might have no impact if the cancer cells' microenvironment is protecting them. Two main issues that affect a drug's effectiveness are (1) the physical environment in which the cancer cells live and whether the treatment can reach them, and (2) the behavior of the non-cancer cells that live alongside the cancer cells. For example [95]:

- Growth factors and other proteins released by non-cancer cells such as fibroblasts, white blood cells, endothelial cells, and adipoctyes (fat cells) can protect cancer cells from the effects of various treatments.
- In some cancers, the cancer cells' microenvironment contains a dense network of structural proteins (called desmoplasia) that compresses blood vessels and prevents cancer drugs from reaching the cancer cells.

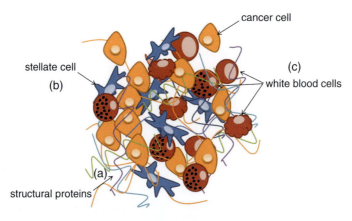

Figure 1.14 **The pancreatic cancer microenvironment can protect cancer cells from the effects of treatment. (a)** Pancreatic cancers often contain a dense, fibrous network of proteins that compresses any blood vessels that are present and prevents cancer drugs from penetrating the tumor. **(b)** Stellate cells (modified fibroblasts) produce fibrous proteins and release pro-survival proteins such as growth factors. **(c)** White blood cells secrete many small proteins and chemicals that protect cancer cells from treatments.

The classic example of the problems posed by the cancer microenvironment is pancreatic cancer. Many scientists have found combinations of chemotherapy and other treatments that can successfully kill pancreatic cancer cells grown in a lab, or grown in mice (called xenografts). However, these same treatments have failed to improve the survival times of most pancreatic cancer patients [96]. And one of the chief obstacles that stop treatments from working against pancreatic cancer is its microenvironment (Figure 1.14). It's not unusual for non-cancer cells to outnumber the cancer cells in these tumors, and the environment is awash with a diverse array of cells and proteins that together prevent drugs from penetrating and protect the cancer cells from death [96].

1.9 FINAL THOUGHTS

In this chapter, I have tried to give you a good idea of why cancers come about, what drives them, how they behave, and why we can't yet cure everyone who develops this disease. Do be aware, though, that this chapter covers just a small percentage of all that scientists have discovered about cancer cells. There are some big areas of science that I have missed out, such as epigenetics, micro-RNAs, the role of metabolic pathways and of viruses and infections, the similarities and differences between cancers in different organs, the difference between a benign tumor, a pre-cancerous lesion and an invasive cancer... Therefore, this chapter is just a selection of information that I have chosen because I think it might come in handy when you read later chapters.

Throughout the rest of this book, I'll be focusing on cancer treatments that target just one protein, or one cell process that is faulty in cancer cells. However, the proteins and processes that are targeted by these treatments represent just a small proportion of all the faulty proteins and processes that drive cancer cells and are responsible for the way they behave. I hope in this chapter I have given you a sense of this – that there are many genetic faults in cancer cells that aren't targeted by even the most recent cancer treatments.

Even so, the treatments described in the rest of this book target a range of different features of cancer cells. These include treatments that target aspects of cell communication, the cell cycle, DNA repair, angiogenesis, and the interaction between cancer cells and the immune system. As well as mentioning them briefly in this introductory chapter, I will explain these processes in more detail when I come to describe the various treatments in later chapters.

REFERENCES

1 Powledge TM (2014). How much of human DNA is doing something? *Genetic Literacy Project.* [Online] Available at: https://www.genetic literacyproject.org/2014/08/05/how-much-of-human-dna-is-doing-something/ [Accessed April 6, 2017].

2 The Cancer Genome Atlas. National Cancer Institute, National Human Genome Research Institute. [Online] Available at: http://cancer genome.nih.gov/ [Accessed April 6, 2017].

3 The International Cancer Genome Consortium. [Online] Available at: https://icgc.org/ [Accessed April 6, 2017].

4 Stratton MR et al. (2009). The cancer genome. *Nature* **458**: 719–724.

5 For information on the use of Herceptin for both HER2-positive breast and stomach cancer see the NHS Choices website: NHS Choices; Herceptin (Trastuzumab). Last accessed August 2016. http://www.nhs.uk/conditions/herceptin/pages/introduction.aspx

6 For an insight in the controversies and debates around what proportion of cancers can be prevented, see: Yong E (2017). No, We can't say whether cancer is mostly bad luck. The Atlantic. [Online] Available at: https://www.theatlantic.com/science/archive/2017/03/no-cancer-isnt-mostly-bad-luck/521049/ [Accessed April 3, 2017].

7 For a list of carcinogens known to cause cancer, and their relative importance in different cancer types, go to the CancerStats section of the Cancer Research UK website: http://www.cancerresearchuk.org/cancer-info/cancerstats/causes/preventable/

8 For a more comprehensive list of preventable causes of cancer see: Cogliano VJ, Baan R, Straif K et al. (2011). Preventable exposures associated with human cancers. *J Natl Cancer Inst* **103**(24): 1827–1839.

9 Cancer Research UK: Causes of cancer and reducing your risk http://www.cancer researchuk.org/about-cancer/causes-of-cancer

10 Cancer Research UK: Statistics on preventable cancers http://www.cancerresearchuk.org/health-professional/cancer-statistics/risk/preventable-cancers

11 American Cancer Society. Diet and physical activity: What's the cancer connection? http://www.cancer.org/cancer/cancercauses/dietandphysicalactivity/diet-and-physical-activity

12 Jolie Pitt, A (2015). Angelina Jolie Pitt: Diary of a surgery. *The New York Times.* Published online 24 March, 2015.

13 Greaves MF et al. (2003). Leukemia in twins: Lessons in natural history. *Blood* **102**(7): 2321–2333.

14 De Bont R, van Larebeke N (2004). Endogenous DNA damage in humans: A review of quantitative data. *Mutagenesis* **19**: 169–185.

15 Valko M et al. (2004). Role of oxygen radicals in DNA damage and cancer incidence. *Mol Cell Biochem* **266**(1–2): 37–56.

16 Wood RD, Mitchell M, Lindahl T (2005). Human DNA repair genes. *Mutation Res* **577**: 275–283.

17 Frank SA. (2007). *Dynamics of Cancer: Incidence, Inheritance, and Evolution.* Princeton (NJ): Princeton University Press. Chapter 12, Stem Cells: Tissue Renewal.

18 Tomasetti C, Vogelstein B (2015). Variation in cancer risk among tissues can be explained by the number of stem cell divisions. *Science* **347**(6217): 78–81.

19 Thomas F, Roche B, Ujvari B (2016). Intrinsic versus extrinsic cancer risks: The debate continues. *Trends Cancer* **2**(2): 68–69.

20 National Human Genome Research Institute website: http://www.genome.gov/11006943

21 Lange SS, Takata K, Wood RD (2011). DNA polymerases and cancer. *Nat Rev Cancer* **11**(2): 96–110.

22 Roberts SA et al. (2013). An APOBEC cytidine deaminase mutagenesis pattern is widespread in human cancers. *Nat Genetics* **45**: 970–976.

23 Swanton C et al. (2015). APOBEC enzymes: Mutagenic fuel for cancer evolution and heterogeneity. *Cancer Discover* **5**(7): 704–712.

24 Miller K (2003). Estrogen and DNA damage: The silent source of breast cancer? *J Natl Cancer Inst* **95**(2): 100–102.

25 Shacter E, Weitzman SA (2002). Chronic inflammation and cancer. *Oncology (Williston Park)* **16**(2): 217–226, 229; discussion 230–2.

26 Hussain SP et al. (2003). Radical causes of cancer. *Nat Rev Cancer* **3**: 276–285.

27 For an introduction to epigenetics see: Learn. Genetics. The Epigenome at a Glance. [Online] Available at: http://learn.genetics.utah.edu/content/epigenetics/intro/ [Accessed April 19, 2017].

28 Or, for a rather unusual explanation of epigenetics using Beethoven's 5th Symphony see: Smith K (2015). Epigenome: The symphony in your cells. *Nature*. [Online] Available at: http://www.nature.com/news/epigenome-the-symphony-in-your-cells-1.16955 [Accessed April 19, 2017].

29 Baylin SB, Jones PA (2012). A decade of exploring the cancer epigenome — biological and translational implications. *Nat Rev Cancer* **11**(10): 726–734.

30 You can find a helpful illustration on the Cancer Research UK website: Preventable cancers: Overall (2011). [Online] Available at: http://www.cancerresearchuk.org/health-professional/cancer-statistics/risk/preventable-cancers#heading-Zero [Accessed April 19, 2017].

31 Parkin DM, Boyd L, Walker LC (2011). The fraction of cancer attributable to lifestyle and environmental factors in the UK in 2010. Summary and conclusions. *Br J Cancer* **105**(S2): S77–S81.

32 For further information on aneuploidy, see: Gordon DJ, Resio B, Pullman D (2012). Causes and consequences of aneuploidy in cancer. *Nat Rev Genetics* **13**: 189–203.

33 For a nice illustration of this look at the NCI website dictionary of cancer terms and look up "BCR-ABL fusion gene": http://www.cancer.gov/publications/dictionaries/cancer-terms [accessed February 26, 2018].

34 Clark JP, Cooper CS (2009). ETS gene fusions in prostate cancer. *Nat Rev Urology* **6**: 429–439.

35 el-Shami K, Stone RM, Smith BD (2008). FLT3 inhibitors in Acute Myeloid Leukemia. *Expert Rev Hematol* **1**(2): 153–160.

36 Shaw AT, Solomon B (2011). Targeting anaplastic lymphoma kinase in lung cancer. *Clin Cancer Res* **17**(8): 2081–2086.

37 Balko J et al. (2013). HER2 (ERBB2) Amplification in breast cancer. *My Cancer Genome.* [Online] Available at: https://www.mycancergenome.org/content/disease/breast-cancer/erbb2/119/ [Accessed March 30, 2017].

38 For a refresher on gene translation see: Scitable (2014). The information in DNA determines cellular function via translation. *Nature Education.* [Online]. Available at: http://www.nature.com/scitable/topicpage/the-information-in-dna-determines-cellular-function-6523228 [Accessed March 31, 2017].

39 Borg A et al. (2010). Characterization of BRCA1 and BRCA2 deleterious mutations and variants of unknown clinical significance in unilateral and bilateral breast cancer: The WECARE study. *Hum Mutat* **31**(3): E1200–E1240.

40 Cosmic. "COSMIC: Signatures of mutational processes in human cancer." Wellcome Trust Sanger Institute. [Online]. Available at: http://cancer.sanger.ac.uk/cosmic/signatures [Accessed March 31, 2017].

41 Vogelstein B, Papadopoulos N, Velculescu VE et al. (2013). Cancer genome landscapes. *Science* **339**(6127): 1546–1558.

42 Kandoth C et al. (2013). Mutational landscape and significance across 12 major cancer types. *Nature* **502**: 333–339.

43 Prior IA et al. (2012). A comprehensive survey of Ras mutations in cancer. *Cancer Res* **72**(10): 2457–2467.

44 Karakas B et al. (2006). Mutation of the PIK3CA oncogene in human cancers.

45 Wieduwilt MJ, Moasser MM (2008). The epidermal growth factor receptor family: Biology driving targeted therapeutics. *Cell Mol Life Sci* **65**(10): 1566–1584.

46 Dang CV (2013). MYC on the path to cancer. *Cell* **149**(1): 22–35.

47 Leicht DT et al. (2007). Raf Kinases: Function, regulation and role in human cancer. *Biochim Biophys Acta* **1773**(8): 1196–1212.

48 Bieging KT et al. (2014). Unravelling mechanisms of p53-mediated tumour suppression. *Nat Rev Cancer* **14**: 359–370.

49 Hopkins BD et al. (2014). PTEN function, the long and the short of it. *Trends Biochem Sci* **39**(4): 183–190.

50 Giacinti C, Giordano A (2006). RB and cell cycle progression. *Oncogene* **25**: 5220–5227.

51 Yap YS et al. (2015). The *NF1* gene revisited – from bench to bedside. *Oncotarget* **5**(15): 5873–5892.

52 Aoki K, Taketo MM (2007). Adenomatous polyposis coli (APC): A multi-functional tumor suppressor gene. *J Cell Science* **120**: 3327–3335.

53 Marechal A, Zou L (2013). DNA damage sensing by the ATM and ATR kinases. *Cold Spring Harb Perspect Biol* **5**(9): a012716.

54 Hanahan D, Weinburg R (2000). The hallmarks of cancer. *Cell* **100**: 57–70.

55 Hanahan D, Weinberg RA (2011). Hallmarks of cancer: The next generation. *Cell* **144**, 646–674.

56 Gerlinger M et al. (2012). Intratumor heterogeneity and branched evolution revealed by multiregion sequencing. *N Engl J Med* **366**: 883–892.

57 Murugaesu N, Wilson GA, Birkbak NJ (2015). Tracking the genomic evolution of esophageal adenocarcinoma through neoadjuvant chemotherapy. *Cancer Discover* **5**: 821.

58 For a reader-friendly description of the research, see: Arney K, Cataloguing the genetic chaos in oesophageal cancer. Science Blog. Cancer Research UK. First published: August 4, 2015. http://scienceblog.cancerresearchuk.org/2015/08/04/cataloguing-the-genetic-chaos-in-oesophageal-cancer [accessed February 26, 2018].

59 Burrell R et al. (2013). The causes and consequences of genetic heterogeneity in cancer evolution. *Nature* **501**: 338–345.

60 Turner NC, Reis-Filho JS (2012). Genetic heterogeneity and cancer drug resistance. *Lancet Oncol* **13**(4): e178–e185.

61 Balkwill FR et al. (2012). The tumor microenvironment at a glance. *J Cell Sci* **125**: 5591–5596.

62 Reviewed in: Cox R, Erler J (2011). Remodeling and homeostasis of the extracellular matrix: Implications for fibrotic diseases and cancer. *Dis Model Mech* Mar 2011; **4**(2): 165–178.

63 Reviewed in: *Microenvironment and Therapeutic Implications: Tumor Pathophysiology Mechanisms and Therapeutic Strategies*. Edited by Baronzio G, Fiorentini G, Cogle CR (2009). Chapter 2: Tumor Microenvironment: Aspects of Stromal-Parenchymal Interaction. ISBN: 978-1-4020-9575-7 (Print) 978-1-4020-9576-4 [Online]. http://www.springer.com/gb/book/9781402095757

64 Reviewed in: Fridman WH et al. (2012). The immune contexture in human tumours: Impact on clinical outcome. *Nat Rev Cancer* **12**, 298–306.

65 For a discussion of how research is helping us understand how white blood cells impact on breast cancer outcomes, see this article on the breastcancer.org website: http://www.breastcancer.org/research-news/immune-cells-linked-to-neadjuvant-response [accessed February 26, 2018].

66 Kalluri R, Zeisberg M (2006). Fibroblasts in cancer. *Nat Rev Cancer* **6**: 392–401.

67 Reviewed in: Folkman J (2006). Angiogenesis. *Annual Reviews of Medicine*. **57**: 1–18.

68 You can find lots of general information on metastatic cancer on the National Cancer Institute website: Metastatic Cancer (2017). *NIH National Cancer Institute*. [Online] Available at: https://www.cancer.gov/types/metastatic-cancer [Accessed April 4, 2017].

69 Steeg PS (2016). Targeting metastasis. *Nat Rev Cancer* **16**: 201–218.

70 Chaffer CL, Weinberg RA (2011). A perspective on cancer cell metastasis. *Science* **331**(6024): 1559–1564.

71 For an overview of cancer metastasis (including a couple of videos), see: CancerQuest (2016). How cancer spreads (metastasis). *Emory Winship Cancer Institute*. [Online] Available at: https://www.cancerquest.org/cancer-biology/metastasis [Accessed April 4, 2017].

72 For a more complete list, see the National Cancer Institute website: Metastatic Cancer (2017). *NIH National Cancer Institute*. [Online] Available at: https://www.cancer.gov/types/metastatic-cancer [Accessed April 4, 2017].

73 Wan L et al. (2013). Tumor metastasis: Moving new biological insights into the clinic. *Nat Medicine.* **19**(11): 1450–1464.

74 Kalluri R, Weinberg R (2009). The basics of epithelial-to-mesenchymal transition. *J Clin Invest* **119**(6): 1420–1428.

75 Jung HY et al. (2015). Molecular pathways: Linking tumor microenvironment to epithelial–mesenchymal transition in metastasis. *Clin Cancer Res* **21**(5): 962–968.

76 Discussed in: Chang JT, Mani SA (2013). Sheep, Wolf, or Werewolf: Cancer stem cells and the epithelial-to-mesenchymal transition. *Cancer Lett* **341**(1): 16–23.

77 Discussed in: Findlay VJ, Wang C, Watson DK et al. (2014). Epithelial to mesenchymal transition and the cancer stem cell phenotype: Insights from cancer biology with therapeutic implications for colorectal cancer. *Cancer Gene Ther* **21**(5): 181–187.

78 Pattabiraman DR, Weinberg RA (2014). Tackling the cancer stem cells – what challenges do they pose? *Nat Rev Drug Discov* **13**(7): 497–512.

79 Discussed in: Singh A, Settleman J (2011). EMT, cancer stem cells and drug resistance: An emerging axis of evil in the war on cancer. *Oncogene* **29**(34): 4741–4751.

80 Clevers H (2011). The cancer stem cell: Premises, promises and challenges. *Nat Med* **17**(3): 313–319.

81 Holderfield M et al. (2015). Targeting RAF kinases for cancer therapy: BRAF mutated melanoma and beyond. *Nat Rev Cancer* **14**(7): 455–467.

82 Gong J et al. (2016). RAS and BRAF in metastatic colorectal cancer management. *J Gastrointest Oncology* **7**(5): 687–704.

83 Dienstmann R et al. (2017). Consensus molecular subtypes and the evolution of precision medicine in colorectal cancer. *Nat Rev Cancer* **17**(2): 79–92.

84 Giancotti FG (2013). Mechanisms governing metastatic dormancy and reactivation. *Cell* **155**(4): 750–764.

85 Zhang C, Yu D (2011). Microenvironment determinants of brain metastasis. *Cell Biosci* **1**: 8.

86 Nguyen DX et al. (2009). Metastasis: From dissemination to organ-specific colonization. *Nat Rev Cancer* **9**: 274–284.

87 Reviewed in: Swanton S (2012). Intratumor heterogeneity: Evolution through space and time. *Cancer Res* **72**: 4875.

88 Bedard P et al. (2013). Tumour heterogeneity in the clinic. *Nature* **501**: 355–364.

89 Turner NC, Reis-Filho JS (2012). Genetic heterogeneity and cancer drug resistance. *Lancet Oncol* **13**(4): e178–185.

90 For a discussion of this as it relates to bowel cancer, see: Smith M, Targeted cancer therapies doomed to fail? *MedPageToday*. First published: June 13, 2012. https://www.medpagetoday.com/hematologyoncology/coloncancer/33253 [accessed February 26, 2018].

91 Romano E et al. (2013). Identification of multiple mechanisms of resistance to vemurafenib in a patient with BRAFV600E-mutated cutaneous melanoma successfully rechallenged after progression. *Clin Cancer Res* **19**(20): 5749–5757.

92 For an overview of intratumoral heterogeneity and its importance in drug resistance, see: Fisher R et al. (2013). Cancer heterogeneity: Implications for targeted therapeutics. *British J Cancer* **108**: 479–485.

93 Watson IR et al. (2013). Emerging patterns of somatic mutations in cancer. *Nat Rev Genet* **14**(10): 703–718.

94 Topalian SL (2016). Mechanism-driven biomarkers to guide immune checkpoint blockade in cancer therapy. *Nat Rev Cancer* **16**: 275–287.

95 Junttila MR, de Sauvage FJ (2013). Influence of tumour micro-environment heterogeneity on therapeutic response. *Nature* **501**: 346–354.

96 Feig C et al. (2012). The pancreas cancer microenvironment. *Clin Cancer Res* **18**(16): 4266–4276.

CHAPTER 2

Introducing Targeted Cancer Treatments

IN BRIEF

Targeted cancer treatments are treatments that target specific proteins, processes, and pathways known to have gone awry in cancer cells. However, there is no one uniformly agreed-upon list of targeted treatments, and each cancer charity, research institution, and individual researcher uses the term (if they use the term at all) to mean different things.

For the purposes of this book, "targeted treatments" are those that target proteins on the surface of cancer cells, block faulty or overactive enzymes in the cell cytoplasm, take advantage of faulty processes in cancer cells, or that target the patient's immune system and create or boost a cancer-fighting immune response.

Most (but not all) of these treatments fall into two categories: they are either monoclonal antibodies or kinase inhibitors. Hence, before we look at individual drugs and their targets, we are first going to pause and explore what monoclonal antibodies and kinase inhibitors are, and what they can and cannot do.

Monoclonal antibody treatments are based on the antibodies made by B cells of our immune system. They therefore retain many of the properties of antibodies, namely, their ability to attach to proteins and trigger immune responses. Scientists have gradually modified them to maximize their ability to kill cancer cells outright and trigger cancer-fighting immune responses. Monoclonal antibodies are large, complex proteins. In order to manufacture them reliably in large quantities, scientists use living cells as antibody-producing factories.

Kinase inhibitors, in contrast, are tiny chemical compounds, similar in size to chemotherapies. They are manufactured by chemists from their constituent atoms (generally lots of carbon, hydrogen, nitrogen, and oxygen, and maybe one or two other atoms such as chlorine or fluorine). What sets them apart from standard chemotherapies is their target. Instead of attacking any cell that is multiplying, they block enzymes known as kinases. These enzymes are found in our cells, and they cause vital chemical reactions to take place. Many kinases are overactive in cancer cells and they force the cells to grow, multiply, and survive.

This chapter outlines the strengths, weaknesses, and uses of both sets of treatments.

A Beginner's Guide to Targeted Cancer Treatments, First Edition. Elaine Vickers.
© 2018 John Wiley & Sons Ltd. Published 2018 by John Wiley & Sons Ltd.

2.1 INTRODUCTION

Over the past 20 years or so, scientists and doctors have used new scientific knowledge to create cancer treatments that target cancer cells in a more precise way than chemotherapy. These are often referred to as "targeted cancer treatments" (see Figure 2.1 for their place in the history of cancer treatments).

However, at the moment there is no uniformly agreed definition as to what the term "targeted cancer treatments" means. Hence, there is confusion about how and when the term is used. For the purposes of this book, I will use the term "targeted therapy" to describe treatments that target a specific protein, process, or pathway known to play a role in cancer. I will include some of the new immunotherapies that target proteins (called checkpoint proteins) that suppress white blood cells, and those that aim to create a very precise immune response against cancer cells. However, I won't include treatments such as interleukin-2 or interferon-alpha, as these boost the immune system in a very general way [8].

The treatments described in this book include those that:

1. Target cell surface proteins known as growth factor receptors. These are found on almost every cell in the human body, and too much of them, or faulty, overactive versions of them, are found on the surface of many cancers (Figure 2.2a).

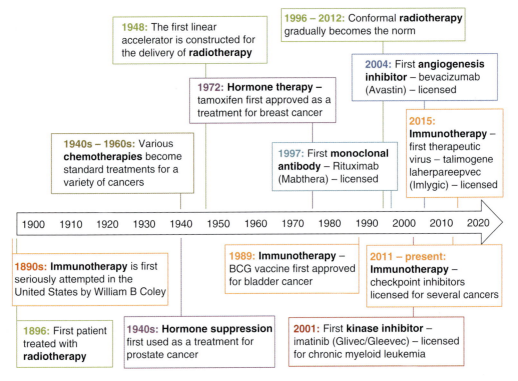

Figure 2.1 A very brief history of some important milestones in the development of non-surgical cancer treatments. The timeline includes milestones in radiotherapy [1], chemotherapy [2], hormone therapy for prostate cancer [3] and breast cancer [4], monoclonal antibody therapies [5], kinase inhibitors [6], and immunotherapies [7].

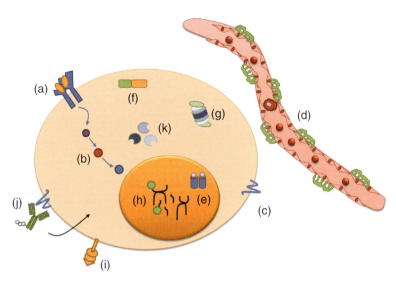

Figure 2.2 Some of the targets of targeted cancer treatments. (a) Cancer cells often overproduce proteins called growth factor receptors, which are found on the cells' surface and are hence accessible to monoclonal antibodies. Sometimes these growth factor receptors are faulty and overactive. **(b)** Growth factor receptors trigger the activity of other proteins inside the cell, many of which are kinases that can be blocked with kinase inhibitors. **(c)** Blood cell cancers (e.g., leukemias and lymphomas) have many proteins on their surface known as CD antigens. Many CD antigens (e.g., CD20, CD38, and CD19) are the targets of antibody-based treatments for blood cancers. **(d)** Tumors need a blood supply, hence they produce signaling proteins that trigger the growth of blood vessels by a process called angiogenesis. These signaling proteins are blocked by a group of treatments known as the angiogenesis inhibitors. **(e)** Some cancers are driven by hormones such as estrogen (breast cancer) or testosterone (prostate cancer). The production of these hormones, or their actions, can be blocked using hormone therapies. **(f)** Some cancers contain fusion proteins. If these fusion proteins are kinases (e.g., Bcr-Abl) they can be blocked with kinase inhibitors. **(g)** Our cells use proteasomes to recycle old and unwanted proteins. Some cancer cells seem dependent on proteasomes for their survival and can be treated with proteasome inhibitors. **(h)** Many cancers have difficulty repairing DNA damage; this vulnerability can be exploited with treatments such as PARP inhibitors. **(i)** Many cancer cells have proteins on their surface such as PD-L1 that directly suppress white blood cells. Cancer cells also persuade other cells in their surroundings to produce the same proteins; hence, they avoid being destroyed by the person's immune system. Immunotherapies called checkpoint inhibitors can overcome this suppression. **(j)** Some antibody-based treatments attach to cell surface proteins and deliver chemotherapy or other toxic substances. **(k)** Cancer cells often contain high levels of proteins such as Bcl-2 that prevent the cell from undergoing apoptosis. Drugs that target Bcl-2 or another of these proteins can force cancer cells to die.

2. Get inside cancer cells and **block kinases**[1] that are normally controlled by growth factor receptors (kinases are depicted in Figure 2.2b and described further in Section 2.1).

3. Target **CD antigens** – This is the collective name for proteins found on the surface of white blood cells and on the surface of cancer cells that cause leukemia, lymphoma, and multiple myeloma (Figure 2.2c).

---

[1] You'll be finding out a lot about kinases in this chapter. For now, I'll just say that kinases are specialized proteins that cause important chemical reactions to take place in our cells and that are often overactive in cancer cells.

4. **Block angiogenesis** – Tumor angiogenesis is the name given to the process through which small blood vessels sprout new side branches that grow to form new blood vessels, enabling blood to reach the tumor's cells and fuel its growth (Figure 2.2d).

5. **Block hormone receptors** found in the cell nucleus or cytoplasm (Figure 2.2e), or **block the production of certain hormones** in the body.

6. **Block fusion proteins**[2] such as Bcr-Abl or ALK fusion proteins; fusion proteins are created by some chromosome rearrangements and translocations (Figure 2.2f).

7. **Block the proteasome** – Proteasomes are our cells' protein-recycling units. Multiple myeloma cells seem particularly dependent on them, therefore proteasome inhibitors are mostly used for this type of cancer (Figure 2.2 g).

8. **Take advantage of some cancer cells' inability to accurately repair DNA damage** by blocking a protein called PARP (Figure 2.2 h).

9. **Overcome cancer's ability to suppress the patient's immune system**. These treatments create or trigger an immune response against cancer cells, and they're called **immunotherapies** (Figure 2.2i).

10. Attach to cell surface proteins and **deliver chemotherapy, radiotherapy, or toxins directly to cancer cells** (Figure 2.2j).

11. **Overcome cancer cells' resistance to apoptosis** (apoptosis is the orderly process by which damaged cells are naturally destroyed) (Figure 2.2 k).

Most targets currently fall into one of two categories: they are either cell surface proteins that can be targeted with **monoclonal antibodies**, or they are kinases that can be blocked with **kinase inhibitors**.

In the rest of this chapter, we are going to explore monoclonal antibodies and kinase inhibitors in a little more detail. However, the individual treatments will really only make sense once we have also looked at their targets, which we will do in later chapters.

Do be aware, though, that some important targeted treatments are not kinase inhibitors or antibodies. For example, the hormone therapies used to treat breast and prostate cancer are chemical compounds that mimic the shape of a hormone or that block an enzyme involved in hormone production. I will discuss these treatments when I come to describe treatments for breast and prostate cancer in Chapter 6.

Other non-kinase non-antibody treatments include some of the new immunotherapies described in Chapter 5 (such as genetically modified T cells, DNA and peptide vaccines, and virus-based treatments). They also include PARP inhibitors (Chapter 4, Section 4.3), hedgehog pathway inhibitors (Chapter 4, Section 4.4), proteasome inhibitors (Chapter 7, Section 7.6), and Bcl-2 inhibitors (Chapter 7, Section 7.9).

2.2 MONOCLONAL ANTIBODIES

Many targeted cancer treatments are monoclonal antibodies (often abbreviated to mAbs). They are based on the naturally occurring antibodies created by our immune system in response to infections (Figure 2.3). All antibodies share a common structure (Figure 2.4), with a **variable region** (called the Fv) that attaches to an antigen, and a **constant region** (called the Fc) that attracts white blood cells.

The word "**monoclonal**" refers to the fact that all the antibodies found in a monoclonal antibody treatment are identical to one

---

[2] Fusion proteins are proteins made from two separate proteins (or bits of proteins) that have been fused together by the cell to create a single protein that should not normally exist.

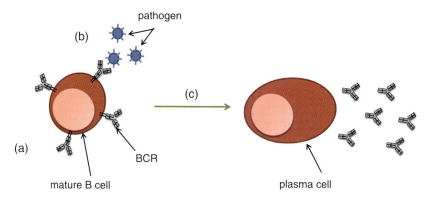

Figure 2.3 **Antibodies are made by specialized B cells. (a)** Our bodies contain many millions of white blood cells known as B cells, each of which has thousands of copies of a unique B cell receptor (BCR) on its surface. **(b)** B cells use their BCRs to recognize and connect with proteins and other complex molecules on the surface of invading pathogens such as bacteria and viruses. Anything that a BCR can connect with is known as an antigen. **(c)** When a B cell's BCRs connect with an antigen, they are activated. After numerous further activation steps, the B cell may become a plasma cell and release millions of copies of its BCR into the blood. BCRs released into the blood are known as antibodies or immunoglobulins.

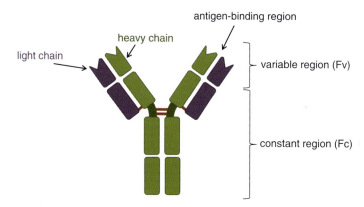

Figure 2.4 Antibodies are large proteins put together in a particular way. Each antibody contains four separate proteins: two **heavy chain** proteins and two **light chain** proteins. These four proteins are held together by chemical bonds (shown in dark red). Each B cell makes an antibody with a unique antigen-binding region, which is created from the ends of the heavy and light chains. Because the antigen-binding regions vary, they are called the "variable region" of the antibody.

another. (If the antibodies in a treatment were different from one another, this would be a polyclonal antibody treatment.)

The idea of using monoclonal antibodies as treatments first became popular in the 1970s, but it was in the 1980s that the first antibody was approved for use as a cancer treatment. Rituximab (Rituxan) is now a widely used treatment for some leukemias and lympho-

mas. (For an overview of the history of monoclonal antibody development, I would recommend Schrama D, 2006 [9].)

Antibodies have a number of properties that make them an ideal starting point for use as cancer treatments, but they also have important limitations [9–12].

There's also confusion and disagreement among medical staff and scientists as to

---

Box 2.1   Should all antibody-based cancer treatments be classed as immunotherapies?

This is a perpetual area of confusion, with different people (and organizations) coming to different conclusions. Let us first take a look at three antibody-based cancer treatments and their mechanisms of action as examples:

- **Trastuzumab (Herceptin)** – This antibody attaches to a protein called HER2 found on the surface of some cancer cells. HER2 forces these cells to grow and multiply, and when HER2 is blocked by trastuzumab, the cells die. Trastuzumab also has the ability to attract and activate white blood cells, which destroy cancer cells. (See Chapter 3, Section 3.4.1 and Chapter 6, Section 6.2.3 for more on trastuzumab.)
- **Rituximab (Mabthera)** – This antibody attaches to a protein called CD20, which is found on the cancer cells of some leukemias and lymphomas. When rituximab attaches to CD20, this is unlikely to kill the cell. Instead, rituximab attracts and activates white blood cells, and it's these white blood cells that kill the CD20-producing cancer cells. (See Chapter 7, Section 7.3.3 for more about rituximab.)
- **Nivolumab (Opdivo)** – This antibody attaches to a protein called PD-1 which is found on activated T cells (a type of white blood cell). It prevents PD-1 from being activated by its ligands (called PD-L1 and PD-L2), which prevents the T cell from being suppressed. The active T cell then (hopefully) kills lots of cancer cells. (See Chapter 5, Section 5.3.5 for more about nivolumab.)

You can see that although these three antibodies share the same structure, that of an antibody, they have different mechanisms of action. My decision when writing this book was to only include treatments that directly target or use the patient's immune system in the chapter on immunotherapies (Chapter 5). For this reason, trastuzumab is described in Chapter 3 under treatments that target signaling pathways, and rituximab is covered in Chapter 7, which is about treatments that are used against hematological cancers. Only nivolumab is in the immunotherapy chapter. But this is a gray area, and I can understand why some people would say that all antibody-based treatments can be classed as immunotherapies.

---

whether all immunotherapy treatments should be described as immunotherapies or not (see Box 2.1).

2.2.1 Useful Properties of Antibodies as Cancer Treatments

Antibodies have various properties that make them effective as cancer treatments:

1. They are **incredibly precise**; an antibody designed to attach to one antigen[3] on the surface of cancer cells will almost never attach to anything else.
2. If an antibody attaches to a protein on the surface of a cell, for example, HER2 or the epidermal growth factor receptor (EGFR), it can **block the receptor directly**, or **prevent the receptor's ligand[4] from binding to the receptor**, and prevent its activation (Figures 2.5a and b).
3. Antibodies can also **prevent receptors from pairing up**; many of the receptors on

---

[3] An antigen is anything (such as a protein, a fragment of a protein, or other large molecule) that an antibody can attach to. The precise location on the antigen where the antibody binds is known as an epitope.
[4] A ligand is something that binds to a receptor. For example, EGF (epidermal growth factor) is a ligand for the EGF receptor.

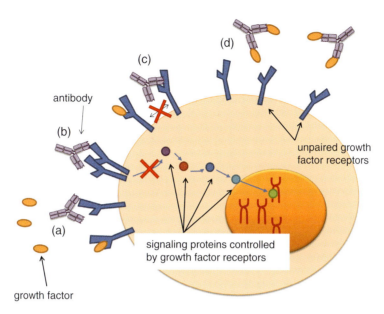

Figure 2.5 Antibodies can block growth factor receptors in several different ways. Many of the proteins targeted by monoclonal antibody treatments are growth factor receptors; these are complicated proteins that attach to growth factors and activate signaling proteins within the cell. Antibodies can block growth factor receptors by: **(a)** attaching to growth factor receptors and preventing growth factors from gaining access; **(b)** directly blocking the receptor's activity; **(c)** preventing receptors from pairing up (receptors are only active when in pairs); **(d)** attaching directly to the growth factor and preventing it from binding to its receptor. Blocking the growth factor receptors on the surface of cancer cells is sometimes sufficient to kill them.

the surface of our cells are only active in pairs (Figure 2.5c).

4. They **can attach to growth factors or other signaling proteins** and prevent them from binding to their receptors (these are called neutralizing antibodies), thereby preventing activation of a receptor (Figure 2.5d).

5. They can attract white blood cells and **trigger an immune response** against cells they are attached to (Figures 2.6a and b).

6. They can **attract complement proteins** [13], which attach to antibodies and either directly kill the cell or attract white blood cells such as macrophages (Figure 2.6c).

7. They **can be used as transportation devices** to deliver toxic drugs, radioactivity, or toxins to cancer cells (there is more about these "conjugated antibodies" in Section 2.2.3).

8. They can be **broken into pieces and stitched back together** to create entirely new proteins with tailor-made functions (see Section 2.2.3).

9. Many millions of identical copies of an antibody can **be reliably manufactured** using living cells.

10. Antibodies are **very stable** and last in the body a long time. They can therefore be given to patients as weekly or even monthly treatments.

2.2.2 Limitations of Antibody Treatments and Reasons for Side Effects

1. Antibodies used as cancer treatments are foreign to the patient's body; the person's immune system therefore sometimes reacts to them, causing **allergy-type reactions**, such as fever, chills, headaches, and red and itchy skin.

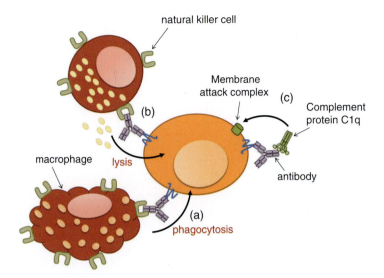

Figure 2.6 **Antibodies can kill cancer cells by attracting white blood cells and complement proteins**. When an antibody attaches to a protein on a cancer cell, it can attract white blood cells such as macrophages and natural killer (NK) cells. **(a)** Macrophages can engulf and digest cancer cells through phagocytosis. **(b)** NK cells release cell-killing enzymes that lyse (destroy) the cell. Together these mechanisms are called "antibody-dependent cell cytotoxicity" (ADCC). **(c)** Antibodies attached to cancer cells also attract complement proteins that come together to form a membrane attack complex (MAC) that can punch holes through the cell's membrane and kill the cell. This is called "complement-dependent cytotoxicity" (CDC).

2. Because antibodies are large proteins, they cannot cross the cell membrane in the way that small drugs can; **therefore, their target must be on the cell's surface.** This severely limits the range of proteins in cancer cells that can be targeted with these treatments.

3. Again, because of antibodies' size, **they can have difficulty getting into all the body's tissues and organs and penetrating the blood-brain barrier.**[5] An additional problem arises if there are regions within a tumor that contain few blood vessels – antibodies are often unable to penetrate these parts of a tumor [14].

4. Because antibodies are proteins, they would be **digested by gut enzymes and degraded by stomach acids** if given to patients as oral treatments. Therefore, they have to be **given by intravenous infusion or subcutaneous injection** to ensure that they enter the bloodstream intact.

5. If an antibody's main mechanism of action is to attract white blood cells, its ability to do this will depend on the types of white blood cells present in the cancer, and whether or not they can be provoked into action. **Many tumors contain an immune-suppressing environment** in which any white blood cells that try to destroy them are suppressed via numerous different mechanisms. Because of this, many antibody treatments are used against blood

---

[5] In our brain, the cells lining the blood vessels are slightly different and closer together than in the rest of the body. This makes it harder for things to get through the blood vessel wall and into the brain. This less permeable lining to our brain's blood vessels (known as the blood-brain barrier) protects our brain from many infections and toxins, but it also makes it difficult for cancer treatments to get into our brain and can prevent them from reaching any cancer cells that are hiding there.

cancers (such as leukemias and lymphomas), in which the cancer cells' environment is less immune-suppressive.

6. Antibodies are very precise, but sometimes the protein that they target on the surface of cancer cells is also present on healthy cells, meaning that healthy cells as well as cancer cells are killed, causing side effects. For example, cetuximab (Erbitux) and panitumumab (Vectibix) block a protein called EGFR, which is found on the cells of many cancers affecting the digestive system and on other cancers too. However, EGFR is also found on healthy cells of the skin, liver, pancreas, bladder, small and large intestines, and many other locations in a healthy human body [15, 16]. Therefore, treating people with an EGFR-targeted antibody such as cetuximab often results in side effects such as skin rashes, nausea, diarrhea, and liver and hair changes [17].

2.2.3 How to Improve Monoclonal Antibody Cancer Treatments

Mouse, Chimeric, Humanized, and Fully Human Antibodies

The first methods scientists used to create monoclonal antibodies meant that it was only possible to create mouse antibodies. Since that time, new technologies mean it is now possible to create a variety of antibody types. These include mouse antibodies, part-human part-mouse antibodies (known as chimeric antibodies), humanized antibodies, and fully human antibodies (see Figure 2.7 for a summary). As the amount of mouse protein is reduced, the antibody becomes less likely to trigger immune reactions.[6]

Making Slight Tweaks

It is also possible to modify antibodies by tweaking a handful of their amino acids or by

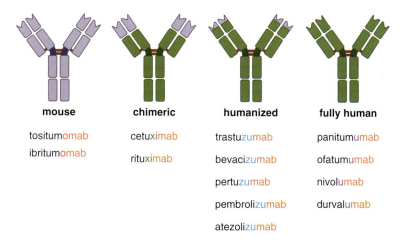

mouse	chimeric	humanized	fully human
tositumomab	cetuximab	trastuzumab	panitumumab
ibritumomab	rituximab	bevacizumab	ofatumumab
		pertuzumab	nivolumab
		pembrolizumab	durvalumab
		atezolizumab	

Figure 2.7 **Different types of antibodies used as cancer treatments.** The scientific name (i.e., not the marketing name) of monoclonal antibodies always ends in **mab** to denote it as a monoclonal antibody. Letters within the name tell you whether it is a mouse antibody (**o**), a chimeric (part mouse, part human) antibody (**xi**), a humanized (almost completely human) antibody (**zu**), or a fully human antibody (**u**). The letters "li" or just "l" in pembrolizumab, atezolizumab, nivolumab, and durvalumab denote that these are immunotherapies that target the immune system.

---

[6] Do remember, though, that even a fully human antibody is still foreign to the patient's immune system. Thus, fully human antibodies such as ofatumumab can still cause dangerous infusion reactions.

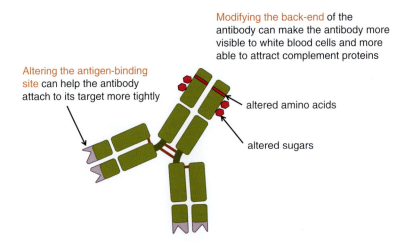

Figure 2.8 **An antibody's effectiveness can be improved by tweaking its structure.** Some antibodies have been improved upon by making slight changes to the antibody's antigen-binding site. Other modifications include altering the constant region of the antibody (either by changing the amino acid sequence or adding sugar molecules) to improve the antibody's ability to attract white blood cells and complement proteins.

altering what sugar molecules get attached to them during construction [11]. These subtle modifications can have an enormous impact on the antibody's effectiveness. For example, slight changes to the antigen-binding region can hugely improve the antibody's ability to attach to its target. And changes to the sugar molecules fused to the constant region can increase the antibody's ability to attract and activate white blood cells (Figure 2.8).

Creating Antibody Conjugates

A conjugated antibody is one that is fused or linked to something that is toxic to human cells – this toxic particle is sometimes referred to as the antibody's payload (Figure 2.9a). The antibody first attaches to a protein on the surface of a cell; it then enters the cell and delivers its payload[7] (Figures 2.9b–f). The toxic payload is commonly chemotherapy (if it's a **drug-linked antibody**), a radioactive

particle (if it's a radiolabeled antibody; **radio-immunotherapy**), or a toxin from a bacterial cell (if it's an **immunotoxin**). One of the crucial things to get right with an antibody conjugate is the linker that holds together the antibody and its payload. This linker has to be stable enough that the conjugate stays together as it travels through the patient's blood and enters their tissues. But the linker needs to break once the conjugate has entered a cancer cell.

Conjugated antibodies have been in development for many years, but there have been a variety of obstacles to their development (reviewed in [18, 19]). As of December 2017, three antibody–drug conjugates: brentuximab vedotin (Adcetris), trastuzumab emtansine (T-DM1; Kadcyla), and inotuzumab ozogamicin (Besponsa) had been licensed in the United States and Europe as treatments for lymphoma, breast cancer, and acute lymphoblastic leukemia, respectively. In addition,

---

[7] I've told you that antibodies are too big to diffuse across the cell membrane. However, when they attach to their target on the cell's surface, this often triggers the membrane to fold inward and create an internal compartment that contains both the antibody and its target (see Figure 2.9c).

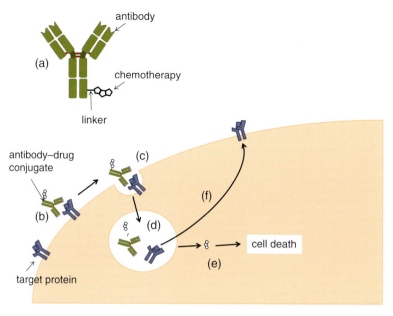

Figure 2.9 **Mechanism of action of antibody–drug conjugates (ADCs). (a)** ADCs are made from an antibody, a linker, and one or more molecules of a chemotherapy. Two commonly used chemotherapies are calicheamicin and auristatins. **(b)** An ADC attaches to its target protein on the surface of a cell. **(c)** The cell's membrane folds inward to create a compartment (an endosome) containing the ADC. **(d)** The ADC's linker is broken, releasing toxic chemotherapy. **(e)** The chemotherapy is released into the cell cytoplasm, where it kills the cell by destroying its microtubules (auristatins) or by causing DNA breaks (calicheamicin). **(f)** The antibody's target protein may be destroyed or recycled back to the cell surface.

two antibodies that are fused to radioactive particles (sometimes called radiolabeled antibodies or radioimmunotherapies) are licensed treatments (although only very rarely used) for lymphoma: ibritumomab tiuxetan (Zevalin) and ^{131}I tositumomab (Bexxar).[8] Many more conjugated antibodies are being investigated in clinical trials for a variety of different cancers.

Complete Reconstruction

For several decades, scientists have been able to chop up genes, switch them around, and put them back into living cells (called recombinant DNA technology). These cells then used the modified gene to manufacture the corresponding protein.

Using recombinant technologies, scientists can create proteins that contain segments of two or more different antibodies, or that are made from part of an antibody fused to part of a completely unrelated protein. One way of applying this technology is to create back-to-back fusions of antibodies to create "bi-specific" antibodies. However, if you took two complete antibodies and fused them back to back, the resulting protein would be enormous and (a) would be difficult to manufacture and (b) would probably get stuck in blood vessels and never make it into a tumor. For these reasons, scientists tend to just use the antibodies' variable regions to make a much more manageable-sized protein.

---

[8] Zevalin is licensed in the United States and Europe, whereas Bexxar is licensed in the United States only.

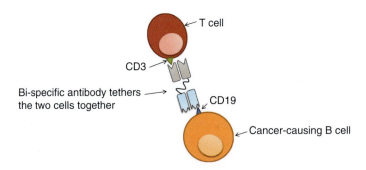

Figure 2.10 **A bi-specific antibody**. The antibody is constructed from the variable regions of an anti-CD19 antibody and an anti-CD3 antibody, which are held together by a linker. The bi-specific antibody draws together a CD19-expressing B cell with a CD3-expressing T cell.

One example of a bi-specific antibody is blinatumomab (Blincyto) (Figure 2.10). This treatment is made from the variable regions of two antibodies: one that targets a protein called CD19 and another that targets CD3. CD19 is a protein found on the surface of B cells, including the cancer cells of B cell leukemias and lymphomas. CD3 is found on the surface of T cells. The goal of blinatumomab is to draw together the two cell types and compel the T cell to destroy the cancer-causing B cell.

Another example where an antibody has been completely reconstructed is in CAR-modified T cell therapy. In this therapy, the variable region of an antibody has been fused to bits taken from a variety of other proteins and inserted into the surface of T cells (there is lots more about CAR-modified T cells in Chapter 5, Section 5.4.2).

2.2.4 Uses of Monoclonal Antibody Treatments for Cancer

The first monoclonal antibody used to treat cancer was rituximab (Mabthera; Rituxan). It was licensed in the United States in 1997 (and in Europe in 1998), and it's now a standard treatment for various leukemias and lymphomas [20]. It attaches to a protein known as CD20, which is found on many of the body's B cells.[9] Other targets of monoclonal antibody treatments are listed in Table 2.1.

In general:
- Antibodies that target CD antigens on the surface of white blood cells (e.g., CD20, CD19, CD38) are used in the treatment of leukemias, lymphomas, and multiple myeloma (cancers caused by faulty white blood cells). They primarily kill cancer-causing white blood cells by recruiting and activating healthy white blood cells (see Figure 2.6). However, these treatments also cause the death of many healthy white blood cells, and as a consequence they suppress the patient's immune system. (These treatments are described in greater detail in Chapter 7.)
- Antibodies that attach to growth factor receptors (such as EGFR and HER2) are used for the treatment of solid tumors such as bowel and breast cancer. These antibodies block the receptors' activity, and because the cancer cells are dependent on the receptor for their survival, this is often sufficient to kill the cancer cells. (These treatments are described in greater detail in Chapter 3, Sections 3.3.1 and 3.4.1). These antibodies can also attract nearby white blood cells,

---

[9] B cells (also called B lymphocytes) are antibody-producing white blood cells.

Table 2.1 Common targets of monoclonal antibody treatments.

Target protein	Where is it found?	Examples of treatments that target the protein	What cancers are these antibodies most commonly used to treat?
Targeted against blood cancers (leukemias, lymphomas, multiple myeloma)			
CD20	On cancer cells from B cell leukemias and lymphomas; on the majority of the body's healthy B cells [21]	Rituximab (MabThera/Rituxan/Zytux) Ofatumumab (Arzerra) Obinutuzumab (Gazyva) Veltuzumab Ocrelizumab Ibritumomab tiuxetan (Zevalin)	B cell leukemia and lymphoma
CD30	On cancer cells from Hodgkin lymphoma and anaplastic large cell lymphoma; also found on healthy, activated B and T cells [22]	Brentuximab vedotin (Adcetris) SGN-30	Hodgkin lymphoma and anaplastic large cell lymphoma
CD33	On cancer cells of acute myeloid leukemia; found on a variety of immature myeloid white blood cells [23]	Gemtuzumab ozogamicin (Mylotarg)	Acute myeloid leukemia
CD38	On a variety of white blood cells, including the cancer cells of multiple myeloma [24]	Daratumumab (Darzalex)	Multiple myeloma
CD52	On all B- and T-cells and a wide range of other white blood cells. On the cancer cells of chronic lymphocytic leukemia, non-Hodgkin lymphoma, acute lymphoblastic leukemia, and some other rare leukemias [25]	Alemtuzumab (MabCampath; Campath)	B cell chronic lymphocytic leukemia (CLL)
CS1 (SLAMF7)	A receptor protein found on the surface of plasma cells (these are antibody-releasing B cells), on natural killer (NK) cells and a subgroup of other white blood cells [26]	Elotuzumab (Empliciti)	Multiple myeloma
Targeted against solid tumors			
EGF receptor	On cells of many cancers, including those of the bowel, ovaries, lungs, head and neck, esophagus, brain [27]; found on healthy cells of many tissues and organs [48, 49]	Cetuximab (Erbitux) Panitumumab (Vectibix) Necitumumab (Portrazza)	Bowel cancer, head and neck cancer, non-small cell lung cancer
HER2[a]	On about 20% of breast cancers and stomach cancers; also a proportion of lung, bladder, bowel, biliary, ovarian, pancreatic, and prostate cancers [28]; found in lower levels than EGF receptor on a variety of healthy cells and tissues [29, 30]	Trastuzumab (Herceptin) Pertuzumab (Perjeta) Trastuzumab emtansine (T-DM1; Kadcyla)	HER2-positive breast cancer, stomach cancer and gastro-esophageal junction cancer

(Continued)

Table 2.1 (Continued)

Target protein	Where is it found?	Examples of treatments that target the protein	What cancers are these antibodies most commonly used to treat?
GD2	Found on neuroblastoma and melanoma cells [31]	Dinutuximab (Unituxin)	Neuroblastoma
VEGF receptor	Found on endothelial cells engaged in angiogenesis, such as healthy cells involved in wound healing and the formation of the placenta during pregnancy; also found on endothelial cells that form tumor blood vessels	Bevacizumab (Avastin) Aflibercept (Zaltrap) Ramucirumab (Cyramza)	Bowel cancer, ovarian cancer, kidney cancer, cervical cancer, breast cancer
Targeted against white blood cells (immunotherapies)			
CTLA-4	Found on T cells [32]	Ipilimumab (Yervoy) tremelimumab	Malignant melanoma
PD-1	Found on T cells, B cells, natural killer T cells, dendritic cells [33]	Nivolumab (Opdivo) Pembrolizumab (Keytruda) Pidilizumab	Malignant melanoma, non-small cell lung cancer, kidney cancer, bladder cancer, head and neck cancer, Hodgkin lymphoma (in trials for many other cancer types)
PD-L1	Found on T and B cells, dendritic cells, macrophages, and other white blood cells. Also on the cancer cells of many tumors, and on myeloid-derived suppressor cells, dendritic cells, macrophages and lymphocytes in the tumor microenvironment [33]	Atezolizumab (Tecentriq) Durvalumab (Imfinzi) Avelumab (Bavencio)	Bladder cancer, non-small cell lung cancer, (in trials for many other cancer types)

[a] HER2 (human epidermal growth factor receptor 2) is also known as Neu and ErbB2.

Source: Scott A et al. (2012). Antibody therapy of cancer. *Nat Rev Cancer* 12(4): 278–287.

which might kill lots of cancer cells. But it's difficult to know how important this is in the overall effectiveness of the drug – the number of white blood cells recruited by the antibody probably varies from cancer to cancer and patient to patient.

- **Antibodies that block activity of VEGF receptors** (either by attaching to VEGF or its receptors) are used to block angiogenesis. These antibodies are used for a range of solid tumors. (These treatments are described in greater detail in Chapter 4.)
- **Antibodies fused to chemotherapy (drug-linked antibodies) appear promising for a variety of cancers.** For example, trastuzumab emtansine is licensed as a breast cancer treatment, and brentuximab vedotin is licensed for Hodgkin lymphoma and anaplastic large cell lymphoma.
- **Antibodies fused to radioactive particles** (radiolabeled antibodies; radioimmunotherapies) are used to treat hematological cancers (mostly leukemias and lymphomas) **but not solid tumors**. All white blood cells are extremely sensitive to radiation and the cancer cells of leukemias and lymphomas retain this characteristic. This means that radiolabeled antibodies are ideal treatments for leukemias and lymphomas but cause too much immune suppression to be useful treatments for solid tumors [34]. Radiolabeled antibodies can also be used to suppress the patient's immune system prior to their receiving a stem cell transplant, though this is only relevant for hematological cancers in which stem cell transplants are used [35].
- **Antibodies that boost the activity of healthy white blood cells** (e.g., those that target checkpoint proteins such as CTLA-4, PD-1, or PD-L1) have so far mostly been used to treat solid tumors; however they are also licensed for people with Hodgkin lymphoma, and their use will no doubt expand in the coming years. These treatments work by "waking up" some of the body's white blood cells (usually the cytotoxic T cells) by blocking the activation of proteins on their surface that would otherwise suppress their activity. (These treatments are described in greater detail in Chapter 5.)

Scott et al. wrote a helpful overview of the mechanisms of action of monoclonal antibody therapies and their uses in 2012 [10]. George Weiner also wrote a very useful article (in 2015) about how monoclonal antibody therapies are used currently, and how they might be improved [36].

2.2.5 Antibody Biosimilars

Treatments such as aspirin or chemotherapy have a relatively simple chemical structure. They can therefore potentially be manufactured by many different companies – all the company needs is an understanding of the chemical composition of the compound and the technology to manufacture it. Thus, when a company's patent expires on one of these drugs, rival companies can quickly manufacture identical, generic versions.

However, monoclonal antibodies are much more complicated treatments. They are proteins constructed by living cells from hundreds of amino acids.[10] Once the cell has made the long string of amino acids that makes up the antibody protein, it then has to fold it properly and pin it into shape with chemical

---

[10] Because antibodies are manufactured by living cells, they are sometimes described as "biological therapies," "biological medicines," "biological agents," or "biologic drugs." However, some organizations refer to all targeted cancer drugs, including kinase inhibitors, as being biological therapies, which is very confusing. I therefore generally avoid referring to any treatment as being a biological therapy.

bonds. Finally, the cell adds vital sugar molecules to the antibody's surface that help the antibody attract complement proteins and white blood cells. Thus, even if a company knows the precise amino acid makeup of an antibody such as rituximab, the cells they use to manufacture the antibody will attach a unique combination of sugar molecules to it [37]. Added to this are the complex processes needed to purify and manufacture the final product.

Because of the complexities involved, each drug company is liable to create a subtly different version of the same monoclonal antibody. As a reflection of this diversity, copy-cat versions of antibodies are called "biosimilars" rather than generics [38].

So far, biosimilar versions of bevacizumab and trastuzumab have been approved for use in Europe and the United States on the bases that they are equally safe and effective as the original treatments. Several biosimilar versions of rituximab are also approved in Europe and are likely to gain approval in the United States.

2.3 KINASE INHIBITORS

The second major group of targeted cancer treatments are the kinase inhibitors. These are small chemical compounds (similar in size to many chemotherapies[11]) that block the activity of kinases. In order to understand why kinase inhibitors are used as cancer treatments, it's first necessary to explain what a kinase is.

2.3.1 Kinases

First, kinases are enzymes. **Enzymes are the catalysts** that cause chemical reactions to take place in our body's cells. All our cells contain thousands of proteins that act as

enzymes. The kinases are a group of more than 500 enzymes that cause one particular chemical reaction to occur, namely, **phosphorylation**.

To phosphorylate something is to **add a phosphate chemical group** to it (phosphate is the name for a phosphorous atom surrounded by oxygen atoms). **Many of our cells' proteins are controlled by phosphorylation**. And it's only when you add phosphate to them that they swing into action and start doing their job. Often, what kinases attach phosphate to is another kinase. The added phosphates can also create new bulges and dips in a protein's surface (kinases mostly attach phosphate to proteins). This creates interaction sites through which the phosphorylated protein can interact with other proteins, or with DNA.

Kinases obtain phosphate from a molecule known as **ATP** [39] (**adenosine tri-phosphate** – shown in Figure 2.11), which contains three phosphate groups (hence "tri"). ATP is the energy source in our cells. Our cells manufacture ATP from glucose, which in turn comes from the food we eat. High-energy chemical bonds hold together the phosphates in ATP; thus, **ATP can be used to store and release a cell's energy.**

So, kinases are enzymes that take a phosphate from ATP (which now becomes ADP – adenosine di-phosphate) and transfer it to something else (see Figure 2.12). The most common thing that kinases attach phosphate to is another protein (often another kinase). Kinases usually attach phosphate to three particular amino acids in recipient proteins: tyrosine, threonine, or serine.

The addition (phosphorylation) and removal (dephosphorylation) of phosphates is a common way through which our cells control the activity of many of their proteins.

---

[11] Kinase inhibitors and chemotherapies are generally 300–700 Da in size, whereas monoclonal antibodies are about 150 KDa (i.e., antibodies are roughly 200 to 500 times bigger).

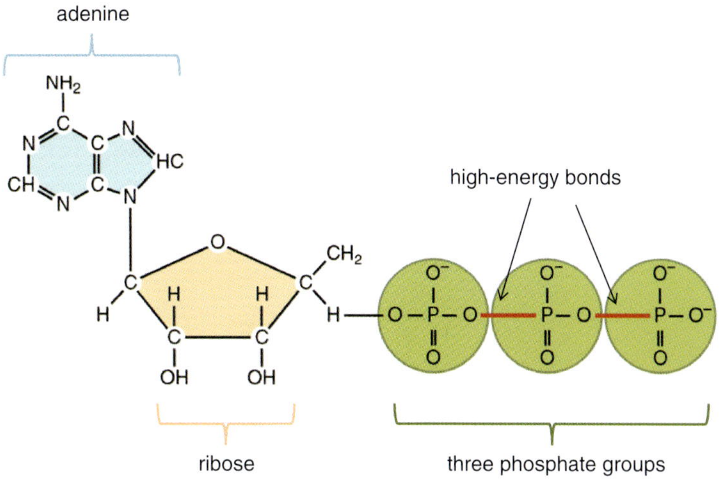

Figure 2.11 **The structure of ATP.** ATP is made from adenine, a sugar molecule called ribose, and three phosphates. The bonds holding together the phosphates release lots of energy when they are broken. When ATP loses one of its phosphates, it becomes a lower-energy molecule called ADP. When it loses two phosphates, it becomes AMP. As well as making up part of the ATP molecule, adenine is also found in DNA and RNA. **Abbreviations:** ATP – adenosine tri-phosphate; ADP – adenosine di-phosphate; AMP – adenosine mono-phosphate *Source:* Image from : https://commons.wikimedia.org/wiki/File:230_Structure_of_Adenosine_Triphosphate_(ATP)-01.jpg Attribution information from http://cnx.org/contents/FPtK1zmh@6.27:zMTtFGyH@4/Introduction. Download for free at http://cnx.org/contents/14fb4ad7-39a1-4eee-ab6e-3ef2482e3e22@8.81.

By adding phosphates to their targets, **kinases exert a huge influence on how our cells behave**.

In many cancers, the cells' abnormal behavior is at least in part due to the presence of overactive kinases. These include many kinases that would normally be under the control of growth factor receptors such as the EGFR, HER2, or VEGF receptors.[12] In addition, **growth factor receptors are themselves kinases** (see Figure 2.13). The part of the growth factor receptor that protrudes inside the cell has kinase activity (you can read more about growth factor receptors and how they work in Chapter 3, Section 3.2). Because kinases play a central role in the behavior of cancer cells, scientists have created many drugs that block them.

Lastly, it's important to know that kinases don't just phosphorylate proteins. In fact, a family of kinases that are overactive in a large proportion of breast, bowel, and lung cancers, and in some blood cancers, are kinases called PI3Ks (phosphatidylinositol 3-kinases). These kinases attach phosphate to a lipid – a fatty molecule – found in cell membranes. A variety of PI3K inhibitors are being developed by scientists, and two drugs, idelalisib (Zydelig) and copanlisib (Aliqopa), are licensed treatments.

---

[12] If you're not sure what a growth factor receptor is, turn to the introduction to Chapter 3 before you go any further.

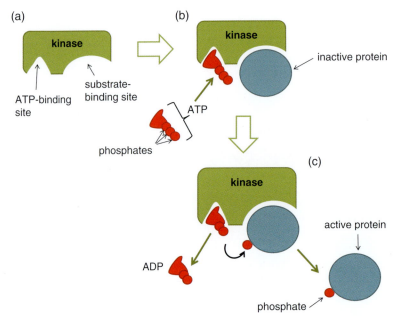

Figure 2.12 Kinases are catalysts that attach phosphates to other proteins and molecules in our cells.
(a) Kinases have docking sites for both ATP and one or more substrates (in this case, an inactive protein).
(b) Both ATP and the inactive protein dock with the kinase. **(c)** The kinase transfers one of the phosphates from ATP to a tyrosine, threonine, or serine amino acid in the protein. This activates the protein. What was ATP is now ADP. The active protein and ADP are released by the kinase.
Abbreviations: ATP – adenosine tri-phosphate; ADP – adenosine di-phosphate

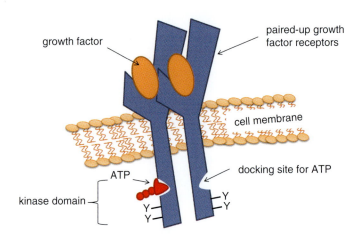

Figure 2.13 Growth factor receptors are kinases. Growth factor receptors are large proteins that sit in our cells' outer membrane. They have three main parts: an extracellular domain that sticks outside the cell, a transmembrane domain that spans the cell membrane, and an intracellular domain that protrudes into the cell cytoplasm. The intracellular domain has two important features: a docking site for ATP and multiple tyrosine (Y) amino acids. When ATP slots into its docking sites, the growth factor receptors phosphorylate each other on tyrosine amino acids. Growth factor receptors become active when phosphorylated.
Abbreviations: ATP – adenosine tri-phosphate

2.3.2 Different Types of Kinase Inhibitors

In order to phosphorylate their targets, kinases need to obtain phosphate from ATP. They therefore have an ATP-binding site, which is normally a pocket in the kinase's surface where ATP will fit (see Figure 2.12a). When the kinase isn't doing anything, this ATP-binding site is hidden by a short series of amino acids known as the activation loop, and ATP can't reach it. However, when the kinase is active (often because another kinase has attached phosphate to it), the activation loop moves, and the ATP-binding site is revealed [40].

Most kinase inhibitors work by mimicking the shape of ATP (see Figures 2.14a and b). The inhibitor slots into the ATP-binding site and prevents ATP from gaining access. However, this means that kinase inhibitors are vulnerable to changes in shape of the binding site, and a common reason for drug resistance is when the gene for a target kinase is mutated and the ATP-binding site has changed shape (Figure 2.14c).

Kinase inhibitors are classified according to how they block a kinase's activity, and whether or not the blockage is temporary or permanent. There are four main types of kinase inhibitors [40], described below and summarized in Figures 2.15a, b, c, and d and Table 2.2. There are also kinase inhibitors that work indirectly by interfering with a separate protein that the kinase interacts with (Figure 2.15e).

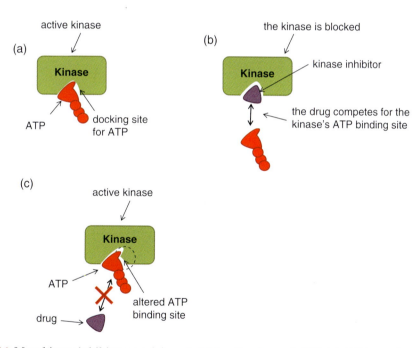

Figure 2.14 Most kinase inhibitors work by mimicking the shape of ATP. (a) All kinases have a binding site for ATP. When the kinase is activated, the ATP-binding site becomes accessible and ATP enters. The kinase is then able to phosphorylate its targets. **(b)** Kinases can be blocked by drugs that mimic the shape of ATP and that compete with ATP for the kinase's ATP-binding site. **(c)** In a cancer cell that is resistant to treatment with a kinase inhibitor, the gene for the target kinase has often sustained a mutation that has changed the binding site's shape. The mutation means that ATP can still enter its binding site, but the drug cannot; therefore, the kinase remains active, and the cancer cell survives.
Abbreviations: ATP – adenosine tri-phosphate

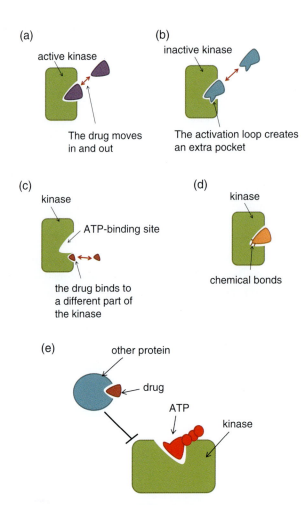

Figure 2.15 There are four classes of kinase inhibitors, and drugs that block kinases indirectly. **(a)** Type 1 kinase inhibitors compete with ATP for the ATP-docking site of active kinases. **(b)** Type 2 kinase inhibitors can enter a kinase's ATP-binding site only when the kinase is inactive. The ATP-binding site of inactive kinases contains an extra pocket created by the kinase's activation loop. **(c)** Allosteric inhibitors bind outside of the ATP-binding site. **(d)** Covalent inhibitors enter the kinase's ATP-binding site and form chemical bonds that hold the drug in place. **(e)** Indirect kinase inhibitors do not bind to the kinase directly; instead, they attach to a separate protein that only inhibits the kinase when the drug is present. **Abbreviations:** ATP – adenosine tri-phosphate

Table 2.2 Comparison of different types of kinase inhibitors.

	Type 1	Type 2	Allosteric inhibitors	Covalent inhibitors
Type of binding	Reversible	Reversible	Reversible	Irreversible
Binding site on the kinase	ATP-binding site	A pocket on one side of the ATP-binding site	Away from the ATP-binding site	ATP-binding site
Competes with ATP?	Yes	No	No	Yes
Relative selectivity	Low	Medium	High	Low
Examples	Gefitinib, erlotinib, sunitinib	Imatinib, nilotinib, sorafenib	Selumetinib, trametinib, cobimetinib	Afatinib, dacomitinib, neratinib

Source: Table adapted from: Blanc J, Geney R, Menet C. (2013). Type II Kinase Inhibitors: An Opportunity in Cancer for Rational Design. *Anticancer Agents Med Chem.* 13(5): 731–747. http://www.ncbi.nlm.nih.gov/pubmed/23094911.

Type 1 Kinase Inhibitors

This is the most common type of kinase inhibitor. These drugs are small molecules that mimic ATP's shape and slot into the ATP-binding site of **active kinases** (see Figure 2.15a.). Thus, they compete with ATP for the binding site, blocking the kinase's activity. This blockage is only temporary – hence they are **reversible** (rather than irreversible) kinase inhibitors. Unfortunately, many of our cells' kinases have similar ATP-binding sites; therefore, these drugs tend to bind to, and block, several different kinases. Some of the drug's targets will be active in cancer cells, and blocking them will hopefully kill the cell. But other (unintended) targets will be active in a range of healthy cells. These drugs therefore often cause a range of toxicities.[13] Examples include lapatinib (Tyverb), sunitinib (Sutent), gefitinib (Iressa), erlotinib (Tarceva), pazopanib (Votrient), vemurafenib (Zelboraf), ruxolitinib (Jakafi; Jakavi), crizotinib (Xalkori), bosutinib (Bosulif), and dasatinib (Sprycel).

Type 2 Kinase Inhibitors

These drugs are small molecules that bind to the ATP-binding site of kinases **when the kinase is inactive** and the activation loop has created an extra pocket (Figure 2.15b). These drugs can **trap their target kinases in an inactive state**. They don't compete with ATP, and they tend to be more selective and cause fewer side effects than the type 1 kinase inhibitors [41]. As with type 1 kinases, these are **reversible** inhibitors; that is, they get into the binding pocket and then drop out again – they don't stick. Examples include imatinib (Glivec; Gleevec), nilotinib (Tasigna), and sorafenib (Nexavar).

Allosteric Inhibitors

These drugs bind to a site on the kinase which is **separate from the ATP-binding site** (Figure 2.15c). Many of these drugs bind to a pocket in the target kinase which is involved in controlling the kinase's level of activity. The allosteric inhibitors that are furthest along in development are the MEK inhibitors [42] (see Chapter 3, Section 3.7.5 for more about MEK inhibitors) such as selumetinib, trametinib (Mekinist), and cobimetinib (Cotellic). However, others are being developed.

Covalent Inhibitors

Some kinase inhibitors are able to chemically bond with the ATP-binding site, making them **"irreversible"** kinase inhibitors (also known as covalent inhibitors) (Figure 2.15d). Because these drugs are able to stick to the ATP-binding site and don't drop out, they are predicted to be more powerful drugs than the reversible kinase inhibitors but may also cause more severe side effects [43]. The most well-known covalent kinase inhibitors are drugs such as afatinib (Giotrif/Gilotrif), neratinib (Nerlynx), and dacomitinib, which block EGFR and two other closely related receptors known as HER2 and HER4 (you can find out more about these receptors in Chapter 3, Section 3.2).

Indirect Inhibitors

Finally, some kinase inhibitors don't physically interact with the kinase they block. Instead, they **work via another protein** (Figure 2.15e). The most well-known examples are everolimus (Afinitor) and temsirolimus (Torisel), which are derivatives of a naturally occurring chemical called rapamycin (everolimus and temsirolimus are sometimes called

---

[13] What side effects they cause depends on their targets. For example, sunitinib blocks a broad range of targets and causes toxicities such as diarrhea, high blood pressure, skin toxicities, hypothyroidisms, fatigue, and nausea (Schmid TA & Gore ME (2016) Ther Adv Urol 8(6):348-371).

"rapalogues"). Rapamycin and rapalogues bind to a protein in our cells called FKBP12, which then interacts with and blocks some of the functions of a kinase called mTOR [44] (there is more about mTOR inhibitors in Chapter 3, Section 3.8.4). So the drug doesn't have to directly come into contact with the target kinase in order to block it.

2.3.3 Common Targets of Kinase Inhibitors

Kinases are very popular with drugs companies as targets of cancer treatments. This is for two main reasons: (1) because lots of kinases are implicated in cancer and (2) because drug companies have become very adept at creating drugs that block them (various kinases and the drugs that block them are summarized in Table 2.3). Because there are so many kinases being targeted for the treatment of cancer, I have grouped them below into three categories according to how the kinase has gone wrong, and how this causes cancer cell growth and survival:

1. **Kinases that are overactive because they are present at abnormally high levels, or because they are faulty due to gene mutations**
Examples include B-Raf, EGFR, ALK, Bcr-Abl, JAK2, HER2, FLT3, KIT, PI3K, AKT, MET, RET, aurora kinases, and polo-like kinases.

   These are all powerful, oncogenic (i.e., cancer-causing) kinases. If there is too much of any of these kinases in a cell, or if they are faulty and overactive, they are capable of forcing cells to take on many properties of a cancer cell.[14] When one of these faulty or overproduced kinases exists in a cancer cell, the cell is commonly "oncogene

addicted"; that is, the cell has become unable to survive without the faulty kinase's activity. Because of this, drugs that block these kinases are capable of killing cancer cells (unless the cell has additional mutations that make it insensitive to treatment).

2. **Kinases that are often overactive because of a mutation affecting another protein, but that aren't themselves abnormal**[15]
Examples include MEK, mTOR, BTK, and CDKs.

   These kinases can be useful drug targets when the protein at fault isn't targetable. For example, mutated, overactive forms of Ras proteins (K-Ras, N-Ras, and H-Ras) can force cells to grow and multiply and are heavily implicated in many cancers. However, we don't have any Ras inhibitors (Ras isn't a kinase, and it has proved very difficult to create drugs that can block it). Ras proteins force cells to multiply via activating kinases such as MEK, Raf, PI3K, and CDKs. Laboratory experiments on cancer cells suggest that by blocking these kinases, you can kill cancer cells with faulty Ras proteins [67]. This type of approach is called **synthetic lethality**[16] – where you try to find a lethal combination of a mutation in one protein, and a drug that targets another protein (illustrated in Figure 2.16).[17]

3. **Kinases found in/on non-cancer cells in the cancer's microenvironment**
Examples include VEGF receptors, PDGF receptors, and FGF receptors.

   These kinases are growth factor receptors found on the surface of endothelial cells that line the body's blood vessels. These receptors are necessary for tumor angiogenesis, and the drugs that block them are

---

[14] Do bear in mind that in a healthy cell the abnormal presence of a powerful, oncogenic protein such as these would trigger apoptosis. So, in a cancer cell, there must be other mutations, perhaps affecting the apoptosis machinery, that permit the cell to survive.

[15] This isn't black and white. Occasionally, the genes for these proteins are affected by mutations, but they're very rare.

[16] In this instance, the word "synthesis" is being used to mean the combination of two things to form something new.

[17] Another example of synthetic lethality is the use of PARP inhibitors to treat BRCA-mutated cancers, described in Chapter 3, Section 3.6.

Table 2.3   Targets and uses of kinase inhibitors as cancer treatments.

Target protein/s	What is it? Where is it found?	Examples of treatments that target the protein	What cancers are these drugs most commonly used to treat?
Kinases found on the surface of blood cancer cells (leukemias, lymphomas, multiple myeloma)			
FLT3	A growth factor receptor mutated in the cancer cells of around a third of people with acute myeloid leukemia (AML) and almost always overproduced by AML cells; also found on the surface of some immature white blood cells [45]	Midostaurin (Rydapt) Lestaurtinib Quizartinib (AC220) Crenolanib Gilteritinib	AML
KIT	A growth factor receptor mutated in the cancer cells of 2-14% of people with acute myeloid leukemia (AML) [46]	Dasatinib (Sprycel) Pazopanib (Votrient) Quizartinib	AML (but none licensed yet)
Intracellular kinases in blood cancer cells (leukemias, lymphomas, multiple myeloma)			
JAK2	A signaling protein found in cells throughout the body. It activates a family of transcription factors known as STATs [47]	Ruxolitinib (Jakafi; Jakavi) Momelotinib Pacritinib	Myeloproliferative neoplasms[a]
BTK (Bruton's tyrosine kinase)	A signaling protein controlled by the B cell receptor, which is found on the surface of B cells [48]	Ibrutinib (Imbruvica) Acalabrutinib (Calquence)	Chronic lymphocytic leukemia, non-Hodgkin lymphoma, Waldenstrom's macroglobulinemia
ABL	Phosphorylates many different proteins involved in cell growth and survival; in chronic myeloid leukemia, the *ABL* gene is accidently fused to another gene called *BCR*, and the cells make a Bcr-Abl fusion protein [49]	Imatinib (Glivec; Gleevec) Dasatinib (Sprycel) Bosutinib (Bosulif) Nilotinib (Tasigna) Ponatinib (Iclusig)	Chronic myeloid leukemia (and a minority of acute lymphoblastic leukemias and acute myeloid leukemias)
PI3Kσ (this form of PI3K is found exclusively in white blood cells)	Controlled by the B cell receptor Implicated in various B cell leukemias and lymphomas [48]	Idelalisib (Zydelig) Copanlisib (Aliqopa) Duvelisib	Chronic lymphocytic leukemia, non-Hodgkin lymphoma
Kinases found on the surface of solid tumor cells			
EGF receptor[b]	A growth factor receptor implicated in many cancers; the kinase domain is sometimes mutated and overactive in lung cancer cells [50]	Gefitinib (Iressa) Erlotinib (Tarceva) Afatinib (Giotrif; Gilotrif)* Dacomitinib* Neratinib (Nerlynx)*	Non-small cell lung cancers containing various EGF receptor mutations
T790M mutated EGF receptor	This mutated form of the EGF receptor is resistant to gefitinib and erlotinib; drugs have been created that specifically target this version of the receptor	Osimertinib (Tagrisso) Rociletinib	Non-small cell lung cancers containing EGF receptor with the T790M mutation
HER2[c]	A growth factor receptor often found in excessive amounts on breast cancer cells and stomach cancer cells; found in small amounts in other cancers [28]	Lapatinib (Tyverb) Afatinib (Giotrif; Gilotrif)* Dacomitinib* Neratinib (Nerlynx)*	Breast cancer, stomach cancer, EGFR-mutated non-small cell lung cancer

(Continued)

Table 2.3   (Continued)

Target protein/s	What is it? Where is it found?	Examples of treatments that target the protein	What cancers are these drugs most commonly used to treat?
IGF-1R, MET, FGF receptors	Growth factor receptors implicated in a range of solid tumors [51–53]	Many are in development	No treatments licensed yet for any cancer
RET	A growth factor receptor implicated in thyroid cancer [54]	Cabozantinib (Cometriq)** Vandetinib (Caprelsa)** Lenvatinib (Lenvima)** Sorafenib (Nexavar)**	Thyroid cancer
KIT, PDGF receptor alpha	Mutated versions of these growth factor receptors are found on the surface of cancer cells in gastrointestinal stromal tumors (GISTs). PDGF receptors are also involved in angiogenesis [55]; KIT is implicated in acute myeloid leukemia [56]	Imatinib (Glivec) Sunitinib (Sutent) Regorafenib (Stivarga) Pazopanib (Votrient)	Gastrointestinal stromal tumors (GISTs)

Intracellular kinases in solid tumor cells

ALK	The normal protein is a growth factor receptor. In some cancer cells, the protein is broken and fused to another protein (such as EML4) to create a hyperactive intracellular kinase. ALK is also overactive in some neuroblastomas [57]	Crizotinib (Xalkori) Ceritinib (Zykadia) Alectinib (Alacensa) Brigatinib (Alunbrig) Entrectinib Lorlatinib	Non-small cell lung cancer, anaplastic large cell lymphoma
mTOR	Involved in cell-signaling pathways and implicated in many cancers [58]	Temsirolimus (Torisel) Everolimus (Afinitor) Voxtalisib*** Dactolisib***	Kidney cancer, breast cancer, PNETs,[d] SEGA[e]
AKT (also known as protein kinase B)	Involved in cell-signaling pathways and implicated in many cancers [59]	Perifosine MK2206 Ipatasertib	No treatments licensed yet for any cancer
B-Raf	Involved in cell-signaling pathways and mutated in around 50% of malignant melanomas [60]	Vemurafenib (Zelboraf) Dabrafenib (Tafinlar)	Malignant melanoma
MEK	Involved in cell-signaling pathways and controlled by B-Raf [61]	Trametinib (Mekinist) Selumetinib Cobimetinib (Cotellic)	Malignant melanoma
PI3Ks (phosphatidyl-inositol-3-kinases)	Involved in cell-signaling pathways and implicated in many cancers [62]	Buparlisib Pictilisib Alpelisib Copanlisib (Aliqopa) Apitolisib	No treatments licensed yet for any solid tumour

Table 2.3   (Continued)

Kinases implicated in angiogenesis

VEGF receptors, (PDGF receptors, FGF receptors)	These growth factor receptor are found on endothelial cells that line normal blood vessels and those found in tumors; they are also sometimes found on cancer cells, although the significance of this is unclear [63]. Because the ATP-binding sites of VEGF, PDGF and FGF receptors are similar to one another, many of the drugs listed have some ability to block all three sets of receptors	Sunitinib (Sutent) Sorafenib (Nexavar) Pazopanib (Votrient) Axitinib (Inlyta) Regorafenib (Stivarga) Cabozantinib (Cometriq) Vandetinib (Caprelsa) Cediranib (Recentin) Lenvatinib (Lenvima) Vatalanib Motesanib Tivozanib	Various solid tumors including bowel cancer, ovarian cancer, cervical cancer, and kidney cancer

Kinases implicated involved in the cell cycle (inhibitors may be useful in solid tumors and blood cancers)

Aurora kinases	Involved in the process of cell division – they are necessary for the correct separation of chromosomes during mitosis; implicated in many cancers [64, 65]	Barasertib Alisertib Danusertib	No treatments licensed yet for any cancer
Polo-like kinases	Involved in several stages of mitosis including the formation of the spindle; implicated in many cancers [60]	Volasertib Rigosertib	No treatments licensed yet for any cancer
CDK 4 & CDK6 (CDK: cyclin-dependent kinase)	Control progression through the cell cycle; implicated in many cancers – often overactive due to faults in other genes such as those for growth factor receptors, Raf, PI3K, or overproduction of cyclin D [66]	Palbociclib (Ibrance) Ribociclib (Kisqali) Abemaciclib (Verzenio) Dinaciclib	Hormone therapy-resistant breast cancer; also in trials for other cancers

Note: *Afatinib, dacomitinib, and neratinib block EGFR, HER2, and HER4.
**All of these drugs RET and VEGF receptors; therefore, they probably have a dual mechanism of action: blocking both RET and angiogenesis.
***These drugs block both mTOR and PI3K.
[a]According to Bloodwise, these are "are a group of blood disorders related to leukaemia in which the body makes too many blood cells."
[b]Also known as human epidermal growth factor receptor-1 (EGFR; HER1).
[c]HER2 stands for human epidermal growth factor receptor-2; it is closely related to HER1 (EGF receptor), HER3, and HER4.
[d]Pancreatic neuroendocrine tumors (PNETs) are rare, slow-growing pancreatic cancers.
[e]Subependymal giant cell astrocytomas (SEGAs) – these are slow-growing brain tumors that occur almost exclusively in people with a rare genetic disease called tuberous sclerosis complex.

known as angiogenesis inhibitors. Do note, though, that some of these receptors are sometimes found on the surface of cancer cells. For example, FGF receptors are involved in angiogenesis, but they are also present on cancer cells in some lung, breast, and stomach cancers and participate in these cancers' development [68].

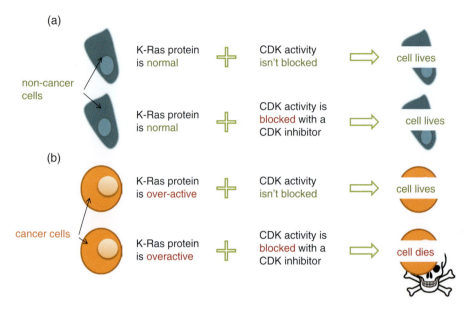

Figure 2.16 **The idea behind synthetic lethality.** **(a)** In healthy cells, K-Ras is normal, and CDK enzymes are not overactive. Blocking CDKs should have little impact on the cells. **(b)** In many cancer cells, K-Ras is faulty and overactive, and this in turn forces the cells' CDK enzymes to be overactive. The combination (synthesis) of faulty K-Ras plus a CDK inhibitor is lethal to the cancer cells.
Abbreviations: CDK – cyclin-dependent kinase

2.3.4 Useful Properties of Kinase Inhibitors as Cancer Treatments

- **Kinase inhibitors can block kinases that are driving the growth and survival of cancer cells**. They are therefore able to kill cancer cells and are useful as cancer treatments.

- Because they are physically much smaller than mAbs, **kinase inhibitors can cross the cell membrane and enter into the main body of the cell – the cytoplasm**. It is thus possible to use kinase inhibitors to block intracellular kinases (such as B-Raf, MEK, and mTOR) that are inaccessible to mAbs.

- Also, because of their small size, **kinase inhibitors can travel around the body and through our organs and tissues much more easily than mAbs**. This means that they can penetrate parts of tumors that are inaccessible to mAbs. In addition, whereas mAbs and most chemotherapies are unable to cross the blood-brain barrier,[18] kinase inhibitors are sometimes able to do so and therefore may be useful against brain metastases from several solid tumors, including lung cancer and HER2-driven breast cancer [69, 70].

- Kinase inhibitors are chemical compounds rather than proteins. This means that many of them **can be taken in tablet form**, making them much easier, and less time consuming, to administer.

- These drugs commonly **block more than one kinase**. For example, drugs that block

---

[18] See footnote 5 about the blood brain barrier.

VEGF receptors will almost always block some PDGF receptors and FGF receptors because the ATP-binding sites of these kinases are similar to one another. The ability to block multiple kinases means that kinase inhibitors can be more potent treatments than monoclonal antibodies, which will only ever block one target. This same characteristic can also lead to unexpected additional uses for kinase inhibitors. For example, imatinib was created as a Bcr-Abl inhibitor for the treatment of chronic myeloid leukemia. However, imatinib was later discovered to block both PDGF receptors and KIT – both of which are involved in gastrointestinal stromal tumors (GISTs). Imatinib is now an important treatment for GISTs.

2.3.5 Limitations of Kinase Inhibitors and the Reason They Cause Side Effects

- Kinase inhibitors, particularly type 1 inhibitors, are very imprecise compared to antibody treatments. For example, in laboratory experiments, sunitinib and pazopanib are each able to block the activity of at least 30 different kinases [71]. As mentioned above, the ability of kinase inhibitors to block more than one target can be an advantage. But this same ability also leads to a greater number of side effects.
- Similar to the antibody treatments, these drugs' targets will be present in healthy cells as well as cancer cells; destruction of these cells causes additional side effects.
- Drug resistance is an issue with kinase inhibitors as with all cancer treatments. Resistance to kinase inhibitors is commonly due to mutations that alter the shape of the kinase's ATP-binding site.

- Kinase inhibitors tend to be broken down by the body very quickly (far more quickly than monoclonal antibodies), and they therefore have to be taken by the patient daily, or even twice daily.
- There is a high degree of drug-to-drug and patient-to-patient variation in the concentration of these treatments in the blood, how long they remain there, how they get broken down, and what proportion is floating free (rather than being stuck to blood proteins). This can make it difficult to find the optimum dose for an individual patient [72, 73].

2.3.6 How Kinase Inhibitors Are Being Improved

In recent years, a range of new technologies has been enabling scientists to proactively design new kinase inhibitors that fit target kinases exactly (rather than testing thousands upon thousands of chemicals for their ability to block kinases in laboratory tests and then trying to improve on the most promising-looking compounds[19]). This is helping scientists create more precise kinase inhibitors, which will hopefully cause fewer side effects than some of the so-called multi-kinase inhibitors such as sorafenib and dasatinib. In addition, allosteric inhibitors seem to be more precise than other types of inhibitors. Efforts are therefore under way to create allosteric inhibitors that can block a wider variety of kinase targets, including creating allosteric inhibitors of growth factor receptors [74].

We are also seeing the creation of kinase inhibitors that can block mutated versions of kinases known to be resistant to other inhibitors. For example, lung cancers that are resistant to EGFR inhibitors such as gefitinib and erlotinib

---

[19] This approach is known as high-throughput screening and lead optimization.

often contain a faulty version of EGFR known as the T790M mutant. New EGFR inhibitors, such as osimertinib (Tagrisso), have been created to block this mutant protein.

Areas for future improvement include predicting patient responses and toxicities more precisely, and a better understanding of how target kinases interact and compensate for one another in different cancer types (for a review, see [15]).

2.4 FINAL THOUGHTS

Although monoclonal antibodies and kinase inhibitors are physically very different from one another, they are often used to block the same targets. For this reason they have an overlapping set of uses and side effects. Monoclonal antibodies have an added dimension to them in that they can attract white blood cells and generate immune responses that can destroy cancer cells. However, their ability to attract white blood cells varies from cancer to cancer and patient to patient, and seems to work best against blood cancers like leukemia and lymphoma. An important limitation of antibody-based treatments is their size and inability to diffuse across cell membranes. This is where the small size of kinase inhibitors and their ability to penetrate the cell cytoplasm and block intracellular targets is an advantage.

As well as having distinct targets, monoclonal antibodies and kinase inhibitors also differ in terms of their specificity for their target. Monoclonal antibody treatments, like the antibodies generated during our body's response to an infection, are incredibly precise. In contrast, most kinase inhibitors

work by entering ATP-binding sites on kinases, and many kinases have very similar ATP-binding sites. Hence, kinase inhibitors tend to block many different kinases alongside the one they've been created to block. This adds to the toxicities caused by kinase inhibitors, but it can also boost their impact on tumors (in which many different kinases may be overactive for different reasons) and be beneficial.

Lastly, we have recently entered a new era in the treatment of cancer in which antibodies that have been designed as powerful immunotherapies are been intensively explored and are generating promising results. Immunotherapies are a distinct group of treatments that directly target white blood cells and create anti-cancer immune responses.[20] Antibodies that target CTLA-4, PD-1, and PD-L1 fall into this category, and we will look at them in much more detail in Chapter 5.

REFERENCES

1　Thariat J et al. (2013). Past, present, and future of radiotherapy for the benefit of patients. *Nat Rev Clin Oncol* **10**: 52–60.

2　DeVita VT, Chu E (2008). A history of cancer chemotherapy. *Cancer Res* **68**(21): 8643–8653.

3　Crawford ED (2004). Hormonal therapy in prostate cancer: Historical approaches. *Rev Urol* **6**(Suppl 7): S3–S11.

4　Jordan VC (1997). Tamoxifen treatment for breast cancer: Concept to gold standard. *Oncology* **11**(2 Suppl 1): 7–13.

5　Liu JKH (2014). The history of monoclonal antibody development – progress, remaining challenges and future innovations. *Annals Med Surg* **3**: 113–116.

---

[20] I am using the term "immunotherapy" to refer to treatments whose primary mechanism of action is that they target the immune system. I am not talking about antibodies that block a protein on cancer cells that is driving their growth (like HER2 or EGFR). However, it is a gray area, as antibodies that target HER2 and EGFR may also attract white blood cells.

6 Cohen P (2002). Protein kinases — the major drug targets of the twenty-first century? *Nat Rev Drug Discov* **1**: 309–315.

7 Lesterhuis WJ et al. (2011). Cancer immunotherapy – revisited. *Nat Rev Drug Discov* **10**: 591–600.

8 For an alternative definition and description of targeted therapies, see: National Cancer Institute. 2014. Targeted Therapy. [Online] Available at: http://www.cancer.gov/about-cancer/treatment/types/targeted-therapies [Accessed February 26, 2018].

9 Schrama D et al. (2006). Antibody targeted drugs as cancer therapeutics. *Nat Rev Drug Discov* **5**(2): 147–159.

10 Mechanisms of action of antibody treatments are summarized in: Scott A et al. (2012). Antibody therapy of cancer. *Nat Rev Cancer* **12**(4): 278–287.

11 Weiner GJ (2015). Building better monoclonal antibody-based therapeutics. *Nat Rev Cancer* **15**(6): 361–370.

12 Chames P et al. (2009). Therapeutic antibodies: Successes, limitations and hopes for the future. *Br J Pharmacol* **157**(2): 220–233.

13 For an introduction to complement proteins, see: Encyclopaedia Britannica. Complement. [Online] Available at: https://www.britannica.com/science/complement-immune-system-component [Accessed February 26, 2018].

14 For an example, see: Lee C, Tannock I (2010). The distribution of the therapeutic monoclonal antibodies cetuximab and trastuzumab within solid tumors. *BMC Cancer* **10**: 255.

15 Fukuyama R, Shimizu N (1991). Expression of epidermal growth factor (EGF) and the EGF receptor in human tissues. *J Exp Zool* **258**: 336–343.

16 Damjanov I, Mildner B, Knowles BB (1986). Immunohistochemical localization of the epidermal growth factor receptor in normal human tissues. *Lab Invest* **55**: 588–592.

17 Macmillan website page on cetuximab http://www.macmillan.org.uk/Cancerinformation/Cancertreatment/Treatmenttypes/Biologicaltherapies/Monoclonalantibodies/Cetuximab.aspx [Accessed February 26, 2018].

18 Reviewed in: Firer MA (2013 June 19). Antibody-drug conjugates in cancer therapy – filling in the potholes that lie ahead. *OA Cancer* **1**(1): 8.

19 Chari R et al. (2014). Antibody–drug conjugates: An emerging concept in cancer therapy. *Angew Chem Int Ed* **53**(15): 3796–3827.

20 National Cancer Institute. 2014. Using the Immune System in the Fight Against Cancer: Discovery of Rituximab. [Online] Available at: http://www.cancer.gov/research/progress/discovery/blood-cancer [Accessed February 26, 2018].

21 Maloney DG (2012). Anti-CD20 antibody therapy for B-cell lymphomas. *N Engl J Med* **366**: 2008–2016.

22 Schirrmann T, Steinwand M, Wezler X et al. (2014) CD30 as a therapeutic target for lymphoma. *BioDrugs* **28**(2): 181–209.

23 Ehninger A et al. (2014). Distribution and levels of cell surface expression of CD33 and CD123 in acute myeloid leukemia. *Blood Cancer J* **4**: e218.

24 Phipps C, Chen Y, Gopalakrishnan S (2015). Daratumumab and its potential in the treatment of multiple myeloma: Overview of the preclinical and clinical development. *Ther Adv Hematol* **6**(3): 120–127.

25 Ginaldi L et al. (1998). Levels of expression of CD52 in normal and leukemic B and T cells: Correlation with in vivo therapeutic responses to Campath-1H. *Leuk Res* **22**(2): 185–191.

26 van de Donk NWCJ et al. (2016). Clinical efficacy and management of monoclonal antibodies targeting CD38 and SLAMF7 in multiple myeloma. *Blood* **127**(6): 681–695.

27 For an overview, see: Hynes NE, Lane HA (2005). ERBB receptors and cancer: The complexity of targeted inhibitors. *Nat Rev Cancer* **5**(5): 341–354.

28 Arguello D et al. (2014). HER2 distribution in diverse tumors: Analysis of 11,493 non-breast, nongastric cancers. *J Clin Oncol* **32**: 2014 (suppl; abstr e22200).

29 Natali PG, Nicotra MR, Bigotti A, Venturo I, Slamon DJ, Fendly BM et al. (1990) Expression of the p185 encoded by HER2 oncogene in normal and transformed human tissues. *Int J Cancer* **45**: 457–461.

30 Press MF, Cordon-Cardo C, Slamon DJ (1990). Expression of the HER-2/ neu proto-oncogene

in normal human adult and fetal tissues. *Oncogene* **5**: 953–962.

31 Yang RK, Sondel PM (2010). Anti-GD2 strategy in the treatment of Neuroblastoma. *Drugs Future* **35**(8): 665.

32 McCoy K, Le Gros G (1999). The role of CTLA-4 in the regulation of T cell immune responses. *Immunol Cell Biol* **77**: 1–10.

33 Ma W et al. (2016). Current status and perspectives in translational biomarker research for PD-1/PD-L1 immune checkpoint blockade therapy. *J Hematol Oncol* **9**: 47.

34 For a great overview of the usefulness of radioactive antibodies see: Larson SM et al. (2015). Radioimmunotherapy of human tumours. *Nat Rev Cancer* **15**(6): 347–360.

35 Zhang M, Gopal AK (2008). Radioimmunotherapy based conditioning regimens for stem cell transplantation. *Semin Hematol* **45**(2): 118–125.

36 Weiner GJ. (2015). Building better monoclonal antibody-based therapies. *Nat Rev Cancer* **15**(6): 361–370.

37 Zheng K et al. (2011). The impact of glycosylation on monoclonal antibody conformation and stability. *MAbs* **3**(6): 568–576.

38 Vulto AG, Jaquez OA (2017). The process defines the product: What really matters in biosimilar design and production? *Rheumatology* **56**(Issue suppl 4): iv14–iv29.

39 For more about ATP, see: Encyclopaedia Britannica. Adenosine Triphosphate. [Online] Available at: https://www.britannica.com/science/adenosine-triphosphate [Accessed February 26, 2018].

40 Zhang J et al. (2009). Targeting cancer with small molecule kinase inhibitors. *Nat Rev Cancer* **9**(1): 28–39.

41 Blanc J, Geney R, Menet C. (2013). Type II Kinase Inhibitors: An Opportunity in Cancer for Rational Design. *Anticancer Agents Med Chem* **13**(5): 731–747.

42 Ohren JF et al. (2004). Structures of human MAP kinase kinase 1 (MEK1) and MEK2 describe novel noncompetitive kinase inhibition. *Nat Struct Mol Biol* **11**: 1192–1197.

43 Boyer MJ et al. (2010). Efficacy and safety of PF299804 versus erlotinib (E): A global, randomized phase II trial in patients (pts) with advanced non-small cell lung cancer (NSCLC)

after failure of chemotherapy (CT). *J Clin Oncol* **28**: 18 s, 2010 (suppl; abstr LBA7523).

44 Shimobayashi M, Hall MN (2014). Making new contacts: The mTOR network in metabolism and signalling crosstalk. *Nat Rev Mol Cell Biol* **15**(3): 155–162.

45 Small D (2006). FLT3 mutations: Biology and treatment. *Hematology Am Soc Hematol Educ Program* 78–84.

46 Yohe S (2015). Molecular genetic markers in acute myeloid leukemia. *J Clin Med* **4**: 460–478.

47 Yamaoka K et al. (2004). The Janus kinases (Jaks). *Genome Biol* **5**(12): 253.

48 Young RM, Staudt LM (2013). Targeting pathological B cell receptor signalling in lymphoid malignancies. *Nat Rev Drug Discov* **12**: 229–243.

49 Pasternak G et al. (1998). Chronic myelogenous leukemia: Molecular and cellular aspects. *J Cancer Res Clin Oncol* **124**: 643–660.

50 Russo A et al. (2015). A decade of EGFR inhibition in EGFR-mutated non small cell lung cancer (NSCLC): Old successes and future perspectives. *Oncotarget* **6**(29): 26814–26825.

51 Reviewed in: Pollak M (2008). Insulin and insulin-like growth factor signalling in neoplasia. *Nat Rev Cancer* **8**: 915–928.

52 Smyth E, Sclafani F, Cunningham D (2014). Emerging molecular targets in oncology: Clinical potential of MET/hepatocyte growth-factor inhibitors. *Onco Targets Ther* **7**: 1001–1014.

53 Wesche J, Haglund K, Haugsten EM (2011). Fibroblast growth factors and their receptors in cancer. *Biochem J* **437**(2): 199–213.

54 Mulligan LM (2014). RET revisited: Expanding the oncogenic portfolio. *Nat Rev Cancer* **14**: 173–186.

55 Heldin CH (2013). Targeting the PDGF signaling pathway in tumor treatment. *Cell Commun Signal* **11**: 97.

56 Lennartsson J, Ronnstrand L (2012). Stem cell factor receptor/c-Kit: From Basic science to clinical implications. *Physiol Rev* **92**(4): 1619–1649.

57 Grande E, Bolos MV, Arriola E (2011). Targeting oncogenic ALK: A promising strategy for cancer treatment. *Mol Cancer Ther* **10**: 569.

58 Yuan R, Kay A, Berg WJ et al. (2009). Targeting tumorigenesis: Development and use of mTOR inhibitors in cancer therapy. *J Hematol Oncol* **2**: 45.

59 Brown JS, Banerji U (2016). Maximising the potential of AKT inhibitors as anti-cancer treatments. *Pharmacol Ther Dec* **2**. pii: S0163-7258(16)30244–3.

60 Davies H, Bignell GR, Cox C et al. (2002). Mutations of the BRAF gene in human cancer. *Nature* **417**: 949–954.

61 Samatar AA, Poulikakos PI (2014). Targeting RAS–ERK signalling in cancer: Promises and challenges. *Nat Rev Drug Discov* **13**(12): 928–942.

62 Yap TA et al. (2015). Drugging PI3K in cancer: Refining targets and therapeutic strategies. *Curr Opin Pharmacol* **23**: 98–107.

63 Harris A, Generali D. (2008). Inhibitors of tumour angiogenesis. In Neidle S (Ed.), *Cancer Drug Design and Discovery*. 2nd ed. London, UK. Elsevier Inc. pp. 275–306.

64 For a review see: Dar AA et al. (2010). Aurora kinases' inhibitors – Rising stars in cancer therapeutics? *Mol Cancer Ther* **9**(2): 268–278.

65 Lens SM et al. (2010). Shared and separate functions of polo-like kinases and aurora kinases in cancer. *Nat Rev Cancer* **10**(12): 825–841.

66 Casimiro MC et al. (2014). Overview of cyclins D1 function in cancer and the CDK inhibitor landscape: Past and present. *Expert Opin Investig Drugs* **23**(3): 295–304.

67 Lamba S et al. (2014). RAF suppression synergizes with MEK inhibition in *KRAS* mutant cancer cells. *Cell Reports* **8**(5): 1475–1483.

68 For a review, see: Katoh M, Nakagama H (2014). FGF receptors: Cancer biology and therapeutics. *Med Res Rev* **34**(2): 280–300.

69 Bartolotti M et al. (2012). EGF receptor tyrosine kinase inhibitors in the treatment of brain metastases from non-small-cell lung cancer. *Expert Rev Anticancer Ther* **12**(11): 1429–1435.

70 Lin N (2013). Breast cancer brain metastases: New directions in systemic therapy. *Ecancermedicalscience* **7**: 307.

71 Kitagawa D et al. (2012). Activity-based kinase profiling of approved tyrosine kinase inhibitors. *Genes Cells* **18**(2): 110–122.

72 van Erp N P, Gelderblom H, Guchelaar H-J (2009). Clinical pharmacokinetics of tyrosine kinase inhibitors. *Cancer Treatment Rev* **35**(8): 692–670.

73 Lankheet N A et al. (2014). Plasma concentrations of tyrosine kinase inhibitors imatinib, erlotinib, and sunitinib in routine clinical outpatient cancer care. *Ther Drug Monit* **36**(3): 326–334.

74 De Smet F, Christopoulos A, Carmeliet P (2014). Allosteric targeting of receptor tyrosine kinases. *Nat Biotechnol* **32**: 1113–1120.

CHAPTER 3

Treatments That Block Proteins Involved in Cell Communication

IN BRIEF

Our cells communicate constantly by releasing small proteins into their surroundings that attach to receptor proteins on their neighbors. These receptors then trigger internal communication pathways that pass on the signal within the cell and make sure it responds appropriately. These communication pathways, and the receptors that control them, have virtually always gone awry in cancer cells. Drugs that block them have become important treatments for many cancers.

In this chapter, I will first provide a general introduction to how cells communicate. I'll then describe how various communication pathways operate, what goes wrong with them in cancer cells, and how these defects are targeted using treatments such as monoclonal antibodies and kinase inhibitors.

Many of the treatments described in this chapter block cell surface receptors called EGFR (epidermal growth factor receptor) and HER2 (human epidermal growth factor receptor-2). EGFR-targeted treatments are important treatments for people with lung cancer and bowel cancer. HER2-targeted treatments are predominantly used against breast cancer.

Other drugs I describe in this chapter target three important signaling pathways triggered by cell surface receptors. These pathways are the MAPK pathway, the PI3K/AKT/mTOR pathway, and the JAK-STAT pathway. The MAPK pathway is perhaps the most well known of the three. It involves proteins such as K-Ras, B-Raf, and MEK. B-Raf and MEK inhibitors are important treatments for malignant melanoma skin cancer.

As yet, treatments that target the PI3K/AKT/mTOR pathway have had only moderate success. mTOR inhibitors are given to some people with kidney cancer or breast cancer, and there are many drugs in trials. Treatments that target JAK2 are used to treat a group of generally slow-growing blood cancers collectively called the myeloproliferative neoplasms (MPNs).

3.1 INTRODUCTION

Our cells are constantly responding to signals from their environment. Depending on the messages they receive, they alter their behavior or might even die. For example, cells use receptor proteins on their surface to detect levels of oxygen, proteins, amino acids, some hormones, and tiny proteins called growth factors. Our cells also have an array of receptors

A Beginner's Guide to Targeted Cancer Treatments, First Edition. Elaine Vickers.
© 2018 John Wiley & Sons Ltd. Published 2018 by John Wiley & Sons Ltd.

inside them that pick up other signals, such as fat-soluble hormones released by the brain, adrenal glands, and sex organs. Also, by forming physical connections with their neighbors, our cells can tell if there are too many, or too few, cells in their neighborhood. In addition, all our tissues and organs contain a network of complex proteins and sugars that our cells make connections with. This "extracellular matrix" (ECM) also provides cells with feedback about their surroundings.

If that wasn't enough, our cells are also programmed to respond to signals sent out by white blood cells. Each type of white blood cell (and there are *lots* of different types) has a repertoire of signaling proteins that it can release into its surroundings to coordinate immune responses and trigger healing. Finally, some of our cells have specialized receptors for light, sound, touch, or electrical signals (for a summary see Figure 3.1).[1]

The largest group of receptors found on the surface of our cells are the **G-protein-coupled receptors** (GPCRs). In fact, there are over 1,000 different GPCRs in the human body [1, 2]. A much smaller group of receptors are the 58 different "**receptor tyrosine kinases**" (RTKs) [3, 4]. These receptors usually respond to growth factors, thus another name for them is "**growth factor receptors**."

Growth factors are tiny proteins that our cells use to communicate with their neighbors. When a growth factor attaches to a growth factor receptor, this triggers a series of events inside a cell. This passing on of a signal from a receptor to the nucleus is called a **signaling pathway, cell communication pathway**, or **signal transduction cascade**.

Many receptors and other proteins involved in signaling pathways are faulty in cancer cells. As a result, over the past 30 years, cell communication has become a major area of cancer research, and a large number of new cancer treatments work by blocking cell communication proteins.

Currently, most cancer drugs that target signaling pathways work by:

1. **Blocking growth factor receptors** on the cell's surface, for example, epidermal growth factor receptor (EGF receptor; EGFR) or human EGF receptor-2 (HER2; Neu; ErbB2)
2. **Blocking kinases inside the cell** that are normally controlled by growth factor receptors (e.g., B-Raf, MEK, mTOR, PI3K, and AKT)
3. **Blocking the production of a hormone**, generally either testosterone or estrogen
4. **Blocking a hormone receptor** – usually either the androgen receptor (the receptor that responds to testosterone) or the estrogen receptor

Because drugs that block hormone receptors are used as treatments for prostate and breast cancer, I'll provide information on drugs that block them in the sections on prostate and breast cancer in Chapter 6.

A handful of cancer drugs work by blocking proteins that are involved in other signaling pathways – ones that aren't controlled by growth factor receptors or hormones. These include drugs that target Hedgehog signaling, which I look at in Chapter 4.

There are yet other signaling pathways that scientists think are very important in some cancers, but that haven't as yet led to any licensed cancer treatments. One example is the WNT/β-catenin pathway, which is overactive in most bowel cancers.

Although human cells contain a vast array of receptors, for the remainder of this chapter

---

[1] The Scitable website from NatureEducation contains a useful ebook, *Essentials of Cell Biology*, which has a chapter on cell communication: http://www.nature.com/scitable/ebooks/essentials-of-cell-biology-14749010/how-do-cells-sense-their-environment-14751787.

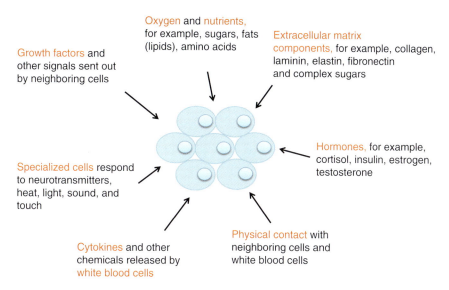

Figure 3.1 Our cells respond to a wide range of short-range and long-range signals. Short-range signals include growth factors, which travel short distances between cells. Our cells also respond to oxygen and nutrients, to complex proteins and sugars in their immediate surroundings (called the extracellular matrix), and to physical contact with neighboring cells. Long-range signals that cells respond to include hormones, which are produced and released by specialized glands throughout the body, such as the adrenal glands, the hypothalamus and pituitary gland in the brain, the testes (in men), and ovaries (in women). Hormones travel throughout the body and affect distant cells. White blood cells that live in the bone marrow and lymphoid tissues, or that patrol the body and accumulate at the site of infections and injuries, send out a wide variety of signals in the form of tiny proteins such as cytokines and chemokines. Finally, specialized cells such as nerve cells (neurons), ear cells, eye cells, and other sensory cells respond to signals such as neurotransmitters, sound, light, and touch.

I will focus on growth factor receptors and the signaling pathways they control. My focus on growth factor receptor signaling is for two reasons:

1. Many of the most common and most powerful genetic mutations that drive the behavior of cancer cells affect growth factor receptor signaling pathways.
2. A large proportion of licensed targeted treatments for cancer work by blocking these pathways.

3.2 INTRODUCING GROWTH FACTOR RECEPTORS

Many targeted cancer treatments target growth factor receptors found on cancer cells[2] such as EGFR and HER2. I'll first explain how these receptors normally function and describe how they have gone wrong in cancer cells. I'll then turn to the treatments that block them.

---

[2] There are treatments that target growth factor receptors on non-cancer cells. Most of these target VEGF receptors on endothelial cells that line blood vessels; they are angiogenesis inhibitors.

3.2.1 Growth Factor Receptors: Some Basics

Growth factor receptors are large, complicated proteins. Thousands of them are embedded in the surface of our cells. Their other name, RTKs, refers to the fact that the part of the receptor that protrudes inside the cell functions as a tyrosine kinase (Chapter 2, Figure 2.13). Each type of human cell is unique in terms of the type and number of RTKs on its surface [5].

The external (extracellular) portion of RTKs – the part that sticks out from the cell's surface – is shaped so that it provides an attachment site for one or more growth factors. Growth factors are typically small proteins produced and released by pretty much all our cells (e.g., FGF1 [fibroblast growth factor-1] is 155 amino acids long; many other growth factors are a similar size [6]). Growth factors travel short distances between cells. When they attach to growth factor receptors on a cell's surface, the receptors pair up, and

this triggers a chain reaction within the cell cytoplasm. Finally, the signal reaches the cell nucleus and transmits an instruction to the cell such as "stay alive," "it's time to multiply," or "it's time to mature and specialize" (Figure 3.2).

At any given time, most of the cells in our body are going about their daily business and have no need to multiply (Figure 3.3a). When this is the case, our cells use growth factors simply to provide a background chatter that keeps them alive [7]. However, cells sometimes become old or damaged and die. If this happens, nearby cells might change or increase the amount of growth factors they produce (Figure 3.3b). Cells close by that have the relevant receptors on their surface will then respond and create extra cells to fill the gap [8].

For many years now, scientists have known that growth factor receptor signaling is seriously awry in cancer cells (Figure 3.3c), and we'll go into this in more detail in Section 3.2.3.

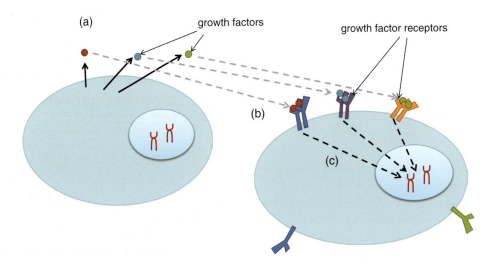

Figure 3.2 Activation of growth factor receptors keeps our cells alive. **(a)** Cells produce and release growth factors into their surroundings. **(b)** Growth factors attach to growth factor receptors and cause them to pair up. This pairing up activates the receptors' kinase domain, and they phosphorylate one another; paired-up receptors activate other proteins in the cell. **(c)** The activated proteins go on to activate more proteins, and more proteins, and this transmits the signal through the cell's cytoplasm (shown with a dotted black line). Eventually, the signal reaches the nucleus.

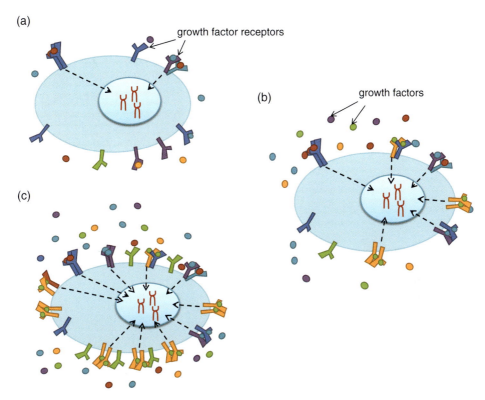

Figure 3.3 Growth factors can have a variety of different impacts on cells. **(a)** Healthy cells need growth factors to stay alive. **(b)** Changes to the amount and type of growth factors present gives this healthy cell a signal to grow and multiply. **(c)** Mutations in cancer cells' DNA, and changes to the amount of growth factors and growth factor receptors on their surface, provide cancer cells with continuous signals to survive, cause them to multiply, increase their mobility, alter their metabolism, and trigger angiogenesis.

3.2.2 Growth Factor Receptors Activate Signaling Pathways

Growth Factor Receptors Become Active When They Pair Up

As I outlined above, the first step in a signaling pathway is when growth factors attach to their receptors. When this happens, the receptors change shape and pair up with one another (a process known as dimerization) (Figure 3.4a and b). Once receptors have paired up, they phosphorylate each other – they take phosphates from ATP and attach them to their partner on tyrosine amino acids.[3] Phosphorylation of the two receptors changes their shape and creates docking sites for other proteins (Figure 3.4c and d). The exact number, and nature, of these docking sites varies from receptor to receptor [9], as does the precise way that the receptors pair up and phosphorylate one another.

Numerous Proteins Attach to Paired-Up Receptors

Various proteins can dock with paired-up, phosphorylated receptors. Many of them are intermediaries that pass on the signal to other

---

[3] Receptors are able pair up even when their growth factor is not present, but they don't seem able to phosphorylate each other until they are attached to a growth factor.

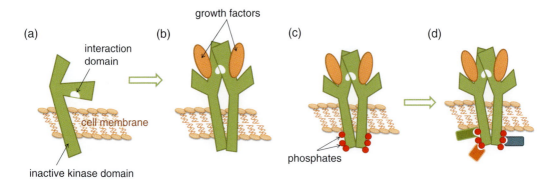

Figure 3.4 **Growth factor receptors phosphorylate one another when growth factors attach to them**. **(a)** An unpaired EGFR. **(b)** When growth factors such as EGF attach to EGFRs, the receptors change shape, thus exposing their interaction domains; they then pair up (dimerize). **(c)** The paired receptors phosphorylate each other. **(d)** The addition of phosphates creates docking sites for other proteins.

proteins. These other proteins are often themselves intermediaries that pass on the signal to others, and so the pathway continues. Finally, the signal is passed to proteins called "transcription factors" in the cell nucleus. These transcription factors then attach to genes and cause gene transcription and protein production.[4] So, when growth factors attach to receptors on a cell's surface, this ultimately causes the cell to alter what proteins it makes, which will impact the cell's behavior.

Activated Receptors Control a Variety of Signaling Pathways

Growth factor receptors control a number of different signaling pathways, such as the MAPK (mitogen-activated protein kinase) pathway, the PI3K/AKT/mTOR pathway, and the JAK-STAT pathway (summarized in Figure 3.5) [10]. These pathways control cell survival, proliferation, and cell movement, and they even influence the creation of blood vessels by angiogenesis. They are commonly overactive in cancer cells for a variety of different reasons and are the target of many new cancer treatments.

A Few Things to Note About Signaling Pathways

There are some general properties of signaling pathways that I think it's useful to know:

- Signaling pathways often involve a variety of different proteins and many small signaling molecules.
- Various pathways interact with and influence one another; this is known as **cross-talk**.
- Sometimes the activation of a pathway triggers a **feedback loop** that later shuts off the pathway or prevents it from becoming overactive.
- The activation of a signaling pathway can be all over in a matter of minutes, or it can last for many hours.
- The end-point of a signaling pathway might be a change that occurs in the cell cytoplasm, such as rearrangement of scaffolding proteins, or it might be the activation of transcription factors in the nucleus that alter what proteins the cell makes.
- Most signaling pathways involve proteins that actively pass on the signal, and proteins that block it; for example, PTEN blocks

---

[4] If you are not sure how transcription factors cause the cell to produce proteins, I recommend looking at this page on the Khan Academy website: https://www.khanacademy.org/science/biology/gene-regulation/gene-regulation-in-eukaryotes/a/eukaryotic-transcription-factors.

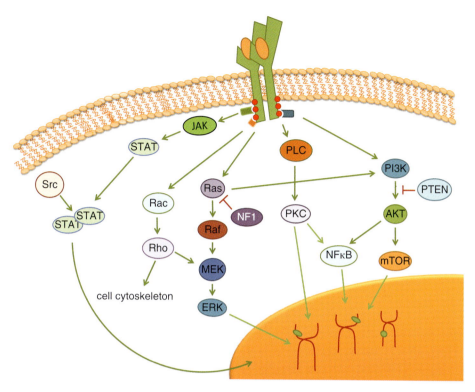

Figure 3.5 **Some of the many proteins and pathways activated by growth factor receptors** [10–12]. When growth factor receptors pair up, they activate many different signaling proteins in the cell, which control processes such as proliferation, survival, growth, and the cell's ability to move. Some of the most important and well-known signaling pathways are those that involve Ras, Raf, MEK, and ERK (known as the MAPK pathway), and PI3K, AKT, and mTOR. This latter pathway is kept under control by PTEN, which prevents the activation of AKT. Rac and Rho control the cell's internal skeleton. ERK, PKC, and mTOR have numerous effects on the cell, including forcing it into cell cycle and enabling it to grow. NFκB is a powerful transcription factor that, once in the nucleus, prevents cell death. STAT is also a transcription factor. As well as being activated by JAK, it is also directly activated by some growth factor receptors. When activated, STAT proteins pair up and enter the nucleus.
Abbreviations: STAT – signal transducer and activator of transcription; mTOR – mammalian target of rapamycin; PI3K – phosphatidylinositol 3-kinase; ERK- extracellular-signal-regulated kinase; PLC – phospholipase C; PKC – protein kinase C; NFκB – nuclear factor kappa-B; JAK – Janus kinase; PTEN – phosphatase and tensin homologue

the PI3K/AKT/mTOR pathway, and a protein called NF1 blocks the MAPK pathway.

- The proteins and pathways activated by a growth factor receptor will depend on: the type of cell it is, where it is, which receptor was activated, how long the receptors remained paired up, which growth factor cased the receptors to pair up, and so on.

- On the basis of which pathways became active, and for how long, the cell will choose its response.

- Many signaling pathways involve a number of kinases. Each kinase phosphorylates one or more other kinases, which then phosphorylate other kinases. Through this process, the signal received at the cell's surface is amplified as it passes through the cell.

- Finally, pathways are generally switched off by removing the activated receptors from the cell surface or removing phosphates from activated kinases.

Before we look further at those pathways, we'll examine some of the different growth factor receptors implicated in cancer and how they've gone wrong in cancer cells. We'll also look at some of the drugs that block these receptors.

EGF Receptors

The first growth factor receptor to be discovered was EGFR in the late 1970s [13], and it's still the one we know most about. This receptor is found on a wide range of cell types in many of our tissues and organs. It responds to the presence of at least seven different growth factors, the main one being EGF [10].

Like other growth factor receptors, when EGF attaches to EGF receptors, the receptors change shape and pair up. However, EGF receptors can also pair up with other members of the EGF receptor family. There are four family members: EGF receptor (also called EGFR, HER1, or ErbB1), HER2 (also called EGF receptor-2, Neu or ErbB2), HER3 (EGF receptor-3; ErbB3), and HER4 (EGF receptor-4; ErbB4).

All four receptors can pair up with themselves or with any other member of the family (Figure 3.6) [14]. However, there are some important differences between them. For example, EGFR, HER3, and HER4 can pair up only when a suitable growth factor is present. In contrast, **HER2 doesn't need a growth factor** to get into the correct shape for pairing – it's in the right shape all the time [15]. Hence, HER2 is constantly pairing up with itself and with other EGF receptors. When it pairs up with other family members, it activates signaling pathways more strongly than pairings that don't contain HER2. HER2 is therefore the most active and most powerful member of the EGF receptor family [14].

As well as EGF receptors, many other growth factor receptors drive cancer cell growth and survival. I've listed some of the most important ones in Table 3.1.

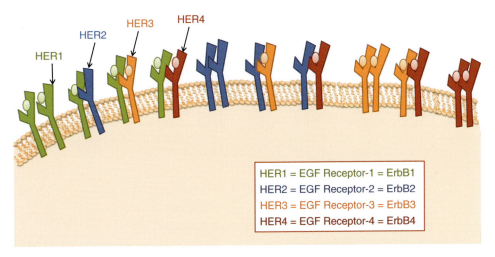

HER1 = EGF Receptor-1 = ErbB1
HER2 = EGF Receptor-2 = ErbB2
HER3 = EGF Receptor-3 = ErbB3
HER4 = EGF Receptor-4 = ErbB4

Figure 3.6 All four EGF receptors can pair up with one another to create homo- and heterodimers.
A homodimer is when two identical receptors have paired up. A heterodimer contains two different receptors. HER2 is different from HER1, HER3, and HER4 in that it doesn't need a growth factor to be present in order for it to pair up.
Abbreviations: HER – human epidermal growth factor receptor; EGF – epidermal growth factor

Table 3.1 Some of the growth factor receptors implicated in cancer.

Receptor	Ligand[a]/growth factor	Main cancers in which the receptor is implicated
EGFR: Epidermal growth factor receptor; ErbB1; HER1	EGF, transforming growth factor alpha (TGF-α), heparin-binding EGF-like growth factor (HB-EGF), amphiregulin, betacellulin, epigen, and epiregulin	Breast cancer, bowel cancer, non-small cell lung cancer (NSCLC), brain tumors, prostate cancer, ovarian cancer, stomach cancer, pancreatic cancer, head and neck squamous cell carcinomas (HNSCCs), anal cancer, esophageal cancer, and many more [16]
HER2: Human EGF receptor-2; ErbB2; Neu	No known ligand	Breast cancer, stomach cancer, esophageal cancer (also some lung, ovarian, uterine, bladder, and bowel cancers) [17]
HER3: Human EGF receptor-3; ErbB3	Heregulin (HRG) (also known as neuregulin)	Thought to be a common reason for drug resistance; frequently present alongside other EGF receptors on cancer cells, for example, those of breast, prostate, ovarian, bowel, and lung [18]
HER4: Human EGF receptor-4; ErbB4	HB-EGF, betacellulin, epiregulin, and heregulin (HRG) (also known as neuregulin)	Melanoma, NSCLC, medulloblastoma [19]
VEGF-R1 and VEGF-R2: vascular endothelial growth factor receptor-1and receptor-2	VEGF-A, -B, -C, -D, and placental growth factor (PlGF)	Any cancer with a blood supply – VEGF-R is on endothelial cells lining blood vessels [20]
PDGFRA and PDGFRB: platelet-derived growth factor receptor alpha and beta	PDGF-A, -B, -C, and -D	Glioblastoma multiforme, gastrointestinal stromal tumors (GIST), bone metastases from prostate cancer; also implicated in angiogenesis [21]
FGF-R1, 2, 3, 4, and 5: fibroblast growth factor receptors	FGFs (there are 22 different fibroblast growth factors)	Bladder cancer, squamous cell NSCLC, cervical cancer, multiple myeloma, prostate cancer, breast cancer, stomach cancer; important in angiogenesis [22]
IGF1-R: insulin-like growth factor-1 receptor	IGF-1 (insulin-like growth factor 1)	Bowel, prostate, breast and lung cancer and probably many others; associated with resistance to EGF-R inhibitors [23]
MET[b]: hepatocyte growth factor receptor	HGF (hepatocyte growth factor)	Kidney, lung, liver and pancreatic cancer and bone metastases from prostate cancer; important in invasion and metastasis; associated with resistance of bowel cancer to EGFR inhibitors and VEGF-R inhibitors [24]
KIT[c]/CD117	SCF (stem cell factor)	Gastrointestinal stromal tumors (GIST), small cell lung cancer (SCLC), acute myeloid leukemia (AML), T-cell lymphoma, testicular germ cell tumors, melanoma skin cancer [25]
FLT3: FMS-like tyrosine kinase 3	FLT3 ligand	Acute myeloid leukemia (AML), acute lymphocytic leukemia (ALL), chronic myeloid leukemia (CML) in blast crisis [26]
RET	Glial cell line-derived neurotrophic factor (GDNF) family ligands (GFLs), including neurturin (NRTN), artemin (ARTN), and persephin (PSPN)	Papillary thyroid cancer, medullary thyroid cancer, NSCLC [27]

[a] A ligand is anything that attaches to a receptor; each receptor has one or more ligands.

[b] MET is sometimes called c-MET. Various other proteins implicated in cancer sometimes have "c-" in front of their name (e.g., c-KIT, c-SRC, c-Myc, and c-Raf). This was historically done in order to distinguish between the human, cellular (c-) version of a gene or protein compared to the viral version (v-) thought to be the cancer-causing version. However, our views of the relationship between viruses and cancer have now changed, and the c- prefix is gradually being dropped. Sadly, adding to the confusion is the fact that sometimes the c- refers to the version of the protein in situations where there are multiple versions. For example, there are three versions of Raf: A-Raf, B-Raf, and C-Raf; so, when you see c-Raf written down, the person might be referring Raf proteins in general or just one of them.

[c] KIT is sometime called c-KIT. See note above about MET for the reason why. Confusingly, KIT is also sometimes called CD117. Every protein found on the surface of white blood cells is allocated a CD number when it is discovered; KIT's number is 117. CD stands for "cluster of differentiation"; it is a historical term coined by the first scientists who examined white blood cells decades ago.

3.2.3 Defects in Growth Factor Receptors in Cancer Cells

One of the most common reasons that growth factor receptor signaling pathways are overactive in cancer cells is because of faults with the receptor (reviewed in [28–30] and summarized in Figure 3.7). For example:

- Many cancers have excess amounts of growth factor receptors on their surface, for example:
  - Excess EGFR on the surface of bowel cancers, lung cancers, and glioblastomas.
  - Around 15%–20% of breast cancers and stomach cancers have extra copies (amplification) of the *HER2* gene [31]. They therefore have more HER2 protein on their surface than normal. This situation is also found in a smaller proportion of ovarian and salivary gland cancer.

- Some cancer cells produce faulty, overactive versions of growth factor receptors, for example:
  - In the cancer cells of around 10% of people with non-small cell lung cancer (NSCLC), the *EGFR* gene is mutated in such a way that the kinase portion of EGFR is overactive [32].
  - FGF receptor genes are mutated in around 50% of bladder cancers and in some cervical cancers, lung cancers, multiple myelomas, and prostate cancers [33].

- Many cancer cells and nearby non-cancer cells make and release large amounts of growth factors, which saturate growth factor receptors on the cancer cells' surface.

The majority of licensed treatments that block growth factor receptors on cancer cells target either EGFR or HER2 (see Table 3.2 and Figure 3.8).

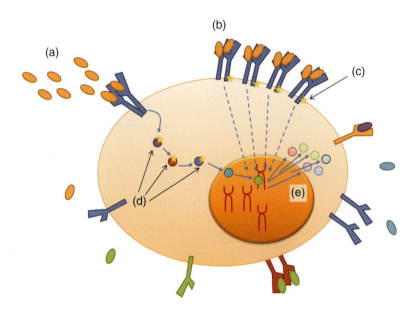

Figure 3.7 Signaling pathways are overactive in cancer cells for a variety of reasons. **(a)** Some cancers produce vast amounts of growth factors that saturate all the available receptors. **(b)** Cancer cells also overproduce growth factor receptors and become hypersensitive to the presence of growth factors. **(c)** The overproduced receptor is often faulty and overactive, sometimes even in the absence of any growth factors. **(d)** Proteins inside the cell that pass on the growth signal are mutated and overactive, for example, Ras (K-Ras, N-Ras, and H-Ras), B-Raf, PI3K, and AKT; proteins that would normally block the pathway (e.g., PTEN) are missing. **(e)** The signaling pathway is constantly active, and this forces the cell to constantly grow and multiply and makes it insensitive to DNA damage.

Table 3.2   EGFR- and HER2-targeted treatments.

Treatment type and licensed examples	Used in what cancers?	Why?
Treatments that target EGFR		
Monoclonal antibodies that block EGFR (e.g., cetuximab/ Erbitux, panitumumab/ Vectibix, necitumumab/ Portrazza)	Cetuximab is a licensed treatment for bowel cancer and head and neck cancer; panitumumab is licensed for bowel cancer; necitumumab is licensed for squamous cell NSCLCs that have high levels of EGFR.	In these cancers, EGFR is normal (wild-type), but there is too much of it.
First- and second-generation kinase inhibitors that block EGFR (e.g., gefitinib/Iressa, erlotinib/Tarceva, afatinib/ Giotrif/Gilotrif[a])	These are licensed treatments for EGFR-mutated non-small cell lung cancer (NSCLC).	In about 10-15% of NSCLCs, the EGF receptor is mutated and overactive; kinase inhibitors are far more likely to be effective when these mutations are present.
Third-generation kinase inhibitors that block EGFR (e.g., osimertinib/Tagrisso, rociletinib[b])	Osimertinib is a licensed treatment for EGFR-mutated NSCLC in which the gene for EGFR contains the T790M mutation.	The T790M mutation causes resistance to first- and second-generation drugs; third-generation drugs have been designed to block EGFR even when the T790M mutation is present.
Treatments that target HER2		
Monoclonal antibodies that block HER2 (trastuzumab/ Herceptin, pertuzumab/ Perjeta, trastuzumab emtansine/Kadcyla)	These are licensed treatments for breast cancers with HER2 gene amplification; trastuzumab is also licensed for HER2-amplified stomach cancer.	The HER2 gene is amplified in 15%–20% of breast cancers and stomach cancers.
Kinase inhibitors that block HER2 (e.g., lapatinib/Tykerb/ Tyverb[c])	Breast cancer.	As above.
Pan-HER inhibitors (these are all irreversible kinase inhibitors)		
Drugs that block EGFR, HER2 and HER4 (e.g., neratinib, dacomitinib, canertinib, afatinib[d])	Afatinib is a licensed treatment for EGFR-mutated NSCLC. Most trials with these agents are in NSCLC and breast cancer.	It is not clear as yet when/where these treatments will be most effective.
Drugs that block EGFR, HER2 and HER3 (e.g., sapitinib/ AZD8931)	In trials for NSCLC, breast cancer and stomach cancer.	EGFR and HER2 are both important in these tumors and resistance to other treatments is sometimes caused by HER3.

[a] Afatinib is a second-generation, irreversible kinase inhibitor. It is actually a pan-HER inhibitor in that it blocks EGFR, HER2, and HER4, but it almost exclusively used in the treatment of lung cancer.
[b] In May 2016, the development of rociletinib was halted due to safety concerns and low response rates: http:// www.onclive.com/web-exclusives/clovis-ends-development-of-rociletinib-in-lung-cancer.
[c] Lapatinib also blocks EGFR.
[d] Afatinib was mentioned earlier as a second-generation EGFR inhibitor.

3.3 DRUGS THAT TARGET EGFR

Drugs that target EGFR can be split into two groups:

1. Monoclonal antibodies that attach to EGFR from outside the cell are most commonly used in the treatment of bowel cancer and head and neck cancer, for example, cetuximab (Erbitux), panitumumab (Vectibix), and necitumumab (Portrazza).

2. Kinase inhibitors that block EGFR from inside the cell are mostly used in the treatment of NSCLC, for example, gefitinib

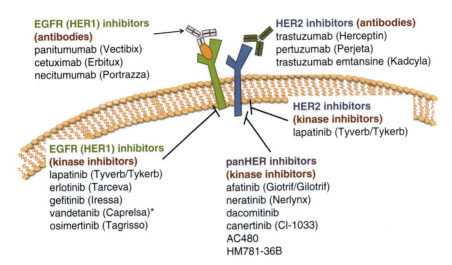

EGFR (HER1) inhibitors (antibodies)
panitumumab (Vectibix)
cetuximab (Erbitux)
necitumumab (Portrazza)

HER2 inhibitors (antibodies)
trastuzumab (Herceptin)
pertuzumab (Perjeta)
trastuzumab emtansine (Kadcyla)

HER2 inhibitors (kinase inhibitors)
lapatinib (Tyverb/Tykerb)

EGFR (HER1) inhibitors (kinase inhibitors)
lapatinib (Tyverb/Tykerb)
erlotinib (Tarceva)
gefitinib (Iressa)
vandetanib (Caprelsa)*
osimertinib (Tagrisso)

panHER inhibitors (kinase inhibitors)
afatinib (Giotrif/Gilotrif)
neratinib (Nerlynx)
dacomitinib
canertinib (CI-1033)
AC480
HM781-36B

* As well as blocking EGFR, vandetanib also blocks VEGF receptors and RET

Figure 3.8 Numerous treatments target either EGFR or HER2. Monoclonal antibodies attach to the external part of the receptors. Kinase inhibitors cross the cell membrane and block the kinase part of the receptors. Many kinase inhibitors have more than one target, and the pan-HER inhibitors block EGFR, HER2 and HER4 or EGFR, HER2 and HER3.
Abbreviations: EGFR – epidermal growth factor receptor; HER2 – human epidermal growth factor receptor-2; VEGF – vascular endothelial growth factor

(Iressa), erlotinib (Tarceva), afatinib (Giotrif; Gilotrif), and osimertinib (Tagrisso).

The goal of all these treatments is to block the receptor and prevent it from activating any internal signaling pathways.

3.3.1 Monoclonal Antibodies That Target EGFR

Physical Make-Up and Differences between Them

As you might have already noticed from the names cetuximab is a chimeric antibody, whereas panitumumab and necitumumab are fully human antibodies[5] (see Figure 3.9 for a comparison between cetuximab and panitumumab). Because of this difference,

panitumumab and necitumumab are theoretically less visible to the patient's immune system and less likely to cause infusion reactions [34].

Another difference between the antibodies is the precise type of antibody that they're made from. Our B cells can produce a variety of different classes of antibodies (called IgA, IgG, IgE, IgD, and IgM[6]), and within each class there are also numerous sub-classes. Panitumumab is made from an IgG2 antibody, whereas cetuximab and necitumumab are made from IgG1 antibodies. Although this might seem like an excessive piece of detail, this subtle difference means that cetuximab and necitumumab are better than panitumumab at attracting and activating

---

[5] The "xi" in cetux**i**mab tells you it is chimeric; the "u" in panit**u**mumab tells you it is fully human.
[6] For a little bit more about what each class of antibody does, see http://www.webmd.com/a-to-z-guides/immunoglobulins.

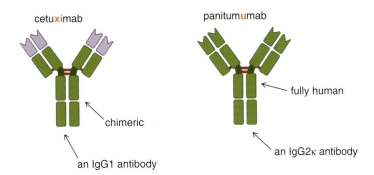

Figure 3.9 Comparison of panitumumab and cetuximab. Both treatments are monoclonal antibodies. However, cetuximab is chimeric – the back part of the antibody is a human IgG1 antibody, whereas the antigen-binding region is from a mouse antibody. Panitumumab is a fully human IgG2κ antibody.

white blood cells. Hence, cetuximab and necitumumab (but not panitumumab) can create a cancer-fighting immune response [35].

Who They Are Given To

Panitumumab and cetuximab are licensed as treatments for people with bowel cancer (see Chapter 6, Section 6.5). Cetuximab is also licensed for head and neck cancer (see Chapter 6, Section 6.8). The cells of both these cancers tend to have lots of EGFRs on their surface. These antibodies have also been tested in clinical trials involving people with many other cancer types. However, even when the cells of those cancers are known to have EGFR on their surface, such as esophageal cancer and ovarian cancer, the antibodies have often had little impact [36, 37]. This could be because the cells of these cancers can swap to using alternative receptors and pathways when EGFR is blocked.

Necitumumab in contrast has been licensed as a treatment for people with squamous cell NSCLC (see Chapter 6, Section 6.4.3). This antibody hasn't been extensively investigated in clinical trials for people with any other type of cancer.

How They Work

Cetuximab, panitumumab, and necitumumab attach to the external part of EGFR and prevent EGF or other EGFR ligands[7] attaching to the receptor. These antibodies also force the cell to internalize and destroy EGFRs [35]. Without any growth factors attached, the receptors can't pair up or become active. As I mentioned before, cetuximab and necitumumab can also attract and activate white blood cells. Despite their differences, cetuximab and panitumumab have given very similar results in clinical trials for people with bowel cancer [34].

Why They Can't Be Given to Everyone

Cetuximab and panitumumab don't work for everyone (neither does necitumumab, but we know a lot less about resistance to necitumumab than we do about resistance to cetuximab and panitumumab). An important discovery has been that in bowel cancer the cancer cells often contain mutations that make treatment with EGFR-targeted antibodies ineffective. These mutations affect proteins involved in the MAPK pathway (there's more about this pathway in Section 3.7). It seems that if intracellular proteins[8] such as Ras or

---

[7] Ligands are molecules such as small proteins that attach to receptors. For example, EGF is a ligand that attaches to EGF receptors.
[8] That is, proteins that exist in the cytoplasm of the cell.

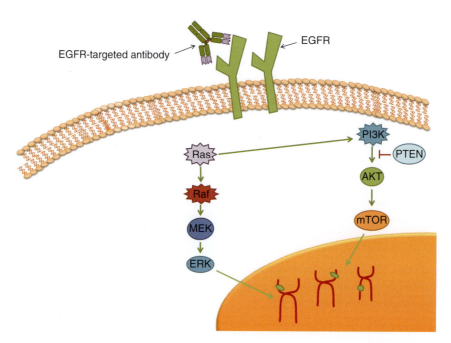

Figure 3.10 **Mutations affecting the MAPK pathway and PI3K pathway cause intrinsic resistance to EGFR-targeted antibodies**. Bowel cancer cells often contain mutated, overactive versions of Ras (particularly K-Ras), Raf (generally B-Raf), or PI3K (mutated proteins are shown as spiky ovals). The presence of any of these mutated proteins causes overactivity of the MAPK pathway (Ras/Raf/MEK/ERK) and the PI3K pathway (PI3K/AKT/mTOR). And, when these pathways are overactive, the receptor on the cell surface becomes redundant. Blocking the activation of EGF receptors using an EGFR-targeted antibody will then have no impact on the cell and will bring no benefit for the patient.
Abbreviations: EGFR – epidermal growth factor receptor; mTOR – mammalian target of rapamycin; PI3K – phosphatidylinositol 3-kinase; ERK- extracellular-signal-regulated kinase; PTEN – phosphatase and tensin homologue

Raf have become overactive, this renders the receptor redundant.[9] If you then block the receptor with an antibody, this won't block the pathway or kill the cell, and the patient doesn't get any better [38] (Figure 3.10).

Faulty Ras proteins are the most common reason why an EGFR-targeted antibody can't be prescribed for a patient with bowel cancer. Around 40% of bowel cancers contain mutated, overactive versions of K-Ras [39], and a further 3% contain mutated N-Ras [40]. Mutations in B-Raf are found in about 6% of bowel cancers [40]. Overactive versions of

any of these three proteins (and probably of other signaling proteins too) cause resistance [38]. Therefore, before prescribing an EGFR-targeted antibody, patients' tumor samples are tested for *KRAS* gene mutations and, if possible, for *NRAS* and *BRAF* gene mutations as well.

Why They Sometimes Stop Working
Even when no *KRAS*, *NRAS*, or *BRAF* gene mutation is found, cetuximab or panitumumab don't help everyone. And if these treatments do work initially, and the cancer

---

[9] There are three main versions of Ras proteins in our cells: K-Ras, N-Ras, and H-Ras; there are also three Raf proteins: A-Raf, B-Raf, and C-Raf.

shrinks or stops growing, this effect doesn't generally last forever.

Many scientists have examined cells from patients whose bowel cancer has stopped responding to cetuximab or panitumumab in order to understand what has happened. They've generally found that resistant cells contain mutations in genes for proteins involved in the MAPK pathway (such as *KRAS* or *BRAF*) or the PI3K/AKT/mTOR pathway (such as *PIK3CA*[10]). Other reasons for resistance include mutations in *EGFR* that destroy EGFR's binding sites for cetuximab and panitumumab, and the overproduction of alternative growth factor receptors such as HER2, HER3, or MET [41, 42]. (You can find more information on the use of EGFR antibodies for bowel cancer in Chapter 6, Section 6.5)

3.3.2 Kinase Inhibitors That Target EGFR

First- and Second-Generation EGFR Inhibitors

EGFR is a cell surface protein accessible to antibodies like cetuximab and panitumumab. But it's also a kinase, and it can therefore be blocked with a kinase inhibitor.[11]

Several kinase inhibitors that block EGFR have been created. Erlotinib and gefitinib were two of the first. They are first-generation, reversible EGFR inhibitors that mimic ATP and block EGFR's kinase activity.[12] Afatinib, dacomitinib, and neratinib, which are second-generation drugs, are slightly different. They are irreversible inhibitors that chemically bond with EGFR's ATP-binding site. As well as blocking EGFR, they also block HER2 and HER4 [43] – because they block multiple human EGF receptors, they are sometimes called pan-HER inhibitors.

All these treatments appear to work best when the cancer cells are producing a mutated, overactive version of EGFR. The cancer in which these mutations are most common is NSCLC. The most common activating mutations are exon 19 deletions and the L858R mutation (there's more about these mutations in Chapter 6, Section 6.4.1).

It seems that when the EGFR is mutated and overactive, lung cancer cells become more reliant on it for their survival than if they simply overproduce the normal, un-mutated (wild-type) version of the protein. Erlotinib, gefitinib, and afatinib are standard treatments for the 10%–15% or so of NSCLCs in which the *EGFR* gene is mutated. (For more about the use of EGFR inhibitors in NSCLC, see Chapter 6, Section 6.4). More recently, neratinib (Nerlynx) has been licensed in the United States as an adjuvant treatment for women with HER2-positive breast cancer (there's more on this in Chapter 6, Section 6.2).

Third-Generation EGFR Kinase Inhibitors

When a patient's cancer becomes resistant to a first- or second-generation EGFR inhibitor, this is commonly due to cancer cells that have a further mutation in their *EGFR* gene [44]. This additional mutation, called the T790M mutation, changes the shape of EGFR's ATP-binding site. Drugs like gefitinib and erlotinib can no longer block the mutated protein.

To overcome resistance, scientists have created third-generation EGFR inhibitors such as osimertinib, which can block T790M mutant EGFR and kill cells that contain it. For a comparison of first-, second-, and third-generation EGFR inhibitors, see Table 3.3. One thing to note in the table is that second-generation

---

[10] Mutations in *PIK3CA* cause PI3K to become overactive.
[11] For more about antibodies and kinase inhibitors, see Chapter 2.
[12] Remember that growth factor receptors are kinases, and they can therefore be blocked with drugs that mimic ATP – see Figures 2.13 and 2.14 for a reminder.

Table 3.3   Comparison of first-, second-, and third-generation EGFR kinase inhibitors.

	First generation	Second generation	Third generation
Type of inhibition	Reversible	Irreversible	Irreversible
Ability to block:			
Wild-type EGFR	Strong	Strong	Weak
Exon 19 deleted EGFR	Strong	Very strong	Very strong
L858R mutated EGFR	Strong	Very strong	Very strong
T790M mutated EGFR	nil	Moderate	Very strong
HER2	nil	Strong	nil
HER4	nil	Strong	nil
Examples of drugs	Gefitinib, erlotinib, and icotinib	Afatinib and dacomitinib	Osimertinib, rociletinib, HM61713, EGF816, and ASP8273

Source: Costa DB (2016).Kinase inhibitor-responsive genotypes in EGFR mutated lung adenocarcinomas: Moving past common point mutations or indels into uncommon kinase domain duplications and rearrangements. *Translational Lung Cancer Res* **5**(3): 331–337.Ke E-E, Wu Yi-Long (2016). EGFR as a pharmacological target in EGFR-mutant non-small-cell lung cancer: Where do we stand now? *Trends Pharmacol Sci* **37**(11): 887–903.

inhibitors also have some ability to block T790M mutant EGFR. However, because second-generation drugs like afatinib are powerful blockers of wild-type EGFR, they cause lots of side effects. And, by the time you've upped the dose of drug sufficiently to block T790M EGFR, you've made life unbearable for the patient. So, it's only the third-generation drugs that can block T790M EGFR at a dose in which they can safely be given to patients [45].

As well as blocking T790M EGFR, third-generation EGFR inhibitors have another strength – their relative inability to block wild-type EGFR. As a result, third-generation drugs like osimertinib cause less severe side effects than first- and second-generation drugs [44, 45].

Who They're Given To

The most common use of EGFR kinase inhibitors is to treat the 10%–15% or so of people with NSCLC whose cancer cells have mutated, overactive EGFRs on their surface.

Erlotinib, a first-generation EGFR kinase inhibitor, has also shown some degree of usefulness against pancreatic cancer, despite a rarity of EGFR mutations in this cancer [46]. It's important to say though that whereas EGFR inhibitors generally hold NSCLC at bay for 9–14 months, in pancreatic cancer they only add a week or two to progression-free survival when combined with chemotherapy compared with chemotherapy alone [47]. The licensing of erlotinib, a first-generation EGFR kinase inhibitor, for people with pancreatic cancer is therefore more of a reflection of how few effective treatment options we have for pancreatic cancer, rather than a belief that erlotinib will provide dramatic benefits [48].

Resistance to EGFR Kinase Inhibitors

Almost all the detailed information we have about resistance mechanisms to EGFR kinase inhibitors comes from people with NSCLC, as these are the people most likely to be treated with one of these drugs. And, as I said earlier, a common reason why a NSCLC becomes resistant to a first- or second-generation EGFR kinase inhibitor is because of cancer cells that contain the T790M mutation in one of their *EGFR* genes. In fact, this T790M mutation is present in about 50%–60% of patients whose cancer has become resistant [45].

Aside from the T790M mutation in the *EGFR* gene, we know about various other

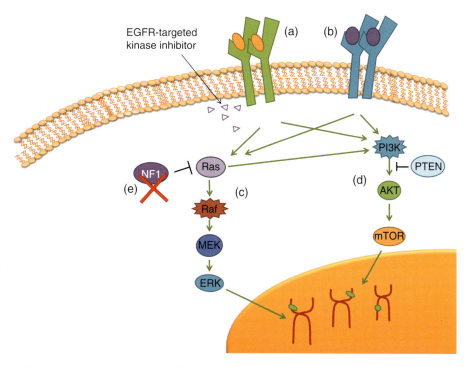

Figure 3.11 Reasons for resistance to EGFR-targeted kinase inhibitors in NSCLC cells. Resistance mechanisms include **(a)** Cancer cells have gained an additional mutation, the T790M mutation, in the EGFR gene, which has altered the ATP-binding site of EGFR such that the drug can no longer block it. **(b)** Cancer cells have additional growth factor receptors on their surface such as HER2, MET, or FGFR. **(c and d)** Cancer cells contain mutated overactive B-Raf or PI3K. **(e)** Cells have lost NF1, which would normally block Ras proteins. **Abbreviations:** EGFR – epidermal growth factor receptor; mTOR – mammalian target of rapamycin; PI3K – phosphatidylinositol 3-kinase; ERK- extracellular-signal-regulated kinase; PTEN – phosphatase and tensin homologue; ATP – adenosine triphosphate; HER2 – human epidermal growth factor receptor-2; FGFR –fibroblast growth factor receptor; NF1 - neurofibromatosis type 1

reasons for resistance. These include overproduction of other growth factor receptors such as HER2, MET, or FGFR; mutations that create overactive versions of PI3K or B-Raf; or loss of NF1 (a suppressor of Ras proteins) (summarized in Figure 3.11). Another reason for resistance is when NSCLC cells change shape and become much more similar to the cells that cause small cell lung cancer (SCLC) [45].

As with bowel cancers resistant to EGFR-targeted antibodies, huge efforts are being made to overcome resistance to EGFR-targeted kinase inhibitors using various targeted drugs.

3.4 DRUGS THAT TARGET HER2

As with EGFR-targeted treatments, the drugs that target HER2 can be split into two groups: monoclonal antibodies and kinase inhibitors. Both of these groups of treatments are primarily given to people[13] with HER2-positive

---

[13] Of course, the vast majority of breast cancers occur in women, but around 400 or so men develop breast cancer in the United Kingdom each year (compared to over 55,000 women)

breast cancer, and sometimes also for HER2-positive stomach cancer[14]:

1. Monoclonal antibodies that block HER2 from outside the cell, for example, trastuzumab (Herceptin), pertuzumab (Perjeta), and trastuzumab emtansine (Kadcyla; T-DM1)
2. Kinase inhibitors that block HER2 from inside the cell, for example, lapatinib (Tyverb; Tykerb)

3.4.1 Monoclonal Antibodies That Target HER2

Physical Make-Up and Differences between Them

Three antibodies that target HER2 are licensed as cancer treatments: trastuzumab, pertuzumab, and trastuzumab emtansine. As you can tell from the names, all three are humanized antibodies, hence the "zu." (That is, the tips of the antibodies – the variable region – come from a mouse antibody, whereas the rest of the antibody is constructed from human antibody protein.)

Although all three antibodies are humanized, they have different mechanisms of action (see Figure 3.12 for a summary).

Trastuzumab was the first HER2-targeted antibody to be licensed. It is thought to have several mechanisms of action, including the following [49]:

• It prevents paired-up HER2s from activating signaling pathways, being most active

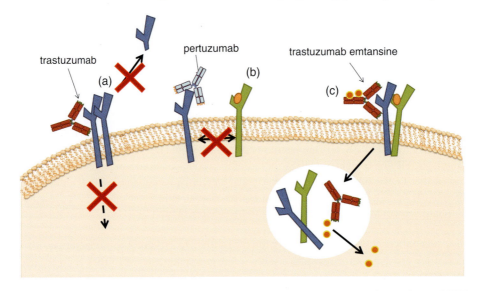

Figure 3.12 Mechanism of action of HER2-targeted antibodies. (a) Trastuzumab attaches to HER2 near the cell membrane. It prevents paired-up HER2 from activating signaling pathways. It also attracts white blood cells and prevents HER2 shedding. **(b)** Pertuzumab prevents HER2 from pairing up with EGFR or HER3, and thereby prevents the activation of signaling pathways (unpaired growth factor receptors cannot activate signaling pathways). Pertuzumab can also attract white blood cells. **(c)** Trastuzumab emtansine (T-DM1) attaches to HER2 and becomes internalized within the cell. The chemotherapy part of T-DM1 then breaks away and attacks the cell's microtubules. T-DM1 can also block signaling pathway activation and attract white blood cells just like the naked trastuzumab antibody.**Abbreviations:** EGFR – epidermal growth factor receptor; HER2 – human epidermal growth factor receptor-2; HER3 – human epidermal growth factor receptor-3

---

[14] About 15%–20% of both breast cancers and stomach cancers have high levels of HER2 on their surface and are considered to be HER2-positive.

against a pairing of HER2 with HER2 (HER2:HER2), and less active against HER2:HER3 or HER2:EGFR [50].

- It recruits white blood cells such as macrophages and natural killer cells, which then destroy HER2-positive cancer cells.
- It prevents the external part of HER2 from breaking off and being shed from the cell – if the HER2 protein is allowed to break, the part of HER2 that remains embedded in the cell membrane (called p95) is extremely active.
- It may have some ability to prevent HER2 from pairing up with one another or with other receptors.
- It causes destruction of HER2.

In contrast, pertuzumab's main mechanism of action is to prevent HER2 from pairing up with EGFR or HER3 [50]. The two antibodies therefore have slightly different, and complementary, mechanisms of action, and some clinical trials have shown that the two antibodies work well in combination [50].

Trastuzumab emtansine (T-DM1) is different again. It is made from trastuzumab linked to a potent chemotherapy called emtansine (also called mertansine or DM1). Like trastuzumab, T-DM1 attaches to HER2. Once attached, the cell membrane folds inward, and HER2 (with T-DM1 still attached) becomes enclosed within a compartment in the cell cytoplasm. Finally, the linker connecting trastuzumab to DM1 breaks, and the DM1 chemotherapy is released. DM1 is a type of chemotherapy that attacks a cell's microtubules. Because microtubules form an essential component of our cells and are necessary for many functions, the cell then dies [51].

From the description of T-DM1, you'd be forgiven for thinking that it would be massively more effective than trastuzumab. However, this is not always the case. Clinical trials have shown T-DM1 to be able to extend survival times in women whose tumors are resistant to trastuzumab [52]. But other trials have failed to show that it is significantly better than standard treatments when given to women whose tumors are still sensitive to trastuzumab [53].

Who They're Given To

Trastuzumab was first licensed in Europe in 2000 for the treatment of HER2-positive breast cancer. In 2010, its license was extended to include HER2-positive stomach cancer. Pertuzumab and T-DM1 are also licensed breast cancer treatments (see Chapter 6, Section 6.2.3 for more about the use of these treatments for breast cancer). HER2-positive cancers are those in which the *HER2* gene is amplified – and this causes the cell to manufacture much more HER2 protein than normal (see Figure 3.13).

Scientists discovered in the mid-1980s that breast cancer cells sometimes have high levels of HER2 on their surface. These cancers were known to be very aggressive and likely to spread and return following treatment [54]. However, this association with poor prognosis has been reversed thanks to HER2-targeted treatments [55].

Why They Sometimes Don't Work

Although HER2-targeted antibodies have proven to be very helpful against HER2-positive cancer, they don't work for everyone. And for people with metastatic cancer, the benefit they bring is generally only temporary (although it can last for many months, if not years) [56].

Much of what we know about mechanisms of resistance to HER2-targeted antibodies comes from studying breast cancers that are resistant to trastuzumab. Various mechanisms of resistance have been found (summarized in Figure 3.14). They include the following [55, 56]:

- Changes to HER2. Sometimes a shortened version of HER2 called p95 is made by cancer cells, which lacks the binding site

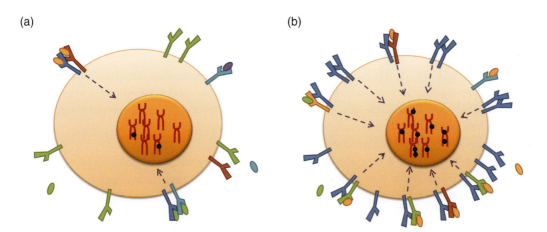

Figure 3.13 **HER2-positive cancers have extra copies of the HER2 gene**. **(a)** Normal cells have two copies of the *HER2* gene and produce very little HER2 protein. **(b)** *HER2* gene amplification leads to overproduction of HER2, which pairs up with itself and other HER-family receptors (namely, EGFR, HER3, and HER4). This causes increased activity of signaling pathways and promotes cell proliferation and survival. **Abbreviations:** EGFR – epidermal growth factor receptor; HER2 – human epidermal growth factor receptor-2; HER3 – human epidermal growth factor receptor-3; HER4 – human epidermal growth factor receptor-4

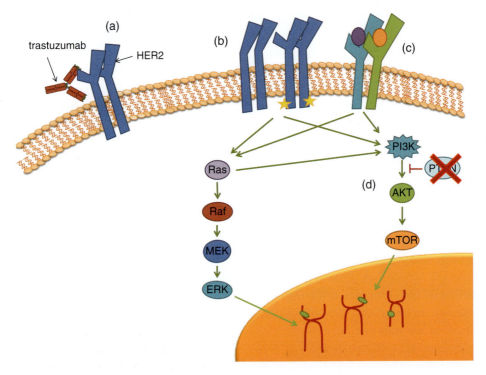

Figure 3.14 **Some reasons for resistance to HER2-targeted antibodies in breast cancer cells**. **(a)** In cells sensitive to trastuzumab, the antibody is able to attach to HER2 and prevent it from activating signaling pathways. **(b)** Some trastuzumab-resistant cells have mutations affecting the HER2 gene. They therefore manufacture overactive HER2, or HER2 that lacks a binding site for trastuzumab. **(c)** Another cause of resistance is the presence of other growth factor receptors on the cell surface. **(d)** Mutations affecting the PI3K pathway, such as those that cause PI3K to be overactive, or loss of PTEN, can also cause resistance. **Abbreviations:** mTOR – mammalian target of rapamycin; PI3K – phosphatidylinositol 3-kinase; ERK-extracellular-signal-regulated kinase; PTEN – phosphatase and tensin homologue; HER2 – human epidermal growth factor receptor-2

for trastuzumab. In other cancers, the kinase portion of HER2 has become overactive.

- The ability of trastuzumab to attract and activate white blood cells is important for maximum benefit – people whose tumors contain low levels of infiltrating white blood cells, or high levels of immune-suppressing proteins (such as PD-L1), seem less likely to benefit from trastuzumab.
- If other growth factor receptors are present on the cancer cells' surface such as EGFR, HER3, MET, IGF-1, and EphA2, these activate signaling pathways even when HER2 is blocked.
- Also, if EGFR or HER3 pairs up with HER2, this creates a pairing that can't be completely blocked by trastuzumab (these pairings can be prevented by pertuzumab, or blocked by lapatinib).
- Mutations that activate the PI3K/AKT/mTOR pathway make HER2 redundant; therefore, blocking HER2 has no impact.
- If there are lots of estrogen receptors (ERs) in the cancer cells, these trigger production of many growth factor receptors, and they activate various signaling pathways that can overcome the effects of trastuzumab.

Thanks to this knowledge, we have seen lots of clinical trials in which treatment combinations have been tried. For example, some trials have tested a combination of trastuzumab with pertuzumab or lapatinib. Other trials have combined trastuzumab with hormone therapies such as anastrozole or letrozole, or with mTOR, AKT, or PI3K inhibitors, or with immunotherapy.

3.4.2 Kinase Inhibitors That Target HER2

Like other growth factor receptors, the intracellular part of HER2 is a kinase. When HER2 pairs up with another HER2 or with an other EGF receptor, the receptors phosphorylate one another and activate various signaling pathways.

In Europe, the only licensed kinase inhibitor targeting HER2 is lapatinib. Lapatinib, like many other kinase inhibitors, mimics ATP and reversibly blocks the ATP-binding site of its targets, EGFR and HER2. And, unlike antibodies targeted against HER2, it can block the broken, constantly active form of HER2 called p95 [57].

In clinical trials investigating lapatinib in combination with other treatments, the addition of lapatinib has generally improved the patient's outlook [57].

Another HER2-targeted kinase inhibitor is neratinib. It is an irreversible inhibitor of EGFR, HER2, and HER4 (it's very similar to afatinib and dacomitinib and is classed as a pan-HER inhibitor). In July 2017 the FDA approved neratinib as an adjuvant treatment for women with early-stage, HER2-positive breast cancer who have already received trastuzumab for a year following surgery.

3.5 DRUGS THAT BLOCK OTHER GROWTH FACTOR RECEPTORS

As well as EGFR and HER2, many other growth factor receptors are found on the surface of cancer cells and on other cells in their immediate environment. Various drugs that target some of these receptors are explained elsewhere in this book. They include the following:

VEGF receptor inhibitors[15] – see Chapter 4, Section 4.1 on angiogenesis inhibitors.

---

[15] Many of the kinase inhibitors that block VEGF receptors also block other growth factor receptors.

KIT and FLT3 inhibitors – see Chapter 7, Section 7.10 on targeted treatments for hematological cancers.

ALK, RET, and ROS1 inhibitors – see Chapter 4, Section 4.2 on drugs that target fusion proteins.

Growth factor receptors such as IGF1R (insulin-like growth factor receptor) and many others have also been implicated in various cancers. However, only PDGFR and KIT inhibitors have been licensed, and I will explain them below.

3.5.1 PDGFR and KIT Inhibitors

Inhibitors of PDGFRα (PDGFR-alpha) and KIT are licensed treatments for a rare type of cancer called GIST (gastrointestinal stromal tumor). Around 60% of GISTs start in the stomach, but they can arise anywhere in the digestive system [58].

Thanks to research in the late 1990s, we know that the vast majority of GISTs (around 90%) contain mutations either in the gene for KIT (80%) or for PDGFRα (5%–10%) [59]. Both PDGFRα and KIT are growth factor receptors and therefore have a kinase domain that protrudes inside the cell.

Many kinases have very similar ATP-binding sites. That's why some kinase inhibitors block the ATP-binding sites of a variety of kinases. And we have several drugs that can block both PDGFRα and KIT alongside their other targets (see Table 3.4).

Imatinib (Glivec; Gleevec) was approved as a treatment for advanced GIST in 2002. As a result, the median survival time for patients with metastatic GIST has improved from about 20 months to 60 months[61].

However, most patients with metastatic GIST do eventually relapse. The most common reason why imatinib stops working is that the gene for KIT has picked up another mutation. The extra mutation generally alters the shape of KIT's ATP-binding site [59]. Thankfully, various forms of KIT that are resistant to imatinib can still be blocked by sunitinib (Sutent) or regorafenib (Stivarga). Both these drugs are licensed treatments for imatinib-resistant GIST and other PDGFRα and KIT inhibitors are in trials.

3.6 INTRODUCTION TO SIGNALING PATHWAYS AS A TARGET FOR CANCER THERAPY

Communication pathways controlled by growth factors normally help our tissues and organs maintain a balance between cell life, death, and proliferation. These same pathways

Table 3.4   Kinase inhibitors that block PDGFRα and KIT.

Drug	Targets include	Stage of development as a treatment for GIST
Imatinib (Glivec; Gleevec)	KIT, PDGF receptors, BCR-ABL, FLT3, and CSF1R	Licensed
Sunitinib (Sutent)	KIT, PDGF receptors, VEGF receptors, and FLT3	Licensed
Regorafenib (Stivarga)	KIT, PDGF receptors, VEGF Receptors, RET, Raf, TIE2, and FGF receptors	Licensed
Nilotinib (Tasigna)	KIT, PDGF receptors, and BCR-ABL	Phase 3 trials
Masitinib	KIT and PDGF receptors	Phase 3 trials
Crenolanib	KIT, PDGF receptors, VEGF receptors, TIE-2, FGF receptor-2, EGFR, HER2, and Src [60]	Phase 3 trials

Source: Bauer S, Joensuu H (2015). Emerging agents for the treatment of advanced, imatinib-resistant gastrointestinal stromal tumors: Current status and future directions. *Drugs* **75**(12): 1323–1334.

are imbalanced and defective in cancer cells. Defects in cell communication pathways help cancer cells grow and multiply rapidly and protect them from self-destructing. Overactive signaling pathways also help cancer cells become more mobile, trigger angiogenesis, and influence the behavior of the cells around them. In fact, **overactive signaling pathways cause cells to take on many of the properties of cancer cells.**

In the first half of this chapter, we looked at growth factor receptors on the surface of our cells that control signaling pathways. But often the reason a signaling pathway is over-active has nothing to do with the receptor on the cell surface. Instead, **the culprit is a faulty protein within the cytoplasm** that would nor-mally only be active in response to a receptor, but for some reason has become active inde-pendently, perhaps because of a mutation.

For the remainder of this chapter, we'll look at three signaling pathways that are often

faulty in cancer cells because of faults in par-ticular proteins within the cell. They are
1. The MAPK pathway
2. The PI3K/AKT/mTOR pathway
3. The JAK-STAT pathway

The drugs that I'm going to mention are those that block B-Raf, MEK, mTOR, PI3K, AKT, and JAK2. There are drugs that block other kinases (such as SRC and ERK), but they're not yet licensed cancer treatments.

3.7 TARGETING THE MAPK SIGNALING PATHWAY

One of the most important signaling path-ways controlled by growth factor receptors is the MAPK (mitogen-activated protein kinase) pathway (Figure 3.15). This involves growth factor receptors, docking proteins, a series of enzymes in the cell cytoplasm (Ras, Raf, MEK, and ERK), and a variety of transcription

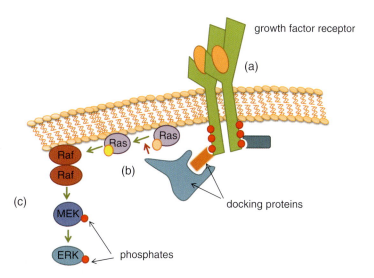

Figure 3.15 Ras, Raf, MEK, and ERK activation. (a) Paired-up growth factor receptors phosphorylate one another, which allows a series of docking proteins to attach. **(b)** These docking proteins activate Ras (K-Ras, N-Ras, or H-Ras) by causing it to let go of GDP (orange circle) and take hold of GTP (yellow circle) instead. Ras is constantly in contact with the cell membrane. **(c)** Ras attracts Raf proteins to the cell membrane where they pair up and become active. Raf proteins are kinases; they phosphorylate MEK, which in turn phosphorylates ERK.
Abbreviations: GDP – guanosine di-phosphate; GTP – guanosine triphosphate

factors in the nucleus, such as ELK-1, Fos, and Myc [62].

3.7.1 The Mechanics of MAPK Pathways

Do note that there are, in fact, multiple MAPK pathways, but I'm going to focus on the pathway that involves Ras, Raf, MEK, and ERK, because this is the one that is overactive in many cancers.

Step 1: Growth Factor Receptors Activate Ras

Once two growth factor receptors have paired up and phosphorylated each other, docking proteins can now attach to them (Figure 3.15a). These docking proteins activate Ras by causing it to change shape. Ras then lets go of a low-energy molecule called GDP and grabs hold of a higher-energy molecule called GTP [63] (see Figure 3.15b; for more about Ras, see Box 3.1).

Step 2: Ras Activates Raf, MEK, and ERK

Once Ras has grabbed a GTP, it becomes active, and it can now activate Raf. Raf, in turn, activates MEK, which activates ERK (Figure 3.15c) [64]. ERK is a member of the MAPK family of kinases.

Step 3: ERK Activity

ERK then phosphorylates some proteins in the cell cytoplasm (such as components of the cell's internal skeleton and various receptors), and it also moves into the cell's nucleus, where it activates transcription factors such as Elk-1 and Myc [65]. (In fact, ERK can phosphorylate over 200 different proteins.) It takes just a few minutes for the activation of

---

Box 3.1   Ras

Ras proteins are immensely powerful; they can compel cells to grow and multiply and are the driving force in many cancers. Ras proteins are present in every cell in our body – similar proteins exist in everything from yeast to insects, birds, plants, and mollusks.

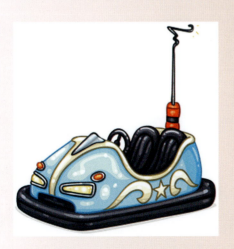

I tend to think of Ras proteins a bit like bumper cars, in that they have a stalk, which constantly tethers them to the internal surface of the cell membrane. While attached by their stalk, they are free to buzz around, looking for activated receptors with docking proteins that they can attach to. If they become detached from the membrane, they can no longer do their job. Some scientists have tried to take advantage of this, and attempted to create drugs that prevent Ras proteins from attaching to the membrane. These drugs did at one point look exciting, but scientists have since discovered that our cells have other ways of attaching Ras to the membrane, so the search for effective Ras inhibitors continues.

Source of image: http://boe.wallab.ee/variant/20130718-43d1b7f35e73cce941e23f2c130f9adcd00ebeb4 b1047d50c653d1b-1024.png.

a growth factor receptor on the surface of the cell to culminate in the activation of Elk-1 and Myc in the nucleus [66].

Depending on the amount and type of growth factors that attached to the receptors, the cell might merely stay alive, or it might start growing and multiplying.

Things to Remember

I've described the MAPK pathway as a linear series of events with one protein activating another and then another. In fact, the MAPK pathway has many branches and loops, and it interacts with other signaling pathways. For example, ERK can activate the JAK/STAT pathway, and the estrogen receptor can activate ERK.

It's important to remember how complicated and nuanced cell signaling is when we look at drugs that block various proteins involved. Although the drug might do its job properly and block the protein it is designed to, this can have unforeseen consequences. Some of these consequences can make the drug less effective, such as if it accidently triggers a feedback loop that activates or blocks another pathway.

It is also important to note that there are often several different versions of each protein. For example, there are four different Ras proteins in human cells (N-Ras, H-Ras, K-Ras4A, and K-Ras4B), three Raf proteins (A-Raf, B-Raf, and C-Raf), and seven MEKs (MEK 1-7). In addition, there are at least 13 MAPKs: ERK1, 2, 3, 4, 5, 7, and 8, JNK1, 2, and 3, and p38α, β, and γ [62].[16] Each cell type uses different versions of these proteins for different purposes and in response to different signals.

Box 3.2 The Greek Alphabet

Scientists are forever using letters from the Greek alphabet to distinguish between different versions of proteins. For example, in this chapter we meet PDGFRα; p38α, β and γ; p110α, β, γ, and δ; and PI3Kα, β, γ, and δ. So it's useful to know how to say them.

α – alpha
β – beta
γ - gamma
δ - delta

3.7.2 Defects in the MAPK Signaling Pathway in Cancer Cells

There are three main ways that the MAPK signaling pathway (i.e., Ras/Raf/MEK/ERK) becomes overactive in cancer cells [67]:

1. **Because of the overactivity of growth factor receptors, and other receptors, on the cell surface** [covered in the first half of this chapter].

2. **Because a Ras protein is overactive** [68]. *RAS* genes (*KRAS, NRAS,* and *HRAS*) are mutated in around a third of all human cancers, causing Ras proteins (K-Ras,[17] N-Ras, or H-Ras) to be overactive. *KRAS* is the most commonly mutated. For example, *KRAS* is mutated in 30%–50% of bowel cancers, up to 90% of pancreatic cancers, and 30% of NSCLCs (particularly in smokers). *NRAS* mutations appear to be most common in malignant melanoma (occurring in 15%–25%), but generally only occur in melanomas in which the *BRAF* gene is normal. You

---

[16] In general, ERK proteins coordinate a cell's response to mitogens – substances that cause cells to grow and multiply, whereas JNK and p38 proteins respond to stress signals, such as low oxygen or nutrient levels.
[17] Although there are two versions of K-Ras – K-Ras4A and K-Ras4B – they are almost identical, so I'll just refer to K-Ras.

also find *NRAS* mutations in various leukemias and lymphomas. *HRAS* mutations are pretty rare in comparison, occurring in only 3% of cancers (compared to 25%–30% for *KRAS* and 8% for *NRAS*). Ras proteins can also become overactive if a protein that would normally control them is missing. For example, neurofibromin is a protein that blocks Ras proteins and prevents activation of Raf. The gene for neurofibromin (*NF1*) is commonly mutated in lung cancer, knocking out its function [69].

3. **Because B-Raf is faulty**. There are three different Raf proteins (A-Raf, B-Raf, and C-Raf), but it is usually just B-Raf which is faulty in human cancers; for example, B-Raf is faulty and overactive in around 50% of malignant melanoma skin cancers, in 8%–10% of bowel cancers, and in some papillary thyroid, biliary, eye, lung, and ovarian cancers [70]. It is also at fault in almost all cases of a rare type of leukemia called hairy cell leukemia. The most common fault in B-Raf affects just one amino acid, which in the normal protein is a valine (V), and in the cancer-causing version of B-Raf is a glutamic acid (E). It is known as the **V600E mutation**.

Mutations in the genes for MEK and ERK proteins are very rare in cancer cells. However, mutations in *MEK* genes are occasionally present in malignant melanoma cells, mainly in cells from people whose cancer has become resistant to B-Raf inhibitors. *MEK* mutations are also found occasionally in lung cancers, bowel cancer, and ovarian cancer [71].

3.7.3 Drugs That Block the MAPK Pathway

The MAPK pathway requires four proteins: Ras, Raf, MEK, and ERK. However, only two of them are the target of licensed cancer treatments: Raf and MEK. (Table 3.5 summarizes how and why MEK and Raf inhibitors are used to treat cancer.)

Ras proteins have so far proved almost impossible to block (see Box 3.1). But, because *KRAS* is the most commonly mutated oncogene in human cancers, scientists continue to strive to make effective K-Ras inhibitors.

Scientists are also working on ERK inhibitors, although it's still early days. For many years, scientists didn't see any point in making ERK inhibitors because they didn't think they'd be any different in their effects from a MEK inhibitor. But, they've since decided that an ERK inhibitor might be worth having because (a) cell signaling is so complicated that scientists' predictions have often been proved wrong, and (b) cancer cells that are resistant to both B-Raf and MEK inhibitors have often found a way to reactivate ERK [64].

Table 3.5 Summary of licensed drugs that block the MAPK pathway.

Drug target and examples	Used in what cancers?	Why?
B-Raf inhibitors: vemurafenib (Zelboraf), dabrafenib (Tafinlar), encorafenib	Predominantly used for B-Raf-mutated malignant melanoma, but also licensed for B-Raf-mutated NSCLC; may eventually be used in a small proportion of bowel cancers and in other cancer types.	50% of malignant melanomas are driven by a mutated B-Raf protein (V600E B-Raf); these cancers are sensitive to B-Raf inhibitors. The same mutation exists in a smaller proportion of bowel and lung cancers.
MEK inhibitors: trametinib (Mekinist), cobimetinib (Cotellic), selumetinib, binimetinib [72]	B-Raf-mutated malignant melanoma. Also licensed in combination with a B-Raf inhibitor for B-Raf-mutated NSCLC. They are also being tested in a wide variety of other cancers.	MEK inhibitors seem able to delay resistance to B-Raf inhibitors and reduce the incidence of secondary skin cancers.

3.7.4 Drugs That Block Raf Proteins

How They Work and Differences between Them

There are four groups of Raf inhibitors at present, which have different strengths and weaknesses and are at different stages of development [64]:

1. **Drugs that block wild-type Raf proteins** (i.e., they block the natural, non-mutated versions of Raf proteins that exist in healthy cells). One example is sorafenib, which can block B-Raf and C-Raf. However, sorafenib also blocks a multitude of other kinases. Sorafenib's effectiveness against kidney and liver cancer (for which it is licensed) may have as much (if not more) to do with its ability to block VEGF and PDGF receptors as to its ability to block Raf proteins.

2. **Drugs that selectively kill cells with V600E mutated B-Raf,** for example, vemurafenib and dabrafenib. In cancer cells with V600E-mutated *BRAF* genes, the mutated B-Raf protein exists as monomers (individual proteins) that potently activate MEK. (If you remember, normal B-Raf is only active when paired up and present as dimers). Vemurafenib and dabrafenib can block the mutated B-Raf monomers, but they can't block healthy B-Raf dimers. Thus, these drugs are active against V600E-mutated cancer cells, but they don't kill healthy cells, and as a consequence they cause relatively few side effects. However, through a strange quirk, vemurafenib and dabrafenib actually stabilize and increase the activity of healthy B-Raf dimers (this is called "the Raf-inhibitor paradox" – explained in Figure 3.16). As a

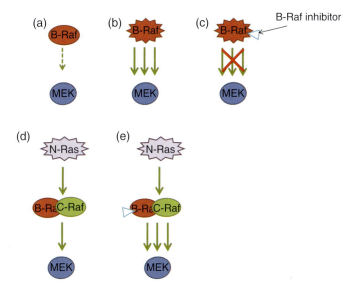

Figure 3.16 The Raf inhibitor paradox. (a) In healthy cells most Raf proteins exist as unpaired monomers that cannot activate MEK. The addition of a Raf inhibitor such as vemurafenib or dabrafenib therefore has little impact. **(b)** In cancer cells in which the B-Raf protein is mutated and overactive, the faulty B-Raf protein strongly activates MEK even as a monomer, which forces the cancer cell to grow and multiply. **(c)** Mutated B-Raf monomers are blocked by the B-Raf inhibitor, causing cell death. **(d)** Non-cancer cells occasionally contain mutated, overactive versions of Ras proteins, such as N-Ras. These faulty Ras proteins activate the cell's Raf proteins, causing them to pair up and form dimers that activate MEK. **(e)** Treatment of these cells with a B-Raf inhibitor actually activates the Raf dimers and causes even greater MEK activity, potentially causing a secondary cancer.

result, cells that contain lots of B-Raf dimers are sometimes forced by the B-Raf inhibitor to become cancer cells and form secondary cancers. This is a problem for people with melanoma because their skin has often been exposed to a lot of sun and contains cells with mutations, such as *NRAS* mutations, which trigger the formation of lots of B-Raf dimers. However, by combining a B-Raf inhibitor with a MEK inhibitor, this problem of secondary cancers is almost completely avoided. Both vemurafenib and dabrafenib are licensed treatments for malignant melanoma, and I describe them in more detail in Chapter 6, Section 6.6.2. A third B-RafV600E inhibitor, LGX818, is in trials.

3. **Drugs that can block B-Raf dimers**, for example, TAK-632 and MLN2480. Unlike vemurafenib and dabrafenib, these drugs can block paired-up Raf proteins. Hence, they can block B-Raf even when the problem does not lie with B-Raf itself, but when B-Raf is instead being controlled by overactive Ras proteins. These drugs might be effective when Ras mutations have caused drug resistance to vemurafenib and dabrafenib. But, because these drugs block healthy B-Raf, side effects could be a problem.

4. **Pan-Raf inhibitors**, for example, CCT196969 and CCT241161. These drugs are designed to block both the normal C-Raf protein found in healthy cells and the V600E mutated B-Raf found in cancer cells. They are still in the early stages of clinical trials. Scientists think these treatments might be helpful in treating melanomas when vemurafenib and dabrafenib have stopped working [73].

Who They're Given To

Raf inhibitors (summarized in Table 3.6) have become important treatments for the 50% or so of people with malignant melanoma whose cancer contains a *BRAF* mutation. I'll therefore discuss them further in Chapter 6,

Table 3.6 Summary of B-Raf inhibitors.

Type of inhibitor	Examples
Drugs that block un-mutated (i.e., wild-type) Raf proteins	Sorafenib (Nexavar)
Drugs that block V600E mutated B-Raf	Vemurafenib (Zelboraf), dabrafenib (Tafinlar), LGX818, and PLX-4720
Pan-Raf inhibitors	TAK-632, MLN2480, CCT196969, CCT241161, and LY3009120

Section 6.6. B-Raf inhibitors have also proven effective against the small proportion of NSCLCs that contain the V600E *BRAF* mutation (see Chapter 6, Section 6.4.5). And they might also be helpful for *BRAF*-mutated bowel cancers (see Chapter 6, Section 6.5.3) and possibly against, other cancers in which *B-RAF* mutations are found (for a list of some cancers in which *BRAF* mutations have been found, see Table 3.7).

Why They Stop Working

When a B-Raf inhibitor is given to patients with *BRAF*-mutated malignant melanoma, the response rate is generally around 50%–60% [74]. Even in treatment-sensitive cancers, the drug tends to only work for a few months (the median duration of response with either dabrafenib or vemurafenib alone tends to be about 5 to 7 months).

Scientists have taken tumor samples from people who didn't benefit at all from a B-Raf inhibitor (those with primary resistance). They've also taken samples from people whose tumor initially responded but is now growing again (secondary resistance).

The reasons behind primary and secondary resistance seem to be a bit different from one another, but many of the mutations found in resistant cells either reactivate the Ras/Raf/MEK/ERK pathway, or they activate the PI3K/AKT/mTOR pathway [75] (see Figure 3.17).

Table 3.7 B-Raf mutations are found in a range of cancer types.

Cancer	% that contain *BRAF* mutations
Melanoma skin cancer	45%
Bowel cancer	11%
Non-small cell lung cancer	2%
Papillary thyroid cancer	41%
Cancers of the central nervous system	8%
Cholangiocarcinoma (bile duct cancer)	4%
Hairy cell leukemia	Up to 100%
Multiple myeloma	5%

Sources: COSMIC; Catalogue of somatic mutations in cancer http://cancer. sanger.ac.uk/cosmic/Tiacci E et al. (2011). BRAF mutations in hairy cell leukemia. *N Engl J Med* **365**(24): 2305–2315.Rustad EH et al. (2015). BRAF V600E mutation in early-stage multiple myeloma: good response to broad acting drugs and no relation to prognosis. *Blood Cancer J* 5: e299.

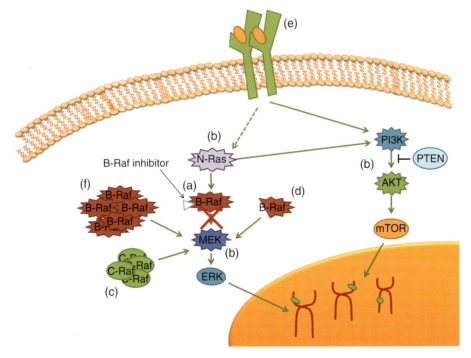

Figure 3.17 Some reasons for resistance to B-Raf inhibitors in malignant melanoma cells. (a) A B-Raf inhibitor blocks mutated B-Raf in a cancer cell. **(b)** Faulty, overactive versions of N-Ras, C-Raf, PI3K, and AKT can activate signaling pathways strongly enough that the cell survives. **(c)** Overproduction of C-Raf reactivates MEK despite B-Raf inhibition. **(d)** Extra mutations in the *BRAF* gene cause the cell to manufacture a shortened (truncated) version of B-Raf that cannot be blocked. **(e)** Cancer cells that have high levels of growth factor receptors on their surface can activate C-Raf and the PI3K/AKT/mTOR pathway to such a degree it can survive B-Raf inhibition. **(f)** Amplification of the mutated *BRAF* gene causes massive production of mutated B-Raf protein, which overwhelms the drug.
Abbreviations: mTOR – mammalian target of rapamycin; PI3K – phosphatidylinositol 3-kinase; ERK- extracellular-signal-regulated kinase; PTEN – phosphatase and tensin homologue

3.7.5 MEK Inhibitors

How They Work

As with many of the other proteins in our cells, there are multiple different MEK proteins – seven in total. But just two of them, MEK1 and MEK2, are activated by the MAPK pathway controlled by growth factor receptors, Ras and Raf.

Unlike drugs that block growth factor receptors and Raf proteins, most MEK inhibitors are allosteric kinase inhibitors. That is, these drugs fit into a small pocket on MEK proteins which is adjacent to the ATP-binding site. When a MEK inhibitor is inside this pocket, MEK is locked into an inactive shape [76].

Who They're Given To

So far, MEK inhibitors have made their greatest impact in treating people with malignant melanoma. Numerous clinical trials have shown that, when used in combination with a B-Raf inhibitor, a MEK inhibitor can delay resistance and avoid secondary cancers caused by the B-Raf inhibitor [77]. (For more information, see Chapter 6, Section 6.6 on malignant melanoma.)

As well as their importance as melanoma treatments, MEK inhibitors are being tested as treatments for a wide variety of other cancers. Scientists are particularly keen to discover whether MEK inhibitors can be effective against cancers that contain Ras mutations [78]. However, it seems unlikely that they will be effective if used on their own [64]. Instead, they're being tested in combination with various other drugs, such as chemotherapy, AKT inhibitors, and EGFR inhibitors for a variety of different cancer types including EGFR inhibitor-resistant lung cancer and *BRAF*-mutated bowel cancer [78].

3.8 TARGETING THE PI3K/AKT/MTOR SIGNALING PATHWAY

So far, I've just described the MAPK signaling pathway, but growth factor receptors also control other pathways. A second is the PI3K/AKT/mTOR pathway (see Figure 3.18 for an overview of this pathway and how it interlinks with the MAPK pathway). In fact, scientists believe that the PI3K/AKT/mTOR pathway is the most common pathway affected by mutations in human cancers [79].

3.8.1 The Mechanics of the PI3K/AKT/mTOR Pathway

Step 1: PI3K Becomes Active

I first mentioned PI3K in Chapter 2, Section 2.3.1 as an important kinase activated by growth factor receptors. However, whereas all the other kinases I've mentioned so far in this book phosphorylate other proteins (which are themselves often kinases), PI3K phosphorylates a lipid molecule found in the cell membrane called PIP_2 (phosphatidylinositol 4,5-bisphosphate). When a growth factor receptor is activated, it recruits PI3K (with additional help from Ras). Once it is connected to the receptor and in close proximity to the cell membrane, PI3K has ready access to supplies of PIP_2 and it can phosphorylate it to produce PIP_3.[18] PIP_3 then activates AKT.[19]

An important feature of PI3K proteins is that they are actually made from two protein parts known as the regulatory subunit and the catalytic subunit. There are four different versions of the catalytic subunit (called p110α, β, δ,[20] and γ), and eight regulatory subunits. These

---

[18] PIP_2 contains two phosphate groups, so when PI3K adds another phosphate it becomes PIP_3 (phosphatidylinositol 3,4,5-triphosphate).
[19] AKT is also called PKB – protein kinase B.
[20] The δ subunit is only found in white blood cells.

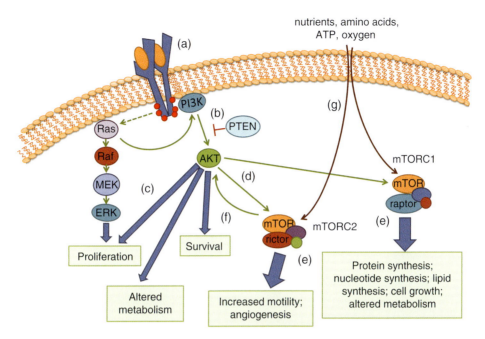

Figure 3.18 The basics of the PI3K/AKT/mTOR signaling pathway. **(a)** As with the MAPK pathway, the PI3K/AKT/mTOR pathway can be triggered by paired-up growth factor receptors that phosphorylate one another (shown by the red circles). **(b)** The paired-up receptors activate P13K, which indirectly activates AKT. **(c)** AKT has numerous impacts on the cell, including triggering cell proliferation, survival, and altered metabolism. **(d)** AKT also activates mTOR, an important controller of cell growth, motility, and angiogenesis. **(e)** mTOR is active when it comes together with other proteins to form mTOR complex-1 (mTORC1) and mTOR complex-2 (mTORC2). mTORC1 and mTORC2 have distinct, but overlapping, effects on the cell. **(f)** mTORC2 also causes further activation of AKT. **(g)** In addition, mTORC is influenced by proteins that respond to the cell's well-being and environment, such as changing levels of glucose, amino acids, ATP, and oxygen.

Abbreviations: mTOR – mammalian target of rapamycin; PI3K – phosphatidylinositol 3-kinase; ERK-extracellular-signal-regulated kinase; PTEN – phosphatase and tensin homologue; ATP – adenosine triphosphate

subunits can pair up in various different combinations[21] to create different versions of PI3K (see Figure 3.19) [80]. I realize this is getting complicated, but it is important because we have pan-PI3K inhibitors that block various different versions of PI3K. And we also have highly selective PI3K inhibitors that only block individual versions of PI3K. Also, different forms of PI3K are implicated in different cancers.

Step 2: PI3K Activates AKT (This Is Blocked by PTEN)

As I've already said, PIP_3 activates AKT. In order to prevent overactivity of AKT, our cells normally contain another protein called PTEN. This protein reverses the actions of PI3K by removing one of PIP_3's phosphates. PTEN is an immensely important protein and a powerful protector against cancer. In fact, loss of PTEN is a common feature of cancer

---

[21] Five of the regulatory subunits (p85α, p85β, p55α, p55γ, and p50α) will pair with p110α, β, and δ. The other three regulatory subunits (p101, p84, and p87PIKAP) will only pair with p110γ.

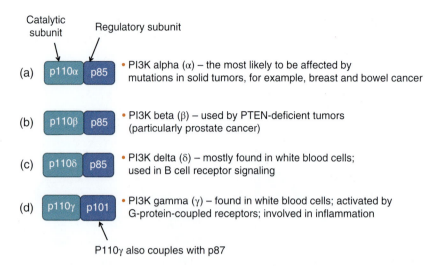

Figure 3.19 PI3K comes in various different forms. There are numerous versions of the two subunits that come together to create PI3K [80]. Each subunit is encoded by a different gene. **(a)** The most commonly-mutated gene for a PI3K subunit in cancer cells is *PIK3CA*, which is the gene for making the p110-alpha subunit of PI3K-alpha. A wide variety of mutations in *PIK3CA* have been found in numerous solid tumors. **(b)** PI3K-beta has overlapping roles with PI3K-alpha and seems to be particularly important to cancer cells that have lost PTEN, which includes the majority of prostate cancers. **(c)** PI3K-delta is predominantly found in white blood cells, in which it is activated by B cell receptors. **(d)** PI3K-gamma is activated by G-protein-coupled receptors rather than by growth factor receptors. **Abbreviations:** PI3K – phosphatidylinositol 3-kinase; PTEN – phosphatase and tensin homologue

cells (see Chapter 3, Section 3.8.2 for more on this).

AKT is yet another powerful kinase that controls numerous other proteins. The net effect of AKT activation is to encourage the cell to multiply, protect it from cell death, and equip it with energy and proteins for growth [80]. Some of AKT's actions are mediated by a kinase called mTOR (mammalian target of rapamycin).

Step 3: AKT Activates mTOR

Many people describe mTOR as a master switch or master regulator. Because, as well as responding to AKT – and therefore to growth factor receptors – mTOR is also influenced by the cell's energy, oxygen, amino acid, and nutrient supplies. And mTOR also responds to a variety of other signaling pathways, such as the Hippo, WNT, and Notch pathways [81]. In fact, it seems that when a cell receives a signal to multiply via its growth factor receptors, it uses mTOR to make sure that it only goes ahead if it's in good health and has the energy and other supplies necessary to do so.

Step 4: mTOR Forms Complexes Which Force the Cell to Grow and Multiply

mTOR's activities are diverse and complicated. Importantly, it can form multi-protein complexes with numerous other proteins. In a grouping known as mTORC1 (mTOR complex 1), which contains a protein called raptor, mTOR can equip cells for rapid growth and proliferation by increasing the production of lipids, mitochondria, and ribosomes. In another grouping, known as mTORC2 (mTOR complex 2), mTOR can further activate AKT and control cell survival, metabolism, proliferation, and the organization of the cell's internal protein skeleton [82].

There is considerable overlap, and some disagreement, over the precise function and control of mTORC1 and mTORC2. And do be aware that the information I've given here is a drastic simplification of the true situation.

3.8.2 Defects in the PI3K/AKT/mTOR Pathway In Cancer Cells

There are various reasons why the PI3K/AKT/mTOR pathway is overactive in cancer cells [83]:

1. **Overactivity of growth factor receptors and other receptors on the cell surface.** Many different growth factor receptors (e.g., EGFR, HER2, MET, and FLT3) are either overproduced or overactive in cancer cells. These receptors all activate PI3K.

2. **Overactivity of the MAPK signaling pathways.** Overactive Ras proteins can trigger PI3K and AKT activity.

3. **Overactivity of PI3K.** *PIK3CA* mutations are common in bowel, breast, brain, liver, stomach, and lung cancers [84]. *PIK3CA* is the gene for the p110α subunit of PI3K, and *PIK3CA* mutations cause PI3K to become overactive[22].

4. **Absence of PTEN.** *PTEN* is now known to be the second most commonly mutated tumor suppressor gene in human cancer cells [85] (the most commonly mutated is *TP53*, the gene for p53). There are many reasons why PTEN is missing in cancer cells, including deletion, suppression, or mutation of the *PTEN* gene and instability of the PTEN protein.

5. **Overactivity of AKT.** Mutations in the three *AKT* genes (*AKT1, AKT2,* and *AKT3*) are less common than *PIK3CA* and *PTEN* mutations. However, amplification of *AKT* genes and other mutations have been found in various cancer types, including head and neck cancer, pancreatic cancer, NSCLC, ovarian cancer, and breast cancer [86].

6. **Absence of mTOR suppressor proteins,** such as the TSC1/TSC2 complex or STK11 (also called LKB1). For example, STK11 is missing from the cells of about 5%–15% of adenocarcinoma NSCLCs [87].

3.8.3 Drugs That Block the PI3K/AKT/mTOR Pathway

Scientists have developed drugs that can block all three of the main proteins in the PI3K/AKT/mTOR pathway. These include drugs that are highly specific and block just one form of PI3K, as well as some that block both PI3K and mTOR together (summarized in Tables 3.8 and 3.9) [88].

So far, two mTOR inhibitors, everolimus (Afinitor) and temsirolimus (Torisel), and two PI3K inhibitors, idelalisib (Zydelig) and copanlisib (Aliqopa), have become licensed treatments. Many more are in trials.

3.8.4 mTOR Inhibitors

The first mTOR inhibitors used as cancer treatments were derivatives of a naturally occurring chemical compound called rapamycin (also known as sirolimus). This chemical is produced by a bacterium discovered on Easter Island over 40 years ago [89]. Rapamycin can suppress our immune system and is used to prevent the body from rejecting transplanted organs. Scientists investigating rapamycin's properties also discovered that it can kill cancer cells. These days, two drugs created from rapamycin, temsirolimus, and everolimus (collectively known as **rapalogues**) are used as treatments for kidney cancer (I discuss their role in kidney cancer in Chapter 6, Section 6.7), pancreatic neuroendocrine cancer (PNET), and mantle cell lymphoma. These drugs are

---

[22] PI3Kδ is the target of some treatments for B cell leukemias and lymphomas. However, it is not PI3Kδ which is at fault in these cancers – the faults rests with the B cell receptor, which controls PI3Kδ.

also sometimes used as breast cancer treatments in combination with hormone therapies (see Chapter 6, Section 6.2.2).

Rapamycin, temsirolimus, and everolimus are thus three closely related drugs that have been created from a natural compound. Unlike many drugs that block kinases, they do not mimic the shape of ATP, nor do they directly inhibit mTOR's kinase activity. Instead, these drugs attach to a protein called FKBP12. The drug–FKBP12 combination then blocks mTORC1 (but not mTORC2) [90].

The inability of rapamycin, everolimus, and temsirolimus to block mTORC2 opens up the possibility that a drug which can block both mTORC complexes might be more effective. Scientists hope that newer mTOR inhibitors (e.g., AZD2014, AZD8055, OSI-027, and INK128) that compete for its ATP-binding site will do just that. They are being evaluated in clinical trials in numerous different cancers, including breast, bowel, liver, ovarian, prostate, and lung cancer.

3.8.5 PI3K Inhibitors

PI3K overactivity is a common feature of cancer cells, and over 30 PI3K inhibitors have been created and tested in clinical trials.

Virtually all PI3K inhibitors are ATP mimics that competitively bind PI3K's ATP-binding site [91].

As of December 2017, two PI3K inhibitors are licensed as cancer treatments: idelalisib, for the treatment of B cell leukemias and non-Hodgkin lymphomas (NHLs), and copanlisib, for the treatment of follicular NHL. Idelalisib is a specific inhibitor that blocks only PI3Kδ, which is almost exclusively found in white blood cells (see Figure 3.19); whereas copanlisib is a pan-PI3K inhibitor (see below). (I'll come back to these treatments in Chapter 7, Section 7.4 on drugs that target B cell receptor signaling).

Pan-PI3K inhibitors block the α, β, γ, and δ forms of PI3K (see Table 3.8). Some of these drugs, such as buparlisib (BKM120), have been the subject of numerous clinical trials. However, side effects have been a problem with pan-PI3K inhibitors. Thus far, only copanlisib has become a licensed treatment, and many trials have been disappointing [79].

Other drugs, such as idelalsib, are able to selectively block just one or two PI3K proteins. Idelalisib is a selective for PI3Kδ, whereas alpelisib is a PI3Kα-selective inhibitor. Alpelisib is currently in trials for breast

Table 3.8 Summary of the specificity of various PI3K inhibitors.

PI3K inhibitor [92]	Isoforms inhibited:				Stage of development
	α	β	γ	δ	
Buparlisib; BKM120	✓	✓	✓	✓	Phase 3 trials for breast cancer
Copanlisib; Aliqopa	✓	(✓)	✓	(✓)	Licensed in the United States for the treatment of follicular NHL
Pictilisib; GDC-0941	✓	✓	✓	✓	Phase 2 trials for breast cancer, NSCLC and glioblastoma
Alpelisib; BYL719	✓				Phase 3 trial for breast cancer
Taselisib; GDC-0032	✓		✓	✓	Phase 3 trials for breast cancer and NSCLC
Duvelisib; IPI-145			✓	✓	Phase 3 trials for NHL and CLL
Idelalisib; CAL-101; Zydelig				✓	Approved for CLL and follicular lymphoma in the United States and Europe

Abbreviations: PI3K – phosphatidylinositol 3-kinase; NHL – non-Hodgkin lymphoma; NSCLC – non-small cell lung cancer; CLL – chronic lymphocytic leukemia

cancer, and there are signs that it will be particularly helpful for patients whose tumors contain a *PIK3CA* mutation and in which PI3Kα is overactive [93].

3.8.6 Dual PI3K and mTOR Inhibitors

The ATP-binding sites on PI3K and mTOR are very similar to one another. So, it has been possible to create chemical compounds that block both of these proteins. Several drug companies have created drugs that do this (see Table 3.9),

but they're still in early phase trials, and toxicity has been a problem [94]. For example, one of the first dual PI3K/mTOR inhibitors created was dactilisib (BEZ235); however, a clinical trial in kidney cancer was halted early due to toxicity and lack of effectiveness [95].

3.8.7 AKT Inhibitors

AKT (also known as protein kinase B – PKB) comes in three main forms: Akt1, Akt2, and Akt3. AKT proteins have a diverse range of uses in human cells, just one of which is to

Table 3.9 Summary of some mTOR, PI3K, and AKT inhibitors.

Drug target and examples	Used in what cancers?	Why?
mTOR inhibitors: **rapamycin, everolimus, temsirolimus, AZD2014, AZD8055, OSI-027, INK128, CC-223**	Kidney cancer, breast cancer, mantle cell lymphoma, and pancreatic neuroendocrine tumors (PNETs); in trials for the treatment of many other cancer types.	Kidney cancers commonly maintain a mutation in the *VHL* gene; this mutation, together with overactive mTOR, drives angiogenesis and the growth of these cancers (see Chapter 6, Section 6.7.1 for more detail); in breast cancer, there is interplay between estrogen receptor signaling and the PI3K/AKT/mTOR pathway; PNETs often contain mutations affecting mTOR activity.
Pan-PI3K inhibitors and selective PI3Kα inhibitors: **Copanlisib (Aliqopa; BAY80-6946), Buparlisib (BKM120), Pictilisib (GDC-0941), Alpelisib (BYL719), XL147, INK1117, PX-866, SAR245408,**	In trials for breast cancer and many other cancer types. Copanlisib is predominantly active against PI3Kα and PI3Kδ and is active against follicular NHL.	PI3Kα is commonly overactive in breast cancer and other solid tumors due to mutations in the *PIK3CA* gene; PI3K is active in other cancers due to overactivity of various cell surface receptors and Ras proteins. Copanlisib's activity against follicular NHL is presumed to be because of its ability to block PI3Kδ.
Selective PI3Kδ inhibitors: **Idelalisib (Zydelig), Taselisib (GDC-0032), Duvelisib (IPI-145), AMG319**	B cell chronic lymphocytic leukemia, and B cell lymphomas.	PI3Kδ is found in white blood cells. It is overactive in many B cell leukemias, lymphomas, and other hematological cancers due to overactivity of B cell receptors.
Dual mTOR/PI3K inhibitors: **Dactilisib (BEZ235), apitolisib (GDC-0980), BGT226, XL765, SF1126, PI103**	Being explored in a variety of cancers.	Many cancers have overactive PI3K/AKT/mTOR pathway; dual targeting of mTOR and PI3K together may overcome some resistance mechanisms to drugs that only target mTOR.
AKT inhibitors: **Perifosine, ipatasertib (GDC-0068), AZD5363, MK2206**	Being explored in a variety of cancers.	Many cancers have overactive PI3K/AKT/mTOR pathway.

activate mTOR. One of their main functions is to promote cell survival by inactivating proteins known to trigger cell death, such as Bad, and activating proteins that promote survival, such as MDM2 [96].

In recent years, scientists have created a wide range of chemical compounds that can block AKT through various different mechanisms of action [96]. However, many of these drugs aren't very specific, and they also block other kinases such as protein kinase A (PKA) and protein kinase C (PKC) [97]. More recently, scientists have managed to make AKT-specific drugs such as ipatasertib (GDC-0068), AZD5363, and MK-2206 [98]. These drugs are still in early phase trials, so it's too early to know whether they work and, if they do, who might benefit from them.

3.9   TARGETING THE JAK-STAT PATHWAY

The JAK-STAT[23] pathway is necessary for normal embryo development, and as an adult it is essential for a healthy immune system, including the production of white blood cells in the bone marrow. The pathway is activated by numerous signaling molecules produced by white blood cells. White blood cells then respond to such signals by perhaps multiplying, moving to the site of an infection, or by producing yet more signaling molecules [99].

3.9.1   The Mechanics of JAK-STAT Signaling

Activation of the JAK-STAT pathway often begins with the activation of a receptor on a cell's surface. Typically, the receptor is a cytokine receptor, but this pathway can also be activated by growth factor receptors [99].

Not surprisingly, cytokine receptors respond to the presence of cytokines. Cytokines are small signaling molecules that our white blood cells use to give one another instructions, such as telling a white blood cell to move to the site of an infection. Cytokines include interferons, interleukins, chemokines, and tumor necrosis factor (TNF) [100].

Cytokine Receptors

Cytokine receptors, like growth factor receptors, are receptors that stick out from the surface of the cell and pick up signals in the form of cytokines and other molecules. They also span the cell membrane and have a portion that protrudes inside the cell, connecting to proteins in the cytoplasm (Figure 3.20) [101].

Activation of the JAK-STAT Pathway by a Cytokine Receptor

When a cytokine attaches to a cytokine receptor, the receptors pair up or form groupings of more than two receptors. Inside the cell, this joining up of the receptors brings JAK proteins together (Figure 3.20a). (JAK proteins are constantly attached to the receptors, so when the receptors come together, JAK proteins come together too.) When brought together, the JAK proteins phosphorylate one another. And, once this has happened, the phosphorylated JAK proteins then phosphorylate STATs (Figure 3.20b). STATs are transcription factors that spend most of the time sitting in the cell cytoplasm. But when JAK phosphorylates them, they pair up and move into the nucleus (Figure 3.20c). Here, they trigger the production of various proteins [99].

Cross-Talk with Growth Factor Receptor Pathways

Growth factor receptors usually communicate with the cell's nucleus via the MAPK signaling

---

[23] In case you were curious, JAK stands for Janus kinase, and STAT stands for signal transducer and activator of transcription.

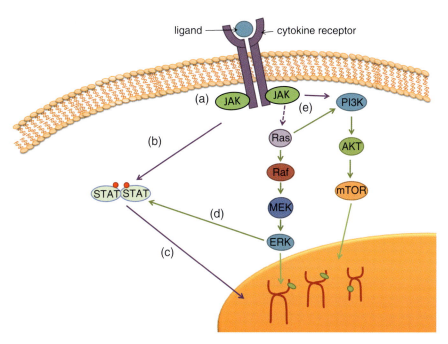

Figure 3.20 The basics of the JAK-STAT signaling pathway. (a) JAK is activated when two or more cytokine receptors come together due to the presence of a ligand, such as a cytokine, growth factor, or hormone. **(b)** JAK phosphorylates STAT transcription factors, which are in the cytoplasm. **(c)** The phosphorylated STATs pair up and move into the nucleus. In the nucleus, STATs control the production of a variety of proteins that together encourage the cell to multiply. **(d)** ERK adds to STAT activity by attaching further phosphates. **(e)** JAK directly activates PI3K and indirectly activates Ras, triggering MAPK pathway and PI3K/AKT/mTOR pathway activity. **Abbreviations:** JAK – janus kinase; STAT – signal transducer and activator of transcription; mTOR – mammalian target of rapamycin; PI3K – phosphatidylinositol 3-kinase; ERK- extracellular-signal-regulated kinase

pathway and the PI3K/AKT/mTOR pathway. However, growth factor receptors are also able to activate the JAK-STAT pathway. For example, ERK, the final protein in the MAPK pathway, directly phosphorylates STAT proteins, increasing their activity.

In addition, when JAK becomes active, it can attach phosphates to growth factor receptors, creating docking sites for proteins that activate the MAPK pathway. And JAK can activate PI3K. Consequently, all three pathways (JAK-STAT, MAPK, and PI3K/AKT/mTOR) add to each other's activity [99, 102].

Additional Complications

As with all other signaling pathways, the JAK-STAT pathway is nuanced and complex. For example, there are four different JAK proteins in our cells (JAK1, JAK2, JAK3, and TYK2) and seven different STATs (STAT1, STAT2, STAT3, STAT4, STAT5a, STAT5b, and STAT6). The four JAK proteins play different but overlapping roles. JAK2 is particularly important in the response of white blood cells to some growth factors and interleukins.

Additional complexity comes from the wide variety of different cytokines and cytokine receptors that our white blood cells use to communicate with one another.

I will come back to the JAK-STAT pathway in Chapter 7, Section 7.8, in which I discuss the usefulness of JAK2 inhibitors as treatments for some hematological cancers.

3.9.2 Defects in the JAK-STAT Pathway in Cancer Cells

There are three main reasons why the JAK-STAT pathway is overactive in cancer cells:

1. **Overactive growth factor receptors, cytokine receptors, and other receptors on the cell surface.** For example, mutated, overactive cytokine receptors have been found on the surface of cancer cells in some myeloproliferative neoplasms (MPNs)[24] and acute leukemias [102].

2. **Mutations affecting *JAK* genes.** *JAK2* mutations are very common in MPNs such as polycythemia vera, essential thrombocythemia, and primary myelofibrosis [103]. Additionally, the *JAK2* gene is amplified in a high proportion of Hodgkin lymphomas [104]. JAK2 fusion proteins and other *JAK2* mutations are found occasionally in acute leukemia and lymphoma cells and in some solid tumors [105]. Mutations in JAK1, JAK3, and TYK2 are mostly found in the cells of T-cell acute lymphoblastic leukemias and lymphomas [102].

3. **Absence of proteins that would normally block the pathway,** such as SOCS1, SOCS2, and SOCS3, in a variety of solid tumors [105, 106].

4. **Mutations in *STAT* genes.** *STAT* gene mutations are relatively rare, but mutations in *STAT3* and *STAT5b* have been found in some T-cell and natural killer cell leukemias. And *STAT6* mutations have been found in primary mediastinal large B cell lymphoma – a rare type of non-Hodgkin lymphoma [107].

3.9.3 JAK2 Inhibitors

The first JAK2 inhibitor created was ruxolitinib (Jakafi;Jakavi), which blocks both JAK1 and JAK2 [108, 109]. As with many of the other JAK inhibitors created so far, ruxolitinib is a reversible inhibitor that competes for the enzyme's ATP-binding site. However, the most common mutation in JAK2 found in MPN cells is the V617F mutation, which does not affect the ATP-binding site. Hence, ruxolitinib does not selectively block the mutated form of the protein. Because of its relative lack of specificity, ruxolitinib suppresses the normal creation of white blood cells in the bone marrow [110].

Ruxolitinib has been the subject of numerous clinical trials and is now licensed in Europe and the United States to treat people with myelofibrosis and other MPNs. Other JAK2 inhibitors in development include pacritinib (a dual JAK2 and FLT3 inhibitor), momelotinib (a JAK1/2 inhibitor) (see Table 3.10), and various drugs that selectively block JAK2, such as XL019 and TG101348 (fedratinib) [111]. (For more about JAK inhibitors see Chapter 7 Section 7.8.)

Table 3.10   Drugs that block the JAK-STAT pathway.

Drug target and examples	Used in what cancers?	Why?
JAK2 inhibitors: **Ruxolitinib (Jakafi; Jakavi),** **pacritinib (SB1518), momelotinib** **(CYT387), fedratinib (SAR302503;** **TG101348), lestaurtinib* (CEP-701),** **AZD1480, BMS911543, LY2784544,** **NS-018, XL019**	Myeloproliferative disorders such as myelofibrosis, polycythemia vera and essential thrombocythemia; also occasionally in trials for other hematological cancers and solid tumors.	Because JAK2 is commonly mutated and overactive in these cancers.

*Lestaurtinib also potently blocks FLT3 and TrkA.

[24] MPNs are a group of often slow-growing cancers affecting white blood cells.

3.10 FINAL THOUGHTS

In this chapter, I have described three signaling pathways that our cells use to communicate with one another and respond to external signals. These signaling pathways are faulty and overactive in cancer cells for a wide variety of reasons, and drugs that block them have become important cancer treatments.

However, as you're probably aware, results from clinical trials with signaling pathway inhibitors don't always give positive results. And, even when someone does benefit from one of these treatments, perhaps even for several years, their cancer almost always returns later, particularly if they have advanced, metastatic cancer. There appear to be many reasons why a cancer might be intrinsically resistant to treatment with a signaling pathway inhibitor, or become resistant over time.

Reasons for this resistance include the following [112–114]:

1. The **cancer was never dependent on the protein being blocked** by the inhibitor. For example, just because EGFR is on the surface of a cancer cell, this doesn't necessarily mean that the cancer cells are reliant on EGFR for their survival.

2. A tumor is made of **multiple populations of cancer cells** that contain different combinations of mutations. It appears to be inevitable that among all those millions of cells, there will be some that contain mutations that enable them to survive a treatment that blocks a single protein or pathway. Given time to grow, these resistant cells cause the cancer to recur.

3. Most kinase inhibitors work by mimicking the shape of ATP and slotting into a kinase's ATP-binding site. Perhaps not surprisingly, these drugs become ineffective if their target's **ATP-binding site changes shape**.

4. Because signaling pathways are so important to our cells, **there's lots of redundancy built into them**. This means that various cell surface receptors and signaling pathways can stand in for one another. And this in turn increases the likelihood that cancer cells will survive treatment with a drug that blocks just one receptor or particular pathway.

5. Signaling pathways are **used by all healthy cells**. Hence, sometimes a signaling pathway inhibitor causes almost as much damage to healthy cells as cancer cells, and it causes so much toxicity that it can't be given in a dose that would eradicate a cancer.

6. Non-cancer cells within the **cancer environment** participate in cell signaling. So they can protect cancer cells from the effects of a signaling inhibitor.

7. Some cancer cells have access to **protective mechanisms** through which they become **dormant and stop multiplying** (called senescence), or through which they become more **resilient** (such as going through the epithelial-to-mesenchymal transition – see Chapter 1, Section 1.6.3). Cells that trigger these mechanisms can often survive treatment.

8. Tumors often contain regions with a **poor blood supply** due to leaky, tangled, and malformed blood vessels. Hence, a drug may simply not be able to get where it's needed.

9. Cancer cells sometimes have proteins in their cell membrane that can **actively pump a drug** out of the cell.

Of course, many of these resistance mechanisms also apply to other treatments included in this book, such as Bcr-Abl inhibitors, PARP inhibitors, and the other approaches covered in Chapter 4. Perhaps the only treatments for which many of these mechanisms don't apply are the immunotherapies: treatments that work by activating or creating immune responses against cancer cells.

Another thing to keep in mind is just how complicated signaling pathways are. Back in Figure 3.5, when I illustrated some of the many proteins and pathways controlled by growth factor receptors, I included a handful of proteins that I haven't mentioned elsewhere in the chapter. These include Rac, Rho, Src, PLC (phospholipase C), and NFκB. Because we don't yet have any licensed treatments that target these proteins, I haven't mentioned them in any detail. However, they are important proteins and often implicated in drug resistance. For example, Src overactivity is a known drug resistance mechanism to HER2-targeted treatments [115].

Thankfully, despite the daunting complexity of signaling pathways, we have seen a huge number of signaling pathway inhibitors become licensed cancer treatments. And efforts continue to make these treatments even more effective, using strategies such as:

- **Combining signaling pathway inhibitors with one another** to shut off feedback loops and to block signaling pathways at multiple points
- Combining treatments that **block different pathways** (although toxicity is always a problem when you do this)
- Combining signaling pathway inhibitors with **immunotherapy** – this approach has several potential advantages: increasing the effectiveness of treatment; overcoming some resistance mechanisms; and minimizing side effects (because the two different sets of treatments cause very different toxicities and can therefore potentially be safely combined)
- Creating kinase inhibitors that are designed to **block kinases** in which the ATP-binding site has changed shape – such as the third-generation EGFR inhibitors
- Using **biomarker tests** to find out which treatment is most likely to work for each patient
- Using **biopsies, or analyzing cancer cells circulating in the blood**, known as circulating tumor cells (CTCs), or **circulating tumor**

DNA (ctDNA), to check for gene mutations likely to cause resistance. It may then be possible to change the person's treatment accordingly

With all these potential strategies, hopefully signaling pathway inhibitors will become even more effective for an even greater number of people with cancer.

REFERENCES

1 Scitable by Nature Education. G-Protein-Coupled Receptors Play Many Different Roles in Eukaryotic Cell Signaling. [online] Available at: http://www.nature.com/scitable/ebooks/essentials-of-cell-biology-14749010/122997540#bookContentViewAreaDivID [Accessed December 13, 2017].

2 For a review of the role of GPCRs in cancer, see: Dorsam RT, Gutkind JS (2007). G-protein-coupled receptors and cancer. *Nat Rev Cancer* **7**: 79–94.

3 Blume-Jensen P, Hunter P (2001). Oncogenic kinase signalling. *Nature* **411**: 355–365.

4 Robinson DR, Wu YM, Lin SF (2000). The protein tyrosine kinase family of the human genome. *Oncogene* **19**: 5548–5557.

5 For a summary of growth factor receptors, see: Scitable by Nature Education. Receptor Tyrosine Kinases Regulate Cell Growth, Differentiation, and Survival [online] Available at: http://www.nature.com/scitable/ebooks/essentials-of-cell-biology-14749010/118241359#bookContentViewAreaDivID [Accessed December 13, 2017].

6 Details of every discovered gene can be found on the GeneCards website: http://www.genecards.org/

7 Heinrichs A (2005). Survival factor. *Nat Rev Mol Cell Biol* **6**: 196.

8 Collins MKL et al. (1993). Growth factors as survival factors: Regulation of apoptosis. *BioEssays* **16**(2): 133–138.

9 For a summary of growth factor receptors, see: Scitable by Nature Education. Receptor Tyrosine Kinases Regulate Cell Growth, Differentiation,

and Survival [online] Available at: http://www.nature.com/scitable/ebooks/essentials-of-cell-biology-14749010/118241359#bookContentViewAreaDivID [Accessed December 13, 2017].

10 For an overview of these signaling pathways, see: Chong CR, Janne PA (2013). The quest to overcome resistance to EGFR-targeted therapies in cancer. *Nat Med* **19**(11): 1389–1400.

11 Harris TJR, McCormick F (2010). The molecular pathology of cancer. *Nat Rev Clin Oncol* **7**: 251–265.

12 Bertotti A, Sassi F (2015). Molecular pathways: Sensitivity and resistance to anti-EGFR antibodies. *Clin Cancer Res* **21**(15): 3377–3383.

13 For a review of the discovery of growth factor receptors and their importance as a target for cancer treatments, see: Gschwind A, Fischer O, Ullrich A (2004). The discovery of receptor tyrosine kinases: Targets for cancer therapy. *Nat Rev Cancer* **4**: 361–370.

14 Rubin I, Yarden Y (2001). The basic biology of HER2. *Ann Oncol* **12**(Suppl.1): S3–S8.

15 Arteaga CL, Engelman JA (2014). ERBB receptors: From oncogene discovery to basic science to mechanism-based cancer therapeutics. *Cancer Cell* **25**(3): 282–303.

16 Reviewed in: Salomon DS, Brandt R, Ciardiello F et al. (1995). Epidermal growth factor-related peptides and their receptors in human malignancies. *Crit Rev Oncol Hematol* **19**(3): 183–232.

17 Reviewed in: Yan M, Parker BA, Schwab R et al. (2014). HER2 aberrations in cancer: Implications for therapy. *Cancer Treatment Rev* **40**(6): 770–780.

18 Reviewed in: Ma J, Lyu H, Huang J et al. (2014). Targeting of erbB3 receptor to overcome resistance in cancer treatment. *Mol Cancer* **13**: 105.

19 Reviewed in: Arteaga CL, Engelman JA (2014). ERBB receptors: From oncogene discovery to basic science to mechanism-based cancer therapeutics. *Cancer Cell* **25**(3): 282–303.

20 Reviewed in: Sharma PS, Sharma R, Tyagi T (2011). VEGF/VEGFR pathway inhibitors as anti-angiogenic agents: Present and future. *Curr Cancer Drug Targets* **11**(5): 624–653.

21 Reviewed in: Heldin CH (2013). Targeting the PDGF signaling pathway in tumor treatment. *Cell Commun Signal* **11**: 97.

22 For a review see: Wesche J, Haglund K, Haugsten EM (2011). Fibroblast growth factors and their receptors in cancer. *Biochem J* **437**(2):199–213.

23 Reviewed in: Pollak M (2008). Insulin and insulin-like growth factor signalling in neoplasia. *Nat Rev Cancer* **8**: 915–928.

24 Reviewed in: Smyth E, Sclafani F, Cunningham D (2014). Emerging molecular targets in oncology: Clinical potential of MET/hepatocyte growth-factor inhibitors. *Onco Targets Therapy* **7**: 1001–1014.

25 Reviewed in: Lennartsson J, Ronnstrand L (2012). Stem Cell Factor Receptor/c-Kit: From Basic Science to Clinical Implications. *Physiol Rev* **92**(4): 1619–1649.

26 Reviewed in: Small D (2006). FLT3 Mutations: Biology and Treatment. *Hematology Am Soc Hematol Educ Program* 178–184.

27 Reviewed in: Mulligan LM (2014). RET revisited: Expanding the oncogenic portfolio. *Nat Rev Cancer* **14**: 173–186.

28 Hynes N, Lane HA (2005). ERBB receptors and cancer: The complexity of targeted inhibitors. *Nat Rev Cancer* **5**: 341–354.

29 Yarden Y, Pines G (2012). The ERBB network: At last, cancer therapy meets systems biology. *Nat Rev Cancer* **12**: 553–563.

30 Tebbutt N, Pedersen MW, Johns TG (2013). Targeting the ERBB family in cancer: Couples therapy. *Nat Rev Cancer* **13**: 663–673.

31 My Cancer Genome. HER2 (ERBB2) in Gastric Cancer [online] Available at: https://www.mycancergenome.org/content/disease/gastric-cancer/erbb2/ [Accessed December 13, 2017].

32 Russo A et al. (2015). A decade of EGFR inhibition in EGFR-mutated non small cell lung cancer (NSCLC): Old successes and future perspectives. *Oncotarget* **6**(29): 26814–26825.

33 Turner N, Grose R (2010). Fibroblast growth factor signalling: From development to cancer. *Nat Rev Cancer* **10**: 116–129.

34 Price TJ et al. (2014). Panitumumab versus cetuximab in patients with chemotherapy-refractory wild-type KRAS exon 2 metastatic colorectal cancer (ASPECCT): A randomised, multicentre, open-label, non-inferiority phase 3 study. *Lancet Oncol* **15**: 569–579.

35 Ciardiello F, Tortora G (2008). EGFR antagonists in cancer treatment. *NEJM* **358**(11): 1160–1174.

36 Helwick C (2014). Cetuximab Fails to Improve Survival in Nonoperable Esophageal Cancer. [online] The ASCO Post. Available at: http://www.ascopost.com/issues/april-15-2014/cetuximab-fails-to-improve-survival-in-nonoperable-esophageal-cancer/ [Accessed December 13, 2017].

37 Teplinsky E, Muggia F (2015). EGFR and HER2: Is there a role in ovarian cancer? *Translational Cancer Res* **4**(1): 107–117.

38 Gong J, Cho M, Fakih M (2016). RAS and BRAF in metastatic colorectal cancer management. *J Gastrointest Oncol* **7**(5): 687–704.

39 Neumann J et al. (2009). Frequency and type of KRAS mutations in routine diagnostic analysis of metastatic colorectal cancer. *Pathol Res Pract* **205**(12): 858–862.

40 Modest DP et al. (2016). Outcome according to KRAS-, NRAS- and BRAF-mutation as well as KRAS mutation variants: Pooled analysis of five randomized trials in metastatic colorectal cancer by the AIO colorectal cancer study group. *Ann Oncol* **27**: 1746–1753.

41 Bronte G et al. (2015). New findings on primary and acquired resistance to anti-EGFR therapy in metastatic colorectal cancer: Do all roads lead to RAS? *Oncotarget* **6**(28): 24780–24796.

42 Dienstmann R et al. (2017). Consensus molecular subtypes and the evolution of precision medicine in colorectal cancer. *Nat Rev Cancer* **17**(2): 79–92.

43 Reviewed in Asami K, Atagi S (2016). Comparing the Efficacy of Gefitinib, Erlotinib, and Afatinib in Non-Small Cell Lung Cancer with Activating Epidermal Growth Factor Receptor (EGFR) Mutations. *Austin J Lung Cancer Res* **1**(1): 1003.

44 Janne PA et al. (2015). AZD9291 in EGFR inhibitor–Resistant non–small-cell lung cancer. *N Engl J Med* **372**: 1689–1699.

45 Cross DAE et al. (2014). AZD9291, an irreversible EGFR TKI, overcomes T790M-mediated resistance to EGFR inhibitors in lung cancer. *Cancer Discov* **4**(9): 1046–1061.

46 Kelley RK, Ko AH (2008). Erlotinib in the treatment of advanced pancreatic cancer. *Biologics* **2**(1): 83–95.

47 Moore MJ, Goldstein D, Hamm J et al. (2007). Erlotinib plus gemictabine compared to gemcitabine alone in patients with advanced pancreatic cancer: A phase III trial of the National Cancer Institute of Canada Clinical Trials Group. *J Clin Oncol* **25**: 1960–1966.

48 For a discussion on the usefulness of erlotinib as a treatment for pancreatic cancer see: Ko AH (2007). Erlotinib in Pancreatic Cancer: A Major Breakthrough? CancerNetwork website. http://www.cancernetwork.com/articles/erlotinib-pancreatic-cancer-major-breakthrough [Accessed December 13, 2017].

49 For a review see: Clifford AH (2007). Trastuzumab — Mechanism of action and use in clinical practice. *N Engl J Med* **357**: 39–51.

50 Harbeck N et al. (2013). HER2 dimerization inhibitor Pertuzumab – Mode of action and clinical data in breast cancer. *Breast Care (Basel)* **8**(1): 49–55.

51 Barok M et al. (2014). Trastuzumab emtansine: Mechanisms of action and drug resistance. *Breast Cancer Res* **16**(2): 209.

52 Verma S et al. (2012). Trastuzumab emtansine for HER2-positive advanced breast cancer. *N Engl J Med* **367**(19): 1783–1791.

53 For an example see: Venkatesan P (2016). Trastuzumab emtansine for HER2-positive breast cancer. *Lancet Oncol* **17**(12): e528.

54 Slamon DJ et al. (1987). Human breast cancer: Correlation of relapse and survival with amplification of the HER-2/neu oncogene. *Science* **235**: 177–182.

55 Luque-Cabal M et al. (2016). Mechanisms behind the resistance to Trastuzumab in HER2-amplified breast cancer and strategies to overcome it. *Clin Med Insights: Oncology* **10**(S1): 21–30.

56 Gu G et al. (2016). Targeted therapy for breast cancer and molecular mechanisms of resistance to treatment. *Curr Op Pharmacol* **31**: 97–103.

57 Segovia-Mendoza M et al. (2015). Efficacy and mechanism of action of the tyrosine kinase inhibitors gefitinib, lapatinib and neratinib in

the treatment of HER2-positive breast cancer: Preclinical and clinical evidence. *Am J Cancer Res* 5(9): 2531–2561.

58 Cancer Research UK. Gastrointestinal stromal tumour (GIST). http://www.cancerresearchuk. org/about-cancer/cancers-in-general/cancer-questions/what-is-the-treatment-for-gist-gastrointestinal-stromal-tumour [Accessed December 13, 2017].

59 Bauer S, Joensuu H (2015). Emerging agents for the treatment of advanced, Imatinib-resistant gastrointestinal stromal tumors: Current status and future directions. *Drugs* 75(12): 1323–1334.

60 Heinrich MC et al. (2012). Crenolanib inhibits the drug-resistant PDGFRA D842V mutation associated with imatinib-resistant gastrointestinal stromal tumors. *Clin Cancer Res* 18(16): 4375–4384.

61 Call J et al (2012). Survival of gastrointestinal stromal tumor patients in the imatinib era: Life raft group observational registry. *BMC Cancer* 12: 90 doi: 10.1186/1471-2407-12-90.

62 For a review of MAPKs and MAPK pathways see: Yang S-H et al. (2013). MAP kinase signalling cascades and transcriptional regulation. *Gene* 513(1): 1–13.

63 Downward J (1996). Control of Ras activation. *Cancer Surv* 27: 87–100.

64 Samatar AA, Poulikakos (2014). Targeting RAS–ERK signalling in cancer: Promises and challenges. *Nat Rev Drug Discov* 13(12): 928–942.

65 Roskoski R Jr (2012). ERK1/2 MAP kinases: Structure, function, and regulation. *Pharmacol Res* 66(2): 105–143.

66 Bahrami S, Drablos F (2016). Gene regulation in the immediate-early response process. *Adv Biol Regulation* 62: 37–49.

67 Santarpia L et al. (2012). Targeting the mitogen-activated protein kinase RAS-RAF signaling pathway in cancer therapy. *Exp Opin Therapeutic Targets* 16(1): 103–119.

68 For a review of the role of faulty Ras proteins in cancer, see: Prior IA et al. (2012). A comprehensive survey of Ras mutations in cancer. *Cancer Res* 72(10): 2457–2467.

69 Redig AJ et al. (2016). Clinical and molecular characteristics of NF1-mutant lung cancer. *Clin Cancer Res* 22(13): 3148–3156.

70 Davies H et al. (2002). Mutations of the BRAF gene in human cancer. *Nature* **417**: 949–954.

71 Bromberg-White JL et al. (2012). MEK genomics in development and disease. *Brief Funct Genomics* 11(4): 300–310.

72 For a fuller list of MEK inhibitors in development, see: Adjei A, Zhao Y (2015). Exploring the Pathway: Inhibiting MEK for Cancer Therapy. ASCO website: https://am.asco.org/exploring-pathway-inhibiting-mek-cancer-therapy-0 [Accessed December 13, 2017].

73 Girotti et al. (2015). Paradox-breaking RAF inhibitors that also target SRC are effective in drug-resistant BRAF mutant melanoma. *Cancer Cell* 27(1): 85–96.

74 Reviewed in Eroglu Z, Ribas A (2016). Combination therapy with BRAF and MEK inhibitors for melanoma: Latest evidence and place in therapy. *Ther Adv Med Oncol* 8(1): 48–56.

75 Reviewed in Spagnolo F et al. (2015). BRAF-mutant melanoma: Treatment approaches, resistance mechanisms, and diagnostic strategies. *Onco Targets Ther* 8: 157–168.

76 Reviewed in Zhao Y, Adjei AA (2014). The clinical development of MEK inhibitors. *Nat Rev Clin Oncol* 11: 385–400.

77 For an overview of the evidence, see: Stenger M (2014). Two Phase III Trials Show Benefit With BRAF/MEK Inhibitor Combination vs BRAF Inhibitor Alone in Advanced Melanoma. The ASCO Post Volume 5, Issue 18. http://www.ascopost.com/issues/november-15,-2014/two-phase-iii-trials-show-benefit-with-brafmek-inhibitor-combination-vs-braf-inhibitor-alone-in-advanced-melanoma.aspx [Accessed December 13, 2017].

78 Martinelli E et al. (2016). Cancer resistance to therapies against the EGFR-RAS-RAF pathway: The role of MEK. *Cancer Treat Rev* Dec 30; **53**: 61–69.

79 For a review, see: Fruman DA, Rommel C (2014). PI3K and Cancer: Lessons, Challenges

and Opportunities. *Nat Rev Drug Discov* **13**(2): 140–156.

80 For an overview of PI3K, see: Thorpe LM et al. (2015). PI3K in cancer: Divergent roles of isoforms, modes of activation and therapeutic targeting. *Nat Rev Cancer* **15**: 7–24.

81 For an overview of the PI3K/AKT/mTOR pathway and development of drugs that target it, see: Rodon J et al. (2013). Development of PI3K inhibitors: Lessons learned from early clinical trials. *Nat Rev Clin Oncol* **10**(3): 143–153.

82 Shimobayashi M, Hall MN (2014). Making new contacts: The mTOR network in metabolism and signalling crosstalk. *Nat Rev Mol Cell Biol* **15**: 155–162.

83 Reviewed in: Watanabe R et al. (2011). mTOR Signaling, function, novel inhibitors, and therapeutic targets. *J Nuclear Med* **52**(4): 497–500.

84 For an overview of PI3K, PTEN and AKT mutations in cancer cells, see: Chalhoub N, Baker SJ (2009). PTEN and the PI3-Kinase Pathway in Cancer. *Annu Rev Pathol* **4**: 127–150.

85 For a review see: Karakas B et al. (2006). Mutation of the *PIK3CA* oncogene in human cancers. *Br J Cancer* **94**: 455–459.

86 For an overview of PTEN and its role in healthy cells and cancer cells, see: Yin Y, Shen WE (2008). PTEN: A new guardian of the genome. *Oncogene* **27**: 5443–5453.

87 Reviewed in: Gill RK et al. (2011). Frequent homozygous deletion of the LKB1/STK11 gene in non-small cell lung cancer. *Oncogene* **30**: 3784–3791.

88 For a comparison of many drugs that block the PI3K/AKT/mTOR pathway, see: Dienstmann R et al. (2014). Picking the point of inhibition: A comparative review of PI3K/AKT/mTOR pathway inhibitors. *Mol Cancer Ther* **13**(5): 1021–1031.

89 For more about the history of rapamycin and temsirolimus (CCI-779) see: Garber K (2001). Rapamycin's Resurrection: A New Way to Target the Cancer Cell Cycle. *J Natl Cancer Inst* **93**(20): 1517–1519.

90 Reviewed in: Yuan R et al. (2009). Targeting tumorigenesis: Development and use of mTOR inhibitors in cancer therapy. *J Hematol Oncol* **2**: 45.

91 Yap TA et al. (2015). Drugging PI3K in cancer: Refining targets and therapeutic strategies. *Curr Opin Pharmacol* **23**: 98–107.

92 For a fuller list of PI3K inhibitors in development, see: Agrawal LS, Mayer AI (2014). Development of PI3K Inhibitors in Breast Cancer. OncLive website. http://www.onclive.com/publications/contemporary-oncology/2014/november-2014/development-of-pi3k-inhibitors-in-breast-cancer/1 [Accessed December 13, 2017].

93 For a discussion of alpelisib see: Inman S (2016). Alpelisib Combo Promising in PIK3CA-Altered, Heavily Pretreated Breast Cancer. [online] OncLive. Available at: http://www.onclive.com/conference-coverage/mbcc-2016/alpelisib-combo-promising-in-pik3ca-altered-heavily-pretreated-breast-cancer [Accessed December 13, 2017].

94 For more about dual PI3K/mTOR inhibitors see: Dienstmann R, Rodon J, Serra V et al. (2014). Picking the point of inhibition: A comparative review of PI3K/AKT/mTOR pathway inhibitors. *Mol Cancer Therapeutics* **13**: 1021.

95 Pongas G, Fojo T (2016). BEZ235: When Promising Science Meets Clinical Reality. [online] The Oncologist. Available at: http://theoncologist.alphamedpress.org/content/21/9/1033 [Accessed December 13, 2017].

96 Nitulescu GM et al. (2016). Akt inhibitors in cancer treatment: The long journey from drug discovery to clinical use (Review). *Int J Oncol* **48**(3): 869–885.

97 Mattmann ME et al. (2011). Inhibition of Akt with small molecules and biologics: Historical perspective and current status of the patent landscape. *Expert Opin Ther Pat* **21**(9): 1309–1338.

98 Davies BR et al. (2012). Preclinical pharmacology of AZD5363, an inhibitor of AKT: Pharmacodynamics, antitumor activity, and correlation of monotherapy activity with genetic background. *Mol Cancer Ther* **11**(4): 873–887.

99 For a wide-ranging review of the JAK-STAT pathway, see: Rawlings JS et al. (2004). The JAK/STAT signaling pathway. *J Cell Sci* **117**: 1281–1283.

100 Zhang J-M, An J (2007). Cytokines, inflammation and pain. *Int Anesthesiol Clin* **45**(2): 27–37.

101 If you want to read more about cytokines and their receptors, I would suggest getting hold of a copy of Janeway's Immunobiology, which is now into its 9th edition: Murphy K, Weaver C (2016). Janeway's Immunobiology. 9th ed. New York, New York: Garland Science.

102 Vainchenker W, Constantinescu SN (2013). JAK/STAT signaling in hematological malignancies. *Oncogene* **32**: 2601–2613.

103 Tefferi A (2016). Myeloproliferative neoplasms: A decade of discoveries and treatment advances. *Am J Hematol* **91**(1): 50–58.

104 Green MR et al. (2010). Integrative analysis reveals selective 9p24.1 amplification, increased PD-1 ligand expression, and further induction via JAK2 in nodular sclerosing Hodgkin lymphoma and primary mediastinal large B-cell lymphoma. *Blood* **116**(17): 3268–3277.

105 Thomas SJ et al. (2015). The role of JAK/STAT signalling in the pathogenesis, prognosis and treatment of solid tumours. *BJC* **113**: 365–371.

106 Buchert M et al. (2016). Targeting JAK kinase in solid tumors: Emerging opportunities and challenges. *Oncogene* **35**(8): 939–51.

107 Springuel L et al. (2015). JAK kinase targeting in hematologic malignancies: A sinuous pathway from identification of genetic alterations towards clinical indications. *Haematologica* **100**(10): 1240–1253.

108 For a review of the development and use of JAK2 inhibitors, see: Sonbol MB et al. (2013). Comprehensive review of JAK inhibitors in myeloproliferative neoplasms. *Ther Adv Haematol* **4**(1): 15–35.

109 Verstovsek S (2009). Therapeutic potential of JAK2 inhibitors. *Hematology / the Education Program of the American Society of Hematology.* **2009**: 636–642.

110 Yacoub A et al. (2014). Ruxolitinib: Long-term management of patients with Myelofibrosis and future directions in the treatment of Myeloproliferative neoplasms. *Curr Hematol Malig Rep* **9**(4): 350–359.

111 Pinilla-Ibarz J et al. (2016). Role of tyrosine-kinase inhibitors in myeloproliferative neoplasms: Comparative lessons learned. *Onco Targets Ther* **9**: 4937–4957.

112 Huang L, Fu L (2015). Mechanisms of resistance to EGFR tyrosine kinase inhibitors. *Acta Pharm Sin B* **5**(5): 390–341.

113 Niederst MJ, Engleman JA (2013). Bypass mechanisms of resistance to receptor tyrosine kinase inhibition in lung cancer. *Sci Signal* **6**(294): 10.1126/scisignal.2004652

114 Lackner MR et al. (2012). Mechanisms of acquired resistance to targeted cancer therapies. *Future Oncol* **8**(8): 999–1014.

115 Peiro G et al. (2014). Src, a potential target for overcoming trastuzumab resistance in HER2-positive breast carcinoma. *Br J Cancer* **111**(4): 689–695.

CHAPTER 4

Drugs That Target: Angiogenesis, Fusion Proteins, PARP, Hedgehog Signaling, and CDKs

IN BRIEF

In Chapter 3, all the drugs I mentioned fitted neatly together under one heading as they all targeted the same process, namely, cell communication. In this chapter, however, I cover a range of treatments that target diverse cell processes and proteins. First, I'm going to walk you through a group of treatments that target angiogenesis – the process through which new blood vessels are formed. Numerous angiogenesis inhibitors have been put through trials – both monoclonal antibodies and kinase inhibitors. Often, the results of these trials weren't as positive as people had hoped. However, the benefits of angiogenesis inhibitors for people with kidney cancer are very clear. And there are lots of ideas as to how these treatments might be improved or used to boost the effects of other treatments.

Our second group of treatments are those that target fusion proteins. Many cancers contain chromosome translocations and rearrangements that cause them to create fusion proteins that contain bits of two different proteins. Most of these proteins can't be blocked using any existing treatments. But, a few of them, such as Bcr-Abl, ALK, ROS1, and RET fusion proteins are kinases, so we can block them with kinase inhibitors.

Next, we'll look at PARP inhibitors. PARP is neither on the cell surface, nor is it a kinase. So, for the first time in this book, we'll be taking a look at a group of treatments that aren't antibodies or kinase inhibitors. Instead, they block a protein called PARP that is involved in DNA repair. PARP inhibitors seem to be particularly effective for women with ovarian cancers that contain defective *BRCA* genes. But, we're now learning that these treatments might be useful for a much broader group of patients – those whose tumors lack an efficient, accurate way of repairing DNA breaks.

A Beginner's Guide to Targeted Cancer Treatments, First Edition. Elaine Vickers.
© 2018 John Wiley & Sons Ltd. Published 2018 by John Wiley & Sons Ltd.

After PARP, we'll turn to the Hedgehog pathway. This pathway is vital for embryonic and adult stem cells. Two cancers, basal cell carcinoma skin cancer and medulloblastoma, commonly contain gene defects that activate this pathway.

Lastly, we'll look at CDK inhibitors. These drugs target a vital component of the cell cycle, so I've included plenty of diagrams that unpack the cell cycle and illustrate how these drugs are designed to work. It's still early days regarding trial results with CDK inhibitors, but there's great optimism that these treatments will be useful for the treatment of people with a variety of cancer types.

4.1 ANGIOGENESIS INHIBITORS: INTRODUCTION

I began explaining angiogenesis in Chapter 1, where I described it as the **sprouting and growth of existing blood vessels**. When this process is triggered by cancer cells, it can help the tumor to grow and spread. In fact, all solid tumors require a blood supply, and they achieve this by triggering angiogenesis (see Chapter 1, Figure 1.10 for an illustration of how angiogenesis takes place).

Back in the early 1970s, scientists started discussing the possibility of **starving a tumor by attacking its blood supply** [1]. Since that time, many companies have created drugs designed to do just that (see Table 4.1 for a summary of licensed angiogenesis inhibitors). These drugs predominantly work by targeting a growth factor called **VEGF (vascular endothelial growth factor)** or its receptor VEGFR.[1] Some of these treatments are now licensed in Europe and the United States for the treatment of a number of different cancers, including kidney cancer,[2] bowel cancer, non-small cell lung cancer (NSCLC),

pancreatic neuroendocrine tumors (PNETs),[3] ovarian cancer,[4] cervical cancer, and liver cancer.

When angiogenesis inhibitors were first proposed, scientists and doctors were extremely hopeful that they would benefit anyone with a solid tumor. However, as with many treatments, the benefits of angiogenesis inhibitors are now known to be more modest than initially predicted [5]. And, although some patients benefit a lot, most patients benefit very little, if at all. Also, the amount of angiogenesis and the characteristics of tumor blood vessels vary greatly from cancer to cancer, from patient to patient, between primary tumors and their metastases, and even from one part of a tumor to another. This means that **angiogenesis inhibitors can have varying degrees of impact** that are difficult to predict [6].

One cancer in which angiogenesis inhibitors have made a big difference is kidney cancer. The survival time of a person with metastatic kidney cancer has improved from a median of one year to two years thanks to currently licensed angiogenesis inhibitors [7].

---

[1] There are actually five versions of VEGF in the human body (VEGF-A, B, C, and D and placental growth factor – PlGF) and three VEGF receptors (VEGF-R1, R2, and R3).

[2] Specifically renal cell carcinoma – the most common type of kidney cancer.

[3] These are very different from the more common, much more aggressive pancreatic cancers; PNETs develop from "exocrine" cells which produce digestive enzymes and fluids.

[4] As it turns out, most "ovarian cancers" do not actually start in the ovaries, so we now tend to describe them collectively as "ovarian epithelial, fallopian tube, or primary peritoneal cancer."

Table 4.1 Angiogenesis inhibitors licensed for use against cancer in the United States and Europe.

Drug name	Mechanism of action [2]	Cancer types it is licensed for [3, 4]
Antibody-based treatments		
Aflibercept (Ziv-Aflibercept; Zaltrap)	A modified (bioengineered) antibody that attaches to three forms of VEGF (VEGF-A, VEGF-B, and placental growth factor) and keeps them away from VEGF receptors	Bowel cancer
Bevacizumab (Avastin)	A monoclonal antibody that attaches to VEGF-A[a] and keeps it away from VEGF receptors	Kidney cancer, bowel cancer, non-small cell lung cancer, ovarian cancer, cervical cancer, breast cancer (Europe only), glioblastoma (United States only)
Ramucirumab (Cyramza)	A monoclonal antibody that attaches to, and blocks, VEGF receptor-2	Stomach cancer,[b] bowel cancer, and non-small cell lung cancer
Small molecule kinase inhibitors		
Axitinib (Inlyta)	Blocks multiple targets including VEGF receptors, PDGF receptors, and KIT	Kidney cancer
Cabozantinib (Cometriq; Cabometyx)	Blocks multiple targets including VEGF receptors, MET, RET, KIT, FLT-3, TIE-2, TRKB, and AXL	Kidney cancer and medullary thyroid cancer[c]
Lenvatinib (Kisplyx; Lenvima)	Blocks multiple targets including VEGF receptors, PDGF receptors, FGF receptors, and RET	Kidney cancer and papillary/follicular/Hürthle cell thyroid cancer
Nintedanib (Vargatef)	Blocks multiple targets including VEGF receptors, PDGF receptors, FGF receptors, Src, Lck, Lyn, and FLT-3	Non-small cell lung cancer (Europe only)
Pazopanib (Votrient)	Blocks multiple targets including VEGF receptors and PDGF receptors; it also has some ability to block FGF receptors	Kidney cancer and soft tissue sarcoma
Regorafenib (Stivarga)	Blocks multiple targets including VEGF receptors and other kinases such as RET, KIT, PDGF receptors, and Raf	Bowel cancer, primary liver cancer, GIST[d]
Sorafenib (Nexavar)	Blocks multiple targets including Raf-1, B-Raf, VEGF receptor-2, VEGF receptor-3, PDGF receptors, RET, FLT3, and KIT	Kidney cancer, primary liver cancer, and papillary/follicular/Hürthle cell thyroid cancer
Sunitinib (Sutent)	Blocks multiple targets including VEGF receptors, PDGF receptors, KIT, and FLT3	Kidney cancer, PNET,[e] and GIST
Vandetanib (Caprelsa)	Blocks multiple targets including VEGF receptors, EGF receptors, and RET	Medullary thyroid cancer
Other angiogenesis inhibitors		
Everolimus (Afinitor)	An indirect inhibitor of mTOR; it binds to FKBP12, which then partially blocks mTOR activity (see Chapter 3, Section 3.8.4 for further details)	Breast cancer, kidney cancer, neuroendocrine tumors, and subependymal giant cell astrocytoma (United States only)
Temsirolimus (Torisel)	As for everolimus	Kidney cancer and mantle cell lymphoma (Europe only)

[a] See footnote 1.
[b] Including cancer that is at the junction between the stomach and the esophagus – called gastro-esophageal junction (GEJ) cancer.
[c] A common theme is that drugs used in thyroid cancer are those that can block RET, a growth factor receptor that is often overproduced, and sometimes mutated, in thyroid cancer cells.
[d] GISTs (gastrointestinal stromal tumors) often contain mutations in KIT (also called CD117) or PDGFRα (platelet-derived growth factor receptor-alpha) – therefore kinase inhibitors that block KIT and PDGFRα are effective against GISTs, irrespective of their impact on angiogenesis.
[e] PNET – pancreatic neuroendocrine tumor.

4.1.1 How Tumors Trigger Angiogenesis

As a cluster of cancer cells grows and multiplies, the cells soon start running short of oxygen. They automatically respond to low oxygen levels (known as hypoxia) in the same way that a healthy cell would; that is, they start to produce a range of growth factors such as VEGF, fibroblast growth factor (FGF), and platelet-derived growth factor (PDGF) [8]. When these growth factors attach to receptors on the surface of nearby endothelial cells (endothelial cells line our blood vessels), the endothelial cells respond. As with other growth factor receptors, attachment of VEGF, FGF, or PDGF to their receptors triggers activity of the MAPK cascade (Ras/Raf/MEK/ERK) and the PI3K/AKT/mTOR pathway. This encourages the cells to survive, but also causes endothelial cells to reorganize themselves, become more mobile, and multiply. In consequence, the blood vessels sprout side branches and grow [9].

The most important and powerful trigger of tumor angiogenesis is VEGF-A, which predominantly attaches to the VEGF receptor-2 (VEGFR2) [1]. However, other forms of VEGF (such as VEGF-C, VEGF-D, and placental growth factor – PlGF) are also released by cancer cells. Instead of attaching to VEGFR2, PlGF attaches to VEGF receptor-1 (VEGFR1) [9]. Many other growth factors and signaling molecules, such as PDGF and FGF, angiopoietins, neurophilins, semaphorins, and ephrins are also involved.

More angiogenesis occurs in some cancers than others. For example, some tumors gain a blood supply by co-opting existing blood vessels or by moving and ordering cancer cells so that they form channels through which blood cells can move [10]. Tumors that are less reliant on angiogenesis (such as pancreatic cancer) are less affected by angiogenesis inhibitors [5].

4.1.2 Tumor Blood Vessels Are Weird

The endothelial cells that line healthy blood vessels are highly organized, well connected to one another, and well supported by pericytes[5]. Healthy blood vessels are also evenly distributed through the tissue to ensure that every cell gets a blood supply. In contrast, the endothelial cells that line a tumor's blood vessels are affected and altered by their cancer neighbors: they are chaotic, irregular in shape, and strangely arranged. In consequence, a tumor's blood vessels are leaky, lumpy, and unstable. They also double-back on themselves, creating areas where there are lots of blood vessels and areas where there are none [11]. The weirdness of tumor blood vessels has a number of consequences [12]:

- Areas of a tumor that completely lack blood vessels become chronically hypoxic (short of oxygen). In the hypoxic areas, cancer cells struggle to survive and, in fact, these areas contain lots of dead and dying cells.
- The blood vessels' leakiness allows cancer cells to squeeze into them and travel elsewhere in the body, eventually causing metastasis.
- The chaotic and leaky arrangement of endothelial cells can impair the blood flow through a tumor and make it difficult for chemotherapy or other drugs to penetrate.

Overall, the number and density of blood vessels in a tumor seems to correlate with the aggressiveness of the cancer. In general, people whose tumors have high density of blood vessels tend to fare worse, and don't live as long as people whose tumors have fewer blood vessels [5].

---

[5] Pericytes wrap themselves around endothelial cells and provide physical support as well as producing a range of growth factors and other molecules.

4.1.3 Why Block VEGF?

VEGF is by far the most powerful trigger of angiogenesis, and it also sustains and supports tumor blood vessels (see Figure 4.1 for a brief overview and Figure 4.2 for an illustration). In summary, VEGF can [5, 13]:

- Cause endothelial cells multiply
- Help endothelial cells survive adverse conditions such as low oxygen or the presence of chemotherapy or radiotherapy
- Help endothelial cells move into new positions
- Increase the permeability of blood vessels
- Attract cells from the bone marrow that cause continual angiogenesis in growing tumors
- Cause tumor blood vessels to dilate
- Prevent white blood cells (specifically dendritic cells) from maturing properly; therefore, VEGF can protect cancer cells from destruction by the immune system [14]

However, sometimes the changes in blood vessel diameter and permeability caused by VEGF seem to disrupt the flow of blood. So, increased VEGF levels don't necessarily help the cancer cells get more blood [15].

4.1.4 Why Angiogenesis Inhibitors Sometimes Work

As I said earlier, most angiogenesis inhibitors target VEGF in some way. There are various reasons why blocking VEGF can be helpful [15]:

- It can **stop the growth of new blood vessels**, hopefully starving cancer cells of oxygen and nutrients and halting further growth and spread.
- It can cause endothelial cells to die and potentially **destroy existing tumor blood vessels**.
- It can cause blood vessels to constrict (become narrower) and **reduce the flow of blood**.
- Some of the strangeness and leakiness of tumor blood vessels is driven by the excessive production of VEGF. So, blocking VEGF can sometimes return the endothelial cells to a more normal arrangement, helping blood to flow through the tumor more easily. This in turn can **improve the**

Why block VEGF?

How important is it?	VEGF is the most important molecule responsible for the sprouting of blood vessels (**angiogenesis**)
How does it work?	**VEGF activates VEGF receptors**, growth factor receptors found on the surface of endothelial cells that line blood vessels
What does it do?	It triggers angiogenesis and keeps existing blood vessels alive
When do tumors need it?	It is needed by tumors throughout their growth and development
Where does it come from?	VEGF is secreted by cancer cells and other cells in the tumor microenvironment, especially white blood cells
What are the benefits of blocking it?	Blocking VEGF or blocking VEGF receptors could destroy existing blood vessels, inhibit metastasis and increase sensitivity to chemotherapy

Figure 4.1 Why block VEGF? This table lists the various properties of VEGF, VEGF receptors, and VEGF signaling pathways, and explains why VEGF and VEGF receptors are the target of the vast majority of angiogenesis inhibitors.

Abbreviations: VEGF – vascular endothelial growth factor

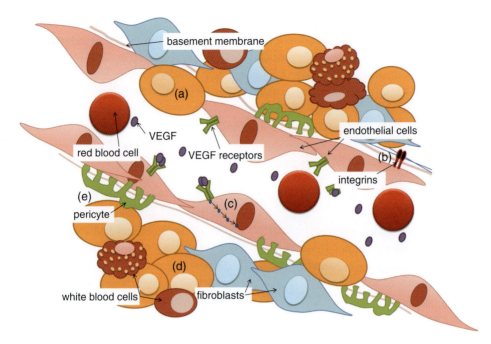

Figure 4.2 **Longitudinal illustration of a cancer blood vessel.** Healthy blood vessels are lined by endothelial cells, which should create an orderly, continuous layer. In a tumor blood vessel, the endothelial cells are less orderly, and there are gaps between them. **(a)** In places, cancer cells take the place of endothelial cells. **(b)** Integrins on the surface of endothelial cells connect with the basement membrane and with proteins in the extracellular matrix. **(c)** Binding of VEGF to its receptors activates the Ras/Raf/MEK/ERK pathway, PI3K/AKT/mTOR pathway, and other pathways. **(d)** The tumor microenvironment contains numerous cell types, including fibroblasts and white blood cells. **(e)** Pericytes provide support to endothelial cells and participate in angiogenesis.
Abbreviations: VEGF – vascular endothelial growth factor; mTOR – mammalian target of rapamycin; PI3K – phosphatidylinositol 3-kinase; ERK – extracellular-signal-regulated kinase

transport and distribution of chemotherapy (or other drugs) and make it more effective [15]. It can also make radiotherapy more effective because it works better when there's more oxygen around.

- **Tumor cells** sometimes have VEGF receptors on their surface; therefore, VEGF blockers might affect them directly.
- Suppression of VEGF might **help the patient's immune system** attack and destroy cancer cells by allowing their white blood cells to mature properly.
- Treatment with chemotherapy or radiotherapy destroys many cancer cells and causes damage to millions of others. It also causes

other stresses, such as a drop in oxygen and poorer nutrient supplies. Cells typically adapt to damage and stress by releasing VEGF. So, treating a patient with a VEGF blocker alongside their other treatment might **prevent the cancer from adapting to its altered environment** and improve the treatment's effectiveness.

Blocking angiogenesis may have different effects on different parts of the tumor. The net result may be very helpful, and bring the patient many months, or even years of additional life. But for other patients, the net result is no improvement at all (see Section 4.1.7 for more about drug resistance mechanisms).

4.1.5 Monoclonal Antibodies and Kinase Inhibitors That Block VEGF or VEGF Receptors

I will group drugs that block angiogenesis into three categories: (1) drugs that prevent VEGF from attaching to its receptors, (2) drugs that directly block the activity of VEGF receptors, and (3) drugs that work through other mechanisms.

However, I will focus my attentions largely on groups 1 and 2, as only two treatments in group 3 are licensed treatments: everolimus and temsirolimus (we met these drugs previously in Chapter 3, Section 3.8.4).

Drugs That Prevent VEGF from Attaching to Its Receptors

There are two licensed drugs that fall into this category: bevacizumab (Avastin) and aflibercept (Zaltrap; ziv-aflibercept). These drugs both attach to VEGF and keep it away from its receptors (see Figure 4.3).

Bevacizumab, as you would expect from its name, is a humanized monoclonal antibody. It attaches to VEGF-A and can't bind to the other forms of VEGF (VEGF-B, C, D, or PlGF). Bevacizumab works by keeping VEGF-A away from VEGF receptor-2 (VEGFR2) – the predominant VEGF receptor on tumor endothelial cells [16]. Because bevacizumab was the first angiogenesis inhibitor created (it first entered trials in 1997), it has been investigated in more trials than any other. It is also licensed for use against more types of cancer than any other angiogenesis inhibitor (see Table 4.1).

Aflibercept is a bioengineered protein – one that would never normally exist in nature. It is made from the back-end of an antibody which has been fused to part of the external, VEGF-binding section of VEGFR1 and a similar section of VEGFR2 (see Figures 4.3 and 4.4). It is made by stitching together the necessary parts

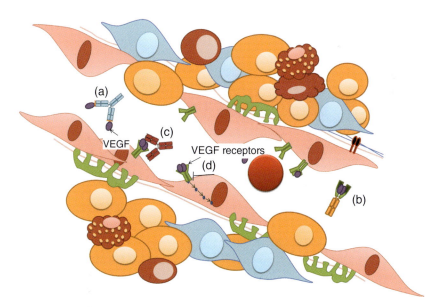

Figure 4.3 **Mechanism of action of various angiogenesis inhibitors. (a)** Bevacizumab, a humanized monoclonal antibody, attaches to VEGF-A and keeps it away from VEGF receptors. **(b)** Aflibercept, a bioengineered protein, attaches to VEGF-A, VEGF-B and PlGF, keeping them away from VEGF receptors. **(c)** Ramucirumab is a humanized antibody that directly attaches to VEGF receptor 2. **(d)** Various kinase inhibitors block the kinase portion of VEGF receptors and of other growth factor receptors. **Abbreviations:** VEGF – vascular endothelial growth factor; PlGF – placental growth factor

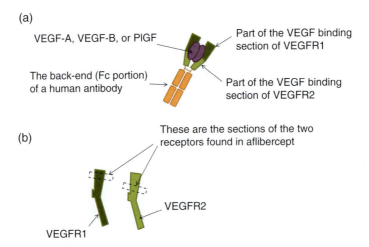

(a)

VEGF-A, VEGF-B, or PlGF

Part of the VEGF binding section of VEGFR1

The back-end (Fc portion) of a human antibody

Part of the VEGF binding section of VEGFR2

(b)

These are the sections of the two receptors found in aflibercept

VEGFR2

VEGFR1

Figure 4.4 Structure of aflibercept (ziv-aflibercept; Zaltrap). (a) Aflibercept is made from parts taken from three separate proteins: VEGFR1, VEGFR2, and an antibody. (b) Diagram showing which parts of VEGFR1 and VEGFR2 are incorporated into aflibercept.
Abbreviations: VEGF – vascular endothelial growth factor; PlGF – placental growth factor; VEGFR – VEGF receptor

of the genes for the three proteins. When the final amalgamated gene is inserted into living cells, they are forced to make the desired aflibercept protein, which is harvested and purified. Because it contains part of VEGFR1 and VEGFR2, aflibercept can attach to VEGF-A, VEGF-B, and PlGF [17].

Mouse experiments to compare the effectiveness of bevacizumab and aflibercept appeared to show that aflibercept is the more powerful treatment [18], presumably because of its ability to block PlGF and other VEGF forms as well as blocking VEGF-A. However, in clinical trials, it seems that these drugs are probably roughly equivalent to one another[6] [19, 20].

Monoclonal Antibodies That Directly Attach to VEGF Receptors

The only licensed monoclonal antibody that directly attaches to VEGF receptors is ramucirumab (Cyramza). Ramucirumab is a fully human monoclonal antibody that attaches to VEGFR2 and prevents any form of VEGF from attaching to it[7] [21]. So far, it has been tested in phase 3 trials in NSCLC, stomach cancer, bowel cancer, liver cancer, and breast cancer. Further phase 3 trials are in progress.

Small Molecule Kinase Inhibitors That Block VEGF Receptors

Many drug companies have created kinase inhibitors that enter cells and block the intracellular, kinase domain of VEGF receptors. There are numerous such drugs and, as of December 2017, nine of them are licensed for use in the United States and United Kingdom (see Table 4.1 for summary information on these drugs).

Most of these treatments are licensed in kidney cancer, and we'll come back to them in Chapter 6, Section 6.7. For now, I'll just say that there is a very precise reason why angiogenesis inhibitors work well in kidney cancer: these

---

[6] It's impossible to get a definitive answer as the drugs haven't been tested against one another in a clinical trial, so the only way of comparing them is by using statistics to compare different trials, which is tricky to do.
[7] VEGF-A, C, and D can all attach to VEGFR2, but VEGF-B and PlGF cannot.

Table 4.2   Summary of licensed kinase inhibitors that block VEGF receptors.

Type	Description	Drugs which fit this category
Type 1	The most promiscuous type of kinase inhibitor; those that compete for the ATP-binding site of the **active** kinase.	Sunitinib [25], axitinib [26], pazopanib [26], cabozantinib [27], and lenvatinib*
Type 2	Slightly less promiscuous drugs; these compete for the ATP-binding site of **inactive** kinases.	Sorafenib [25] and regorafenib [28]
Covalent inhibitors	These attach to the ATP-binding site and then stay there – they chemically attach themselves to the receptor and stay put.	Vandetanib [25]

*Lenvatinib does compete with the ATP-binding site of active VEGFR2 (and other kinases), but it also seems to interact with a neighboring region of VEGFR2, which means that it holds on to the receptor for longer [29].

cancers commonly lack a protein called VHL (von Hippel-Lindau). In healthy cells with sufficient oxygen, VHL causes the cell to destroy a protein called HIF1A, which would otherwise trigger angiogenesis. Kidney cancer cells generally lack VHL, so there's nothing to destroy HIF1A, and hence it triggers the release of VEGF and causes angiogenesis. Because of their lack of VHL, kidney cancers have lots of blood vessels [22] and are the most sensitive of any cancer to angiogenesis inhibitors [5].

Four out of the nine licensed treatments – vandetanib, cabozantinib, sorafenib, and lenvatinib – are licensed for the treatment of people with thyroid cancer. Their usefulness as thyroid cancer treatments probably owes as much, if not more, to their ability to block RET [23] (RET stands for "rearranged during transfection"). RET is a growth factor receptor whose gene is commonly mutated in thyroid cancer cells [24] (I'll come back to the topic of RET in Section 4.2.5).

Back in Chapter 2, I told you a bit about various different types of kinase inhibitors. Kinase inhibitors that block VEGF receptors fit into various categories (see Table 4.2 for a quick summary). As you can see, most of the kinase inhibitors that block VEGF receptors tend to be highly promiscuous drugs; that is, they block numerous kinases and not just VEGF receptors [25] (see Figure 4.5 for an

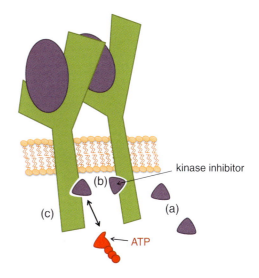

Figure 4.5 Basic mechanism of action of kinase inhibitors that block VEGF receptors. (a) Kinase inhibitors easily enter cells by crossing the cell membrane. **(b)** They mimic the shape of ATP and compete for the receptor's ATP-binding site. This prevents paired-up VEGF receptors from phosphorylating each other. **(c)** Without phosphates, there are no docking sites for other proteins, and hence the receptors cannot activate signaling pathways that would normally cause angiogenesis. **Abbreviations:** VEGF – vascular endothelial growth factor; ATP – adenosine tri-phosphate

illustration of the basic mechanism of action of kinase inhibitors).

The ability of these drugs to block multiple kinases[8] can be helpful as it means you can

---

[8] These drugs are often referred to as "multikinase inhibitors."

block other receptors involved in angiogenesis with a single drug (such as PDGF receptors and FGF receptors). However, it also means that they are likely to block kinases that are essential to healthy cells, causing side effects [30, 31].

4.1.6 Other Angiogenesis Inhibitors

As you can see in Table 4.1, the only licensed angiogenesis inhibitors that don't work by directly blocking VEGF or VEGF receptors are everolimus and temsirolimus. I've mentioned these drugs before (in Chapter 3, Section 3.8.4). They work by blocking some of the actions of mTOR, which is part of the signaling pathway involving PI3K, AKT, mTOR, and PTEN. mTOR is involved both in controlling the growth and survival of cells and in controlling angiogenesis.

mTOR inhibitors seem able to (a) block the growth of cancer cells, (b) prevent cancer cells from releasing VEGF, and (c) block the growth of endothelial cells [32]. In kidney cancers and pancreatic neuroendocrine tumors (PNETs), mTOR inhibitors can improve patients' survival times by many months [33]. Everolimus is also licensed as a treatment for women with hormone-receptor-positive breast cancer (see Chapter 6, Section 6.2.2).

In addition to mTOR inhibitors, scientists and doctors are exploring lots of other ways of blocking angiogenesis or attacking tumor blood vessels. So far, none of these ideas has led to a cancer treatment that has been licensed for use. However, many ideas are still being pursued, such as creating drugs that block FGF receptors, integrins, angiopoietins, ephrins, notch signaling, and TGF-beta [34, 35].

4.1.7 How Cancers Survive Angiogenesis Inhibitors

Angiogenesis inhibitors have substantially improved the survival times of people with kidney cancer, and they have benefited thousands of people with other types of cancer. However, angiogenesis inhibitors haven't been as effective as was initially hoped [5]. Sometimes, it looks as though the treatment is working, and the cancer stops growing, only to start growing again a few weeks or months later. Other times, the tumor seems completely unaffected [36].

One of the main problems with blocking angiogenesis as a strategy to treat cancer is that we currently have no way of knowing who it's going to work for. In a single tumor, there may be areas where there is a good blood supply and areas where there is a very poor supply. There might also be areas where an inefficient blood supply is hindering the tumor's growth, and other areas where the same low oxygen levels are helping the tumor spread and helping it avoid destruction by the patient's immune system. The impact of an angiogenesis inhibitor could therefore go either way: it might starve the tumor and slow its growth; it might normalize some blood vessels and increase blood flow; it might help the delivery of chemotherapy; it might help the cancer spread; it might increase or decrease the cancer's aggressiveness; and it might help or hinder the patient's immune system to destroy cancer cells. As a result, doctors cannot tell what the overall impact of the angiogenesis inhibitor is going to be when they prescribe it for their patient [13].

Sometimes treatment with an angiogenesis inhibitor can be very beneficial to a patient with advanced cancer, and it stops their tumor from growing. However, even then, it is only a matter of time before the effect wears off (do remember, though, that sometimes the beneficial effects can last for many months, especially for people with metastatic kidney cancer).

Scientists have now discovered various ways through which tumors adapt to treatment with an angiogenesis inhibitor and start growing again. I've summarized a few of

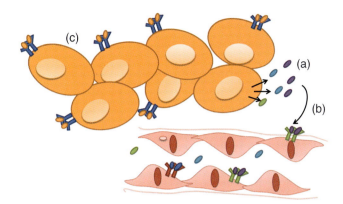

Figure 4.6 Reasons for resistance to angiogenesis inhibitors: rebound growth factor production and survival of hypoxia-resistant cells. **(a)** Angiogenesis inhibitors cause oxygen levels to drop, which triggers tumor cells and endothelial cells to produce even greater quantities of VEGF, PDGF, PlGF, angiopoitins, and other growth factors. **(b)** These growth factors activate receptors on endothelial cells, keeping them alive and triggering yet more angiogenesis. **(c)** Some cancer cells contain DNA mutations and other adaptations that enable them to survive low oxygen levels, making them insensitive to angiogenesis inhibitors. **Abbreviations:** VEGF – vascular endothelial growth factor; PDGF – platelet-derived growth factor; PlGF – placental growth factor

these mechanisms below, but this is by no means an exhaustive list [9]:

1. The tumor cells **produce alternative growth factors** (such as FGF, PDGF, ephrins, and angiopoietins) that trigger and sustain angiogenesis even when VEGF or VEGF receptors have been blocked (see Figures 4.6a and b).
2. Angiogenesis inhibition causes oxygen levels to drop to levels that are toxic to most cells. However, any cells in the tumor that contain **DNA mutations** or other changes that allow them to survive low oxygen levels will survive (see Figure 4.6c).
3. The tumor **finds other ways to gain a blood supply**, for example by co-opting or growing along existing blood vessels.
4. Cancer cells release chemicals that **attract cells from the bone marrow** – these cells produce growth factors and cytokines that support existing blood vessels and help new blood vessels to form (see Figure 4.7a).

5. Low oxygen levels cause cancer cells to **go through the EMT** (the epithelial-to-mesenchymal transition[9]); this causes the cells to become more resilient and mobile, allowing them to move to new locations in the body with a better blood supply (see Figure 4.7b).
6. **Pericytes multiply** and surround the endothelial cells, increasing their stability and reducing their requirement for VEGF (see Figure 4.7c).

4.1.8 The Search for Biomarkers
Since the creation of angiogenesis inhibitors, hundreds of scientists have attempted to discover a **predictive biomarker** for angiogenesis inhibitors (I am using the words "predictive biomarker" to mean something that scientists can measure before, or soon after, giving a patient treatment, which can be used to predict whether the treatment is going to be effective). So far, the search has been unsuccessful.

---

[9] See Chapter 1, Section 1.6.3 for more about the EMT.

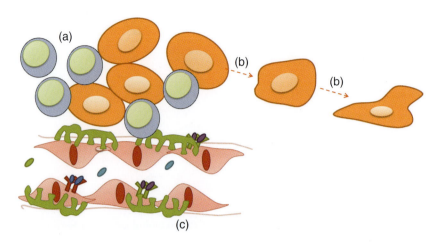

Figure 4.7 **Reasons for resistance to angiogenesis inhibitors: bone marrow cells, the EMT, and increased pericytes. (a)** Low oxygen levels and the presence of some growth factors attract cells from the bone marrow. These cells infiltrate the tumor and produce a variety of cytokines and growth factors that encourage more angiogenesis. **(b)** The drop in oxygen caused by angiogenesis inhibitors can trigger cancer cells to undergo the EMT, leading to increased cancer cell aggression and invasion into neighboring tissues. **(c)** Drug-resistant tumors have greater numbers of pericytes supporting and stabilizing their blood vessels and reducing their requirement for VEGF.
Abbreviations: VEGF – vascular endothelial growth factor; EMT – epithelial-to-mesenchymal transition

However, many possible biomarkers are still being investigated.

Potential biomarkers that scientists have studied include [37]:

1. Using sophisticated scanners to monitor changes to the way blood flows through a patient's tumor
2. Measuring changes in a patient's blood pressure
3. Measuring the levels of various proteins in the patient's bloodstream, such as various forms of VEGF, or measuring the number of tumor cells or endothelial cells that end up in the person's blood
4. Looking for inherited variations in genes that correlate with successful angiogenesis treatment
5. Looking inside tumors – at the levels of various proteins, at the presence or absence of white blood cells, at the number of blood vessels and whether they are healthy

If this search for biomarkers were to be successful, it would bring huge benefits to cancer patients. It would mean that only cancer patients who benefit from angiogenesis inhibitors receive them, allowing other patients to avoid the side effects of unnecessary treatment.

4.2 DRUGS THAT BLOCK FUSION PROTEINS: BCR-ABL, ALK, RET, AND ROS1

4.2.1 What's a Fusion Protein?

As I mentioned in Chapter 1, a fusion protein is a protein made by a cell when two genes, or parts of two genes, have become fused together. This is commonly the result of a chromosome translocation – when two chromosomes have broken, and the cell has put them back together incorrectly. The cell then uses the fused gene to create a fusion protein (see Figure 4.8).

The first translocation ever discovered in cancer cells (in 1973) was the translocation

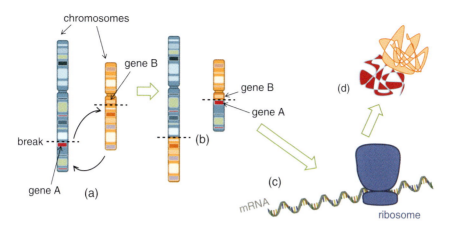

chromosomes

gene B

gene B

gene A

(d)

break

(b)

gene A (a)

(c)

mRNA

ribosome

Figure 4.8 How fusion proteins are created. (a) Each of the 46 chromosome in our cells contains hundreds of genes. Cancer cells often contain broken chromosomes, and sometimes two chromosomes have broken at the location two different genes (labeled A and B). **(b)** As the cell repairs the damage, it might accidently put the chromosomes together the wrong way round so that the two genes end up next to each other. **(c)** When the cell transcribes the fusion gene, it creates a strand of mRNA that contains information from both genes. **(d)** Ribosomes use the information in the mRNA to create a fusion protein. **Abbreviations:** mRNA – messenger RNA

between chromosomes 22 and 9, which causes the creation of a Bcr-Abl fusion protein. Bcr-Abl is an overactive kinase which is virtually always found inside the cancer cells of people with chronic myeloid leukemia [38].

Since the discovery of Bcr-Abl, hundreds of other fusion proteins have been discovered inside cancer cells [39]. At first (in the 1970s and 1980s), scientists thought that chromosome translocations and fusion proteins were much more common in hematological cancers (leukemias, lymphomas, and multiple myeloma) than in solid tumors. But in the past 30 years or so, scientists have discovered translocations in solid tumors like prostate cancer, lung cancer, and thyroid cancer [40].

4.2.2 Why Can We Block Some Fusion Proteins and Not Others?

Fusion proteins that contain a kinase domain are often targetable using a kinase inhibitor. For example, Bcr-Abl, ALK, and ROS1 fusion proteins can all be blocked with kinase inhibitors.

But not all the fusion proteins found in cancer cells are kinases. Fusion proteins found in the cancer cells of many acute leukemias are faulty transcription factors. These fusion proteins include AML1-ETO, TEL-AML1, PML-RARα, and MLL fusions. The normal version of these transcription factors would trigger the production of various proteins that help white blood cells to mature. However, the faulty transcription factor fusions found in acute leukemia cells often suppress genes instead of activating them, or control a completely different set of genes than the normal transcription factor [41].

The faulty transcription factor fusion proteins found in hematological cancers have so far proved to be very difficult to target. The only exception is PML-RARα. This fusion protein is found in the cells of people with a rare form of acute myeloid leukemia called acute promyelocytic leukemia (APL). We now have two very successful treatments for APL: ATRA (all-*trans* retinoic acid) and arsenic trioxide. Both these treatments cause the leukemic cells

Table 4.3 Some of the kinase fusion proteins found in human cancers.

Genes involved	Behavior of the fusion protein	Cancer(s) in which the fusion gene is found
(the gene for the kinase is in bold)		
BCR and **ABL** [38]	The Bcr-Abl protein is a highly active kinase that phosphorylates lots of different proteins, including PI3K.	Virtually all chronic myeloid leukemia (CML) and some acute lymphoblastic leukemia (ALL)
ALK and usually EML4, TFG, KIF5B, KLC1 or STRN (in NSCLC) or NPM (in anaplastic large cell lymphoma) [44, 45]	ALK is a growth factor receptor. The fusion protein retains the normal protein's ability to activate the Ras/Raf/MEK/ERK and PI3K/AKT/mTOR pathways.	Majority of anaplastic large cell lymphoma; 3%–5% of NSCLC; occasionally found in other cancers such as breast, esophageal, kidney, bowel, and diffuse large B cell lymphoma (DLBCL)
ROS1 and CD74 [46] or SLC34A2 [47]	ROS1 is a growth factor receptor very similar to ALK.	1%–2% of NSCLC; occasionally found in other cancers such as cholangiocarcinoma, ovarian cancer, stomach cancer, or bowel cancer
RET and usually CCDC6 (in thyroid cancer) or KIF5B or CCDC6 (in NSCLC) [48]	RET is a growth factor receptor. The fusion protein retains the normal protein's ability to activate the Ras/Raf/MEK/ERK and PI3K/AKT/mTOR pathways.	20% of papillary thyroid cancers and 1%–2% of NSCLCs

Source: For a more complete list of fusion genes and proteins in solid tumors, see: Parker BC and Zhang W (2013). Fusion genes in solid tumors: An emerging target for cancer diagnosis and treatment. Chin J Cancer **32**(11): 594–603. For a review of translocations that create overactive kinases found in solid tumors, see: Shaw AT et al. (2013). Tyrosine kinase gene rearrangements in epithelial malignancies. Nat Rev Cancer **13**(11): 772–787.

to destroy PML-RARα; the cells then rapidly mature and then die [42].

I'm going to spend the rest of this section talking about fusion proteins that are overactive kinases, because these are the ones that we can do most about (see Table 4.3 for a list of some of the most common kinase fusion proteins found in cancer cells). Many of these fusion proteins are pretty rare; for example, ALK fusion proteins are found in around 3%–5% of people with non-small cell lung cancer (NSCLC) [43]. However, the technology to search for these translocations is getting cheaper and quicker all the time, so it's becoming easier to test patients' tumor samples. At the same time, scientists are successfully creating more and more drugs that block kinases. As a result, we are now in an era where it is possible to test a patient's tumor for the presence of a wide number of mutations that create overactive kinases, and treat the patient accordingly.[10]

4.2.3 Bcr-Abl Inhibitors

The Bcr-Abl fusion protein is found in the cancer cells of virtually all people with chronic myeloid leukemia (CML) and in around 25% of people with acute lymphoblastic leukemia (ALL), rising to 50% in people with ALL aged 60 or over [49]. I am therefore going to discuss Bcr-Abl inhibitors in greater detail in Chapter 7, in which I cover targeted treatments for hematological cancers.

Bcr-Abl inhibitors tend to be rather nonspecific, and many of them can block the activity of other kinases such as KIT and PDGF-receptors [50]. Both KIT and – to a lesser extent – PDGF receptors are implicated

---

[10] It will probably be several more years before this becomes standard practice because of the costs and logistics involved.

in a rare type of cancer called GIST (gastro-intestinal stromal tumor). For more about Bcr-Abl inhibitors as treatments for GIST, see Chapter 3, Section 3.5.1.

4.2.4 ALK and ROS1 Inhibitors

Both ALK and ROS1 are growth factor receptors [51]. Like other growth factors, they have an extracellular,[11] ligand-binding section and an intracellular[12] kinase section that activates signaling pathways.

A diverse array of fusion proteins involving these two receptors have been discovered in human cancers, including 30 different ALK fusion proteins [52]. Whatever the partner protein, the section of ALK or ROS1 found in the fusion protein always contains kinase activity [53]. And, because the normal ALK and ROS1 proteins are growth factor receptors that trigger cell communication pathways such as the Ras/Raf/MEK/ERK pathway and the PI3K/AKT/mTOR pathway, the fusion proteins can do the same. However, the fusion proteins contain the kinase portion of ALK and ROS1 and not the external part of the protein where the growth factor would bind. This means that the fusion proteins are uncontrollable; they are active all the time, and force the cell to grow and multiply.

The cancer in which ALK and ROS1 inhibitors are most commonly used is NSCLC (their use in NSCLC is described further in Chapter 6, Section 6.4.4). However, they are only relevant to the small proportion of patients whose tumors contain an *ALK* or *ROS1* gene rearrangement. In NSCLC, the most common ALK fusion protein is ALK-EML4 (EML4 stands for echinoderm microtubule-associated protein-like 4) [54]. Several different ROS1 fusion proteins have been found in NSCLC [55].

Aside from being found as part of fusion proteins in lung cancer, ALK is also known to be important in some other cancers. For example, mutated, overactive versions of ALK have been found in 6%–8% of neuroblastomas (rare cancers that generally affect children). In addition, cancer cells of neuroblastomas and NSCLC occasionally contain extra copies of the *ALK* gene, forcing the cell to make more ALK protein [56] (see Figure 4.9 for a summary of the ways in which ALK can be overactive in cancer cells).

First-Generation ALK Inhibitors

The fist ALK inhibitor was a drug called crizotinib (Xalkori); however, it was actually originally created to block MET (MET is yet another growth factor receptor). Like many other kinase inhibitors, crizotinib works by competing with ATP for its targets' ATP-binding site. It's now known to have three main targets: MET, ALK, and ROS1 [57]. Crizotinib is a licensed treatment for the 3%–5% or so of advanced NSCLCs that contain ALK fusion proteins, and it's also being trialled in other cancers.

As with EGF-receptor inhibitors (such as erlotinib, gefitinib, and afatinib), the benefits from crizotinib don't last forever – typically the cancer starts growing again after about 7–10 months of treatment [58, 59]. One reason for treatment resistance is the presence of cancer cells with an additional mutation in the ALK fusion gene such as the C1156Y and L1196M mutations among others [60]. In other patients, the disease returns in their brain because crizotinib isn't very good at getting into brain tissue [61]. Other resistance mechanisms involve mutations that reactivate the MAPK or PI3K/AKT/mTOR pathways [60].

---

[11] The bit of the receptor that protrudes out of the cell.
[12] The bit of the receptor that protrudes into the cell cytoplasm.

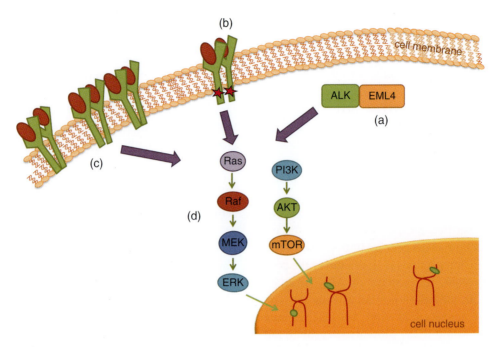

Figure 4.9 Cancer-causing mutations in the *ALK* gene. (a) A translocation or other chromosome rearrangement involving the *ALK* gene forces the cell to make an uncontrollable ALK fusion protein. **(b)** A mutation affecting the kinase part of ALK has made it overactive. **(c)** Amplification (extra copies) of the *ALK* gene forces the cell to make extra ALK protein. **(d)** Overactivity of ALK triggers numerous signaling pathways (not all shown) which force the cell to grow, multiply, and stay alive.

Abbreviations: ALK – anaplastic lymphoma kinase; EML4 – echinoderm microtubule associated protein-like 4; mTOR – mammalian target of rapamycin; PI3K – phosphatidylinositol 3-kinase; ERK – extracellular-signal-regulated kinase

Second- and Third-Generation ALK Inhibitors

Second-generation ALK inhibitors such as alectinib (Alecensa), ceritinib (Zykadia), and brigatinib (Alunbrig) are able to block some of the mutated versions of the ALK fusion protein that cause resistance to crizotinib [62, 63]. And they're also better at penetrating the brain. More recently, we've also seen third-generation drugs, such as lorlatinib (PF-06463922), enter into trials. For a summary of some of the properties of these drugs, see Table 4.4.

ROS1 Inhibitors

As well as blocking ALK, crizotinib (and some of the other ALK inhibitors) is also able to block ROS1 [64]. *ROS1* gene rearrangements are found in about 1%–2% of NSCLCs and almost never coexist with ALK mutations or EGFR mutations [65]. Crizotinib is now licensed for people with a *ROS1*-mutated NSCLC in both the United States and Europe. (I'll talk more about both ALK and ROS1-targeted treatments for lung cancer patients in Chapter 6, Section 6.4.4.)

4.2.5 RET Inhibitors

RET inhibitors such as vandetanib (Caprelsa), cabozantinib (Cometriq; Cabometyx), sorafenib (Nexavar), and lenvatinib (Kisplyx; Lenvima), are all licensed for the treatment of thyroid cancer. As you found out earlier in the chapter (in Section 4.1), as well as blocking RET, all of these drugs also block VEGF receptors and can be classed as angiogenesis inhibitors.

Table 4.4 Comparison of first-, second-, and third-generation ALK inhibitors.

	First generation		Second generation		Third generation
	Crizotinib	**Alectinib**	**Ceritinib [62]**	**Brigatinib**	**Lorlatinib**
Type of inhibition	Reversible	Reversible	Reversible	Reversible	Reversible
Ability to block:					
Wild-type ALK-EML4	Yes	Yes	Yes	Yes	Yes
G1123S mutation	No	Yes	No	N/D	N/D
C1156Y	No	Yes	No	Yes	Yes
L1196M	No	Yes	Yes	Yes	Yes
G1202R	No	No	No	Yes	Yes
G1269A/S	No	Yes	Yes	Yes	Yes
I1171T	No	No	Yes	N/D	N/D
F1174C	No	Yes	No	Yes	Yes
Ability to enter the brain [63]	Poor	Good	Good	Good	Good
Other kinases blocked by this drug [63]	MET, ROS1	LTK, GAK	IGF-1R, INSR, STK22D	ROS1	ROS1

N/D – not determined.
Source: Tran PN, Klempner SJ (2016). Focus on Alectinib and Competitor Compounds for Second-Line Therapy in *ALK*-Rearranged NSCLC. *Front Med (Lausanne)* **3**: 65.

RET, like ALK and ROS1, is a growth factor receptor. It is mostly found on the surface of cells that help create an embryo's nerves, bones, cartilage, and other tissues in the very first few weeks of life [66]. RET fusion proteins are common in papillary thyroid cancer (the most common type of thyroid cancer) [67], and they are also found in around 1%–2% of NSCLCs. As with other kinase fusion proteins, RET fusion proteins always contain the kinase part of the RET protein. So far, 13 different RET fusion proteins have been discovered, including pericentriolar material 1 (PCM1)-RET, ret finger protein (RFP)-RET, and hook protein 3 (HOOK3)-RET [68].

As with ALK, becoming part of a fusion protein is not the only way that RET can become dangerous. Point mutations in *RET* (particularly one known as the M918T mutation) are found in a rare form of thyroid cancer called medullary thyroid cancer. The M918T mutation changes the range of proteins that RET is able to phosphorylate [69].

Drugs that block RET are licensed treatments for medullary and/or papillary thyroid cancer (see Table 4.1). However, as all RET inhibitors also block VEGF receptors and other kinases, it's impossible to know how much of the benefit to patients is from the inhibition of RET. RET inhibitors are also looking promising for people with NSCLCs containing RET fusion proteins [70], although it's still early days.

4.3 PARP INHIBITORS

PARP (poly ADP ribose polymerase) inhibitors were originally designed to benefit one particular group of people: women who have inherited a mutation in one of their *BRCA* genes and who have subsequently developed breast or ovarian cancer. These drugs are now being explored in other cancers, but I'll explain why they might be helpful for women with breast or ovarian cancers that contain *BRCA* mutations first, and then I'll talk about other cancers afterward.

In order to explain PARP inhibitors, I need to go through a few different concepts:

- What is PARP?
- What are BRCA proteins?
- Why do women with BRCA mutations develop cancer?
- Why might PARP inhibitors be effective against cancers with faulty BRCA genes?
- What other cancers might PARP inhibitors be helpful for, and why?
- How do PARP inhibitors work?

4.3.1 What Is PARP?

PARP proteins play a vital role in the **repair of single-strand breaks in our cells' DNA** [71] (see Figure 4.10). These little nicks to our DNA happen every day of our lives in each one of the billions of cells in our body. As I mentioned in Chapter 1, DNA damage

is often caused by oxygen free radicals: high-energy oxygen atoms that are created by our cells as they produce energy. The creation of oxygen free radicals is unavoidable, and they are responsible for these little nicks in our DNA [72].

Happily, our cells have PARP and other proteins, and they're therefore well equipped to repair single-strand DNA breaks. However, if these breaks somehow go unnoticed and unrepaired, this causes problems for the cell. In fact, an unrepaired nick in DNA can later cause a complete break in the chromosome (called a double-strand DNA break) [71]. Double-strand breaks are incredibly toxic to our cells, and they need to be repaired as quickly as possible. This is where BRCA proteins come in.

4.3.2 What Are BRCA Proteins?

There are two BRCA proteins in our cells: BRCA1 and BRCA2. These proteins are physically very different from one another, but they are both involved in the repair of double-strand DNA

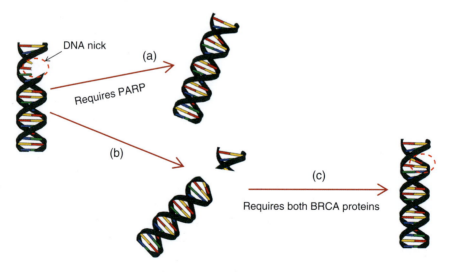

Figure 4.10 The role of PARP and BRCA proteins in repairing DNA damage. **(a)** Thousands of small nicks in our DNA occur every day. They are repaired through a process that relies on PARP proteins. **(b)** If left unrepaired, a single-strand nick ultimately becomes a double-strand break. **(c)** Using homologous recombination, which is dependent on both BRCA proteins, the cell accurately repairs the double-strand break. **Abbreviations:** PARP – Poly(ADP-ribose) polymerase; BRCA – breast cancer susceptibility gene

breaks through a process called **homologous recombination (HR)**. HR is very efficient and very accurate. Hence, it's our cells' preferred method of repairing double-strand DNA breaks [71].

In order to make BRCA1 and BRCA2 proteins, our cells have two genes known as *BRCA1* and *BRCA2* which contain the instructions to make these proteins.

The two *BRCA* genes were discovered by scientists in the mid-1990s when they were trying to work out why breast and ovarian cancers sometimes run in families.[13] We have two copies of every gene – one from our mother and one from our father. The scientists discovered that if a woman inherits a fault in one of her copies of either *BRCA1* or *BRCA2*, then her risk of developing breast cancer and/or ovarian cancer[14] is much higher than for other women. She's also likely to develop cancer at a relatively young age [73]. People who inherit *BRCA1* and *BRCA2* mutations are also slightly more at risk of pancreatic cancer, stomach cancer, laryngeal cancer, and prostate cancer (men only) [74].

4.3.3 Why Do Women with *BRCA* Mutations Develop Cancer?

Both BRCA proteins are involved in HR (BRCA1 is also involved in controlling the cell cycle and has other functions [75]). If a woman has inherited a fault in one of her *BRCA* genes, then **the fault is present in every cell in her body**. But, because we have two copies of every gene, a fault in one copy isn't necessarily disastrous. In fact, even if our cells only have one functioning copy of *BRCA1* or *BRCA2*, then we develop normally. The classic example is the actor and director Angelina Jolie. She has said very publicly that she inherited a faulty copy of *BRCA1* from her mother and has lost many female family members to cancer [76, 77].

However, our cells' DNA is getting damaged every day of our lives, and this damage affects the entire genome. Hence, in a woman with an inherited *BRCA1* or *BRCA2* mutation, there is always a chance that a cell will pick up a second mutation, this time affecting its healthy copy of the *BRCA* gene [78]. If this happens in a breast or ovary (or fallopian tube) cell, the results can be devastating (see Figure 4.11). Cells that were getting on quite happily have now lost their one healthy copy of *BRCA1* or *BRCA2*. And the BRCA1 and BRCA2 proteins, being so different from one another physically, cannot stand in for each other. When either of its BRCA proteins is completely missing, **the cell can't perform HR**. When this is the case, the cell has to rely on other methods to repair double-strand DNA breaks, and these other methods aren't as good.

The main fall-back method that cells have for repairing double-strand DNA breaks is called **non-homologous end joining (NHEJ)**. In NHEJ, the cell essentially takes two ends of DNA and jams them together [79]. A cell that is reliant on NHEJ is liable to make lots of mistakes and accumulates DNA mutations quickly. In fact, cells that lack one of their BRCA proteins and have to rely on NHEJ are **genomically unstable** (see Chapter 1 for more about this). They end up with lots of huge mistakes in their chromosomes and are liable to become cancer cells [80]. In Table 4.5, I've summarized a couple of other characteristics of the cancers that develop in women with inherited faults in *BRCA* genes.

---

[13] *BRCA1* and *BRCA2* are abbreviations for *breast cancer susceptibility gene-1* and *breast cancer susceptibility gene-2*.

[14] I have mentioned before that many "ovarian cancers" actually develop from faulty cells in the fallopian tubes, so I'm using the term "ovarian cancer" to mean a cancer that starts in the ovaries or fallopian tubes. See this Medscape article for more information: http://www.medscape.com/viewarticle/843469 (accessed December 13, 2017).

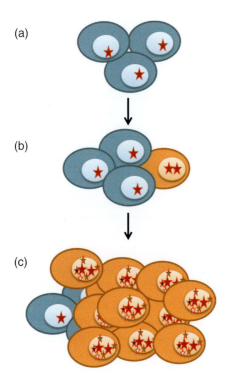

(a)

(b)

(c)

Figure 4.11 The path from BRCA mutations to cancer. (a) If a woman is born with a fault in one of her *BRCA* genes, then every cell in her body will contain the fault. But the second, healthy copy of the gene is enough to keep her healthy. **(b)** If the second copy of the affected *BRCA* gene gets damaged in one of her breast or ovary cells, this cell will be completely unable perform homologous recombination. Instead, the cell will have to rely on an error-prone method (called non-homologous end joining – NHEJ) to repair double-strand breaks to its DNA. **(c)** Because it has to rely on NHEJ, the cell is genomically unstable and accumulates damage to many important genes. **Abbreviations:** NHEJ – non-homologous end joining; BRCA – breast cancer susceptibility gene

Women who have inherited a *BRCA1* mutation have about a 40% risk of developing ovarian cancer and a 57%–65% risk of developing breast cancer by age 70. The respective figures for a woman who has inherited a *BRCA2* mutation are an 11%–18% risk of ovarian cancer and a 45%–49% risk of breast cancer [71].

One aspect of *BRCA* mutations and cancer that puzzles scientists is why mutations in

Table 4.5   Characteristics of *BRCA*-mutated cancers in mutation carriers.

Cancer	Characteristics
***BRCA1*-mutated breast cancers**	The majority (69%) are "triple negative"; that is, they do not contain estrogen or progesterone receptors, nor do they have HER2 on their surface. They are likely to be aggressive and difficult to treat.
***BRCA2*-mutated breast cancers**	Characteristics of these cancers vary a lot from woman to woman, but they generally do contain estrogen and progesterone receptors. Only around 16% are triple negative.
***BRCA1*- or *BRCA2*-mutated ovarian cancers**	These tend to be high-grade (i.e., very aggressive) serous cancers. The cancer sometimes starts in the ovaries, but it could have started in the fallopian tubes. These cancers tend to be very sensitive to chemotherapy, at least to begin with. But they are also genomically unstable and quickly become resistant to treatment.

Source: The information in this table is from the National Cancer Institute website; the page is extensive and contains a lot more detail: Genetics of Breast and Gynecologic Cancers–for health professionals (PDQ®). National Cancer Institute. http://www.cancer.gov/types/breast/hp/breast-ovarian-genetics-pdq/#link/_136 (Accessed December 14, 2017).Concise information can be found here: Salhab M, Bismohun S, Mokbel K (2010). Risk-reducing strategies for women carrying brca1/2 mutations with a focus on prophylactic surgery. *BMC Womens Health* **10**(1).

BRCA genes particularly cause breast and ovarian cancers rather than any other type [81]. But, despite lots of scientists having investigated this, there's still no agreement as to why it is the case.

4.3.4 Why Might PARP Inhibitors Be Effective against Cancers in People with Inherited Faults in *BRCA* Genes?

So far, I've said that both BRCA and PARP proteins are involved in DNA repair. PARP predominantly helps our cells repair single-strand DNA breaks. BRCA proteins, in

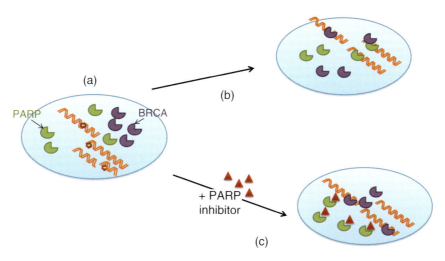

Figure 4.12 **A PARP inhibitor does not kill cells with both PARP and BRCA proteins. (a)** The blue oval represents the nucleus of a healthy cell, in which you find both PARP and BRCA proteins (and all the other proteins necessary for DNA repair). This cell's DNA is constantly getting damaged (represented by yellow spiky circles and broken orange DNA strands). **(b)** Single-strand breaks are repaired by a PARP-dependent process; double-strand breaks are repaired using homologous recombination (HR). **(c)** Exposing the cell to a PARP inhibitor (red triangles) prevents it from repairing single-strand breaks, which ultimately become double-strand breaks. However, double-strand breaks are repaired using HR, and the cell is fine.
Abbreviations: PARP – Poly(ADP-ribose) polymerase; HR – homologous recombination; BRCA – breast cancer susceptibility gene

contrast, are involved in an accurate method (homologous recombination – HR) of repairing double-strand DNA breaks. When a woman with an inherited *BRCA1* or *BRCA2* gene defect develops cancer, the cancer has arisen because a cell has lost its second, healthy copy of the affected *BRCA* gene. As a result, the cancer cells in that woman will be unable to perform HR. However, all the other cells in her body will be able to use HR to repair DNA because they can use BRCA protein made from their healthy version of the affected *BRCA* gene.

So why might a PARP inhibitor kill cancer cells, but leave the woman's healthy cells alone? To answer this, let's first go back to the cells of a woman who hasn't inherited a *BRCA* gene mutation (see Figure 4.12). In her cells, PARP and both her BRCA proteins are functioning normally. When you give her a PARP inhibitor, this blocks PARP activity. With PARP blocked, her cells are likely to accumulate lots of double-strand breaks. But, because her BRCA proteins are normal, these extra double-strand breaks can be swiftly and accurately mended, and her cells survive.

Let's contrast that with the cells of someone like Angelina Jolie. All her cells contain a defect in one copy of *BRCA1* – the copy she inherited from her mother. This means that her cells only have one healthy *BRCA1* gene – the one inherited from her father. However, the one healthy gene she has, does seem to be enough to do the job and create enough BRCA1 protein[15] to keep her healthy.

---

[15] I know that a gene can't directly create a protein, but saying "that the one healthy copy of the *BRCA1* gene is accessed by transcription factors and RNA polymerase frequently enough that there is sufficient BRCA1 mRNA in her cells to create sufficient BRCA1 protein" seems rather long-winded.

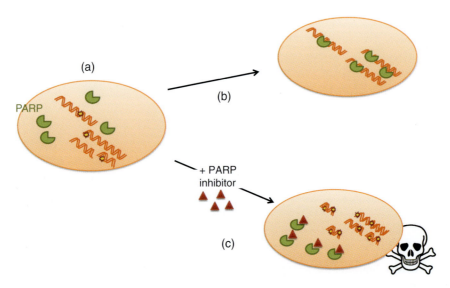

Figure 4.13 **A PARP inhibitor does kill cells that lack either BRCA1 or BRCA2 proteins**. **(a)** The orange oval represents the nucleus of a **cancer cell** in a woman who has inherited a *BRCA* gene mutation. This cell contains PARP, but it is completely missing either the BRCA1 or BRCA2 protein. The cell therefore cannot perform homologous recombination (HR). This has led the cell to become genomically unstable, which has ultimately caused it to become a cancer cell. **(b)** When the cancer cell sustains damage to its DNA, it is forced to repair the damage using PARP (to repair single-strand breaks) or non-homologous end joining (NHEJ) to repair double-strand breaks. **(c)** If the woman is treated with a PARP inhibitor, this prevents her cells from using PARP to repair single-strand breaks. These breaks ultimately become double-strand breaks, which the cancer cell can only repair using an error-prone method such as NHEJ. The cell quickly accumulates DNA damage to critical levels, and the cell dies. The rest of the cells in her body, which still retain a healthy copy of the *BRCA* gene, can perform sufficient HR to stay alive.
Abbreviations: PARP – Poly(ADP-ribose) polymerase; HR – homologous recombination; NHEJ – non-homologous end joining; BRCA – breast cancer susceptibility gene

And, even if she were given a PARP inhibitor, the vast majority of her cells would be fine.[16]

Finally, let's look at the **cancer cells** in a woman who has inherited either a *BRCA1* or a *BRCA2* gene defect. These cells became cancer cells because they lost their second, healthy copy of the affected *BRCA* gene and were therefore unable to perform HR (see Figure 4.13). Consequently, these cells rely on NHEJ to repair double-strand DNA breaks. If this woman is given a PARP inhibitor, her cells accumulate double-strand DNA breaks. But, whereas the vast majority of her cells can

perform HR and are fine, the cancer cells, which have to rely on NHEJ, die. Scientists think that this happens because DNA damage accumulates so quickly in the cancer cells that they self-destruct [71].

Scientists often refer to the use of PARP inhibitors in people with cancers linked to faulty *BRCA* genes as an example of "synthetic lethality." They're referring to the fact that a combination (a synthesis) of the cancer cells' inability to perform HR plus exposure to a PARP inhibitor causes them to die (see Figure 4.14).

---

[16] PARP inhibitors do cause some side effects, but for most women these seem to be relatively mild; see http://www.cancerresearchuk.org/about-cancer/cancers-in-general/treatment/cancer-drugs/olaparib (accessed December 13, 2017).

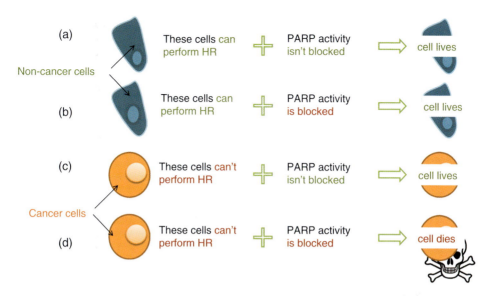

Figure 4.14 The synthetic-lethal situation created by the combination of BRCA mutations and PARP inhibition. **(a)** The non-cancer cells in a person with a *BRCA* mutation can perform homologous recombination. **(b)** Even if PARP is blocked with a PARP inhibitor, these cells stay alive. **(c)** Cancer cells in which both copies of either *BRCA1* or *BRCA2* are faulty cannot perform homologous recombination and rely on non-homologous end joining to repair double-strand breaks in their DNA. **(d)** The combination (synthesis) of the lack of BRCA protein **plus** a PARP inhibitor is lethal to the cancer cells.
Abbreviations: PARP – Poly(ADP-ribose) polymerase; BRCA – breast cancer susceptibility gene

4.3.5 How PARP Inhibitors Block PARP

PARP proteins (there are at least two of them) are not kinases; therefore you can't use a kinase inhibitor to block them. PARP inhibitors are small chemicals that tend to do two things to varying degrees:

1. They compete with a chemical called NAD+[17] for a binding site on the PARP protein. PARP needs NAD+ to do its job; so, without access to NAD+, **PARP is blocked** [82].

2. They prevent PARP proteins from letting go of damaged DNA, trapping them in place [83]. This causes the cell to **run out of available PARP proteins** and causes further DNA damage.

4.3.6 What Other Cancers PARP Inhibitors Might Be Helpful for, and Why

So far, I've only talked about using PARP inhibitors for cancers that arise in women with inherited *BRCA* gene defects. These cancers account for around 5%–10% of breast cancers and 10%–15% of ovarian cancers [84]. However, clinical trials have also proven that PARP inhibitors are effective for women with ovarian cancers that have arisen as a result of **sporadic BRCA mutations**, that is, mutations that have occurred during their lifetime [71]. These cancers behave in a very similar way to cancers in women with inherited (germline) *BRCA* mutations. There's also a lot of interest in using PARP inhibitors much more widely.

[17] NAD+ (nicotinamide adenine dinucleotide) is a complicated chemical found in our cells that is necessary for the function of lots of different enzymes, including PARP. See: http://science.sciencemag.org/content/350/6265/1208.full (accessed December 13, 2017).

For example, they may be useful [84]:

1. For other cancers, such as prostate cancers, malignant melanomas, and pancreatic cancers, occurring in men and women with inherited *BRCA* mutations.

2. For people with cancers that don't necessarily have defective BRCA proteins, but have some other problem that makes them unable to perform HR. These cancers are often said to be "BRCA-like," to exhibit "BRCAness" or be "homologous recombination-deficient." For example, around 20% of prostate cancers have defects in various DNA repair proteins [85]. Also, around 50% of high-grade ovarian cancers contain defects in HR (this figure includes women with inherited *BRCA* mutations) [86].

3. For people whose cancer is known to be sensitive to platinum-based chemotherapy, as this is a sign that the cancer has difficulty in repairing DNA damage and therefore might also be sensitive to a PARP inhibitor.

4. As a way of increasing the effectiveness of chemotherapy and radiotherapy by preventing cancer cells from repairing the DNA damage that these treatments cause.

5. For cancers that lack PTEN (PTEN suppresses the PI3K/AKT/mTOR pathway). This is one of the reasons that PARP inhibitors are being explored for prostate and endometrial cancers: these cancers often lack PTEN.

Not surprisingly, there are many clinical trials currently taking place that are evaluating various PARP inhibitors. The majority of these trials are recruiting women with breast or ovarian cancer. However, trials are also evaluating their usefulness in prostate, lung, pancreatic, cervical, endometrial, gastric, head and neck cancer, and many other cancer types.

As of December 2017, only olaparib (Lynparza) had been licensed for use in both Europe and the United States (niraparib (Zejula) and rucaparib (Rubraca) are licensed in the United States only). Table 4.6 summarizes the current state of development of five PARP inhibitors: olaparib, rucaparib, veliparib, niraparib, and talazoparib. All five drugs seem to give relatively similar response rates and side effects in clinical trials [87]. However, we're still yet to discover exactly which cancers, and which patients, will benefit most from this group of treatments.

4.3.7 Resistance Mechanisms to PARP Inhibitors

As with virtually all cancer treatments, some people's cancers are inherently resistant to PARP inhibitors, and others' respond to treatment initially and then start growing again. Reasons for resistance to PARP inhibitors include the following [71]:

• Further mutations in *BRCA* genes (in addition to whatever mutation caused the cancer in the first place) that restore normal BRCA protein activity.

• Mutations affecting genes such as *53BP1* or *MAD2L2*, both of which are involved in DNA repair.

• There is some evidence that some cancers have protein pumps in their surface membrane that can expel the PARP inhibitor prevent it from reaching a concentration that would trigger cell death.

4.4 HEDGEHOG PATHWAY INHIBITORS

In Chapter 3, I discussed drugs that block cell signaling pathways such as the Ras/Raf/MEK/ERK pathway, the PI3K/AKT/mTOR pathway, and the JAK/STAT pathway. However, many other proteins and pathways influence how cells behave and influence whether they survive.

One such pathway is the Hedgehog pathway (so named because fruit fly larvae in which the Hedgehog pathway is faulty are

Table 4.6 Summary of the state of development of various PARP inhibitors as of December 2017 (listed in alphabetical order).

Drug	Stage of development	Completed and ongoing phase 3 clinical trials
Niraparib (Zejula)	• FDA and EMA: Licensed for women with ovarian cancer who have responded to platinum-based chemotherapy	• Platinum-sensitive ovarian cancer or *BRCA*-mutated ovarian cancer (NCT01847274) • *BRCA*-mutated, HER2-negative breast cancer (NCT01905592) • Platinum-sensitive ovarian cancer (NCT02655016)
Olaparib (Lynparza)	• FDA: Licensed for women with ovarian cancer due to inherited *BRCA* gene mutations, and for women whose ovarian cancer is sensitive to platinum chemotherapy • EMA: Licensed for women with *BRCA*-mutated ovarian cancer (inherited or sporadic mutations)	• *BRCA*-mutated and -unmutated ovarian cancer (NCT03106987, NCT01844986, NCT02282020, NCT03278717, NCT01874353, NCT02477644, NCT02477644, NCT02502266) • *BRCA*-mutated or homologous recombination-deficient breast cancer: (NCT02032823, NCT03286842, NCT02000622, NCT02810743, NCT03150576) • Pancreatic cancer in people with inherited *BRCA* mutations (NCT02184195) • Stomach cancer (NCT01924533) • Prostate cancers with homologous recombination gene defects (NCT02987543)
Rucaparib (Rubraca)	• Granted accelerated approval for BRCA-mutated ovarian cancer by the FDA[a] in December 2016	• *BRCA*-mutated ovarian cancer (NCT02855944) • Platinum-sensitive ovarian cancer (NCT01968213) • Prostate cancers with homologous recombination gene defects (NCT02975934)
Talazoparib	Not licensed yet	• Breast cancer in women with an inherited *BRCA* mutation (NCT01945775) • Homologous recombination-deficient non-small cell lung cancer (NCT02154490)
Veliparib	Not licensed yet	• Ovarian cancers in women with and without inherited *BRCA* mutations (NCT02470585) • *BRCA*-mutated, HER2-negative breast cancer (NCT02163694) • Triple-negative breast cancer (NCT02032277) • Glioblastoma multiforme (NCT02152982) • Non-small cell lung cancer (NCT02106546, NCT02264990)

FDA – US Food & Drug Administration; EMA – European Medicines Agency; HER2 – human epidermal growth factor receptor-2.
Source: For information on FDA-licensed treatments see: Drugs Approved for Ovarian, Fallopian Tube, or Primary Peritoneal Cancer. National Cancer Institute. https://www.cancer.gov/about-cancer/treatment/drugs/ovarian (Accessed December 14, 2017).
For information on EMA-licensed treatments see: Medicines. European Medicines Agency. http://www.ema.europa.eu/ema/index.jsp (accessed December 14, 2017).
For information on clinical trials see: ClinicalTrials.gov. https://clinicaltrials.gov/ct2/home (accessed December 14, 2017).
[a] For more information about different types of FDA approval, see http://www.fda.gov/forpatients/approvals/fast/ucm20041766.htm.

balled-up and extra bristly [88]). This pathway is **highly active in mammalian embryos**. It helps ensure that we have two arms, two legs, two eyes, and so on. And it helps our cells move, and makes sure they all end up in the right place [88]. The pathway is also **active in *adult* stem cells**[18] in our skin, hair follicles, brain, bone marrow, prostate (men only),

---

[18] Adult stem cells are rare cells found in many of our organs and tissues. When they multiply, they can create specialized cells of different types. They can replace dead cells and help our tissues regenerate after sustaining damage. http://www.sciencedaily.com/terms/adult_stem_cell.htm (accessed December 13, 2017).

bladder, and other locations [89]. Lastly, the Hedgehog pathway is **activated when we get injured** – it activates repair pathways and helps tissues regenerate [88].

Faults in various proteins involved in the hedgehog pathway have been found in the cancer cells of basal cell carcinoma (BCC) skin cancer and medulloblastoma. The pathway is also overactive in other cancer cell types [90].

4.4.1 Components of the Hedgehog Pathway

The Hedgehog pathway involves two receptors, Patched and Smoothened, and a ligand called Hedgehog. (As ever, there are multiple versions of each protein; e.g., there are three Hedgehog proteins in our bodies: Sonic Hedgehog, Indian Hedgehog, and Desert

Hedgehog.) Hedgehog proteins activate the Hedgehog pathway by attaching to Patched. When this attachment takes place, Patched can no longer block Smoothened. Hence, Smoothened is now free to act, and it in turn causes activation of GLI transcription factors (see Figure 4.15 for an illustration [91]). Genes controlled by GLI transcription factors include many oncogenes, such as the genes for Cyclin D1, Myc, and Bcl-2.

4.4.2 Hedgehog Pathway Inhibitors

Almost all Hedgehog pathway inhibitors **work by blocking Smoothened**. The first hedgehog pathway inhibitor discovered by scientists was a molecule called cyclopamine. This chemical is found in a poisonous plant common in the United States called the

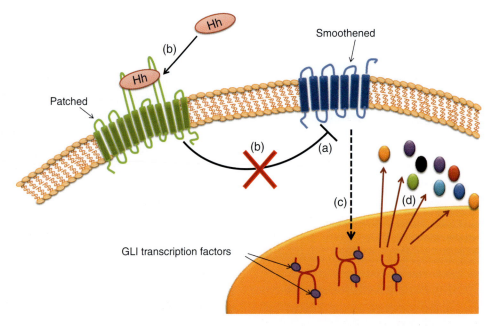

Figure 4.15 The basics of the hedgehog signaling pathway. (**a**| In the absence of hedgehog proteins, the Patched receptor blocks the hedgehog pathway by suppressing Smoothened (another receptor). (**b**) However, when hedgehog (Hh) proteins attach to Patched, it no longer blocks Smoothened, and Smoothened becomes active. (**c**) Increased Smoothened activity indirectly leads to the activation of GLI transcription factors. These transcription factors attach to numerous genes and (**d**) switch on production of various proteins including cyclin D1, Myc, and Bcl-2, which encourage the cell to survive and multiply. **Abbreviations:** Hh – hedgehog; GLI – glioma associated

California false hellebore[19] (*veratrum californicum*). In the 1950s, scientists in Idaho discovered that sheep that ate *veratrum californicum* often gave birth to lambs with only one eye [92].

Cyclopamine fits into a channel in the Smoothened protein. Other Smoothened inhibitors (such as vismodegib and sonidegib), created since cyclopamine was discovered, fit into other pockets and grooves in Smoothened [91].

4.4.3 Hedgehog Pathway Inhibitors for the Treatment of BCC and Medulloblastoma

Mutations that activate the Hedgehog pathway are extremely common in two cancer types: BCC and medulloblastoma.

BCCs are the most common type of skin cancer. They are slow growing and can usually be surgically removed before they have spread; as a result, they cause few deaths. However, if BCC does spread, or if it's in a location where surgery isn't possible, such as on someone's face, then it can be much harder to treat [93]. Around 90% of BCCs have mutations in either the gene for Patched or that for Smoothened [94]. Smoothened inhibitors such as vismodegib (Erivedge) and sonidegib (Odomzo; LDE225) have both proved to be helpful treatments for BCC in large clinical trials and are licensed both in the United States and Europe. However, doctors have cautioned that drug resistance and side effects are a problem for many patients [95].

Medulloblastomas are rare brain tumors that tend to be aggressive and fast growing and affect more children than adults.[20] Around 70%–75% of children are cured with standard treatments, but at the expense of many long-term side effects [96]. Around 30% of medulloblastomas contain mutations affecting the Hedgehog pathway and are known as the SHH-subtype. Hedgehog inhibitors have been put through trials involving children and adults with SHH-subtype medulloblastomas. Although their tumors do shrink to begin with, they quickly become resistant [96]. However, scientists in the United States are now developing a test that can be performed on the cancer cells of children with medulloblastoma to identify children likely to gain the greatest benefit from a Hedgehog pathway inhibitor [97].

4.4.4 Broadening the Uses of Hedgehog Inhibitors

Hedgehog inhibitors are being explored as treatments for various cancer types for a number of different reasons [90]:

1. As described above, hedgehog pathway inhibitors can help people with BCC or medulloblastoma whose cancers are driven by mutations affecting the Hedgehog pathway. This includes being helpful for people with Gorlin Syndrome, which is caused by an inherited mutation[21] in the gene for Patched. People with Gorlin Syndrome tend to develop lots of BCCs and other tumors. Trials in these patients (patients with mutations affecting the Hedgehog pathway) have given the best results achieved with Hedgehog pathway inhibitors so far.

2. In other cancers, the hedgehog pathway is overactive despite there being no mutation affecting the pathway. Sometimes this is because there is autocrine activation of the Hedgehog pathway. "Autocrine

---

[19] It's also sometimes called the Californian corn lily.

[20] For more about medulloblastomas, see http://www.abta.org/brain-tumor-information/types-of-tumors/medulloblastoma.html (accessed December 13, 2017).

[21] The mutation might be inherited from an affected parent, or the mutation might have taken place in a single egg or sperm, or in a newly fertilized embryo.

activation" means that the same cell both produces a ligand and has the receptors to respond to it. For example, in some bowel cancers, the cancer cells overproduce Hedgehog proteins, and they have Patched and Smoothened receptors, which enable them to respond to it.

3. More commonly, there is **paracrine activation** of the Hedgehog pathway. "Paracrine activation" means that one cell produces the ligand, but a different, nearby cell responds to it. For example, in pancreatic cancer, the cancer cells produce lots of Hedgehog proteins but don't have Patched or Smoothened receptors. In this instance, Hedgehog activates the Hedgehog pathway in nearby, non-cancer cells, such as epithelial cells, fibroblasts, and white blood cells. These cells respond to Hedgehog by releasing growth factors and other molecules that help the cancer cells survive and multiply [98] (see Figure 4.16). Scientists have found paracrine Hedgehog signaling in small cell lung cancer, pancreatic cancer, bowel cancer, metastatic prostate cancers, melanomas, and glioblastoma [94]. However, trials of Hedgehog pathway inhibitors in these cancers have been disappointing so far.

4. The final reason to block the Hedgehog pathway is because it is active in **cancer stem cells.** Writing anything about cancer stem cells is fraught with problems because no one can agree what a "cancer stem cell" is [99]. However, as I mentioned in Chapter 1, some cancers seem to contain a population of cells that have some of the properties of healthy stem cells, can survive chemotherapy and radiotherapy, and

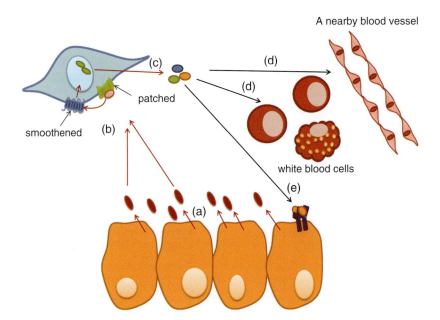

Figure 4.16 Paracrine activation of hedgehog signaling in pancreatic cancer. (a) Around 75% of pancreatic cancers produce hedgehog (Hh) proteins. **(b)** Hh proteins activate the Hh pathway in nearby stromal cells, such as fibroblasts. **(c)** GLI transcription factors are activated, causing stromal cells to release growth factors and cytokines. **(d)** Growth factors released by stromal cells cause angiogenesis and activation of white blood cells. **(e)** Growth factor receptors on the surface of prostate cancer cells are activated, leading to cancer growth, invasion, and metastasis.
Abbreviations: Hh – Hedgehog; GLI – glioma associated

cause a cancer to re-grow even if most of its cells have been killed. Like healthy adult stem cells, cancer stem cells seem to rely on the Hedgehog pathway. However, despite running a variety of clinical trials, scientists haven't yet been able to prove that drug combinations designed to kill cancer stem cells are better than standard treatments.

As I write this, there are many clinical trials taking place around the world in which hedgehog pathway inhibitors are being used on their own, or in combination with other drugs. With time, we will hopefully build up a picture of who should be given these drugs and what improvements we might expect to see.

4.5 CYCLIN-DEPENDENT KINASE (CDK) INHIBITORS

In this final section of the chapter, we turn our attention to the cell cycle: the step-by-step series of events our cells always go through when they multiply (see Figure 4.17 for an overview of the process). Many of you might have learned about the cell cycle in A level biology or an undergraduate degree. Or you might have learned about it when being taught how various forms of chemotherapy exert their effects. However, although many chemotherapies work by targeting one or more aspects of the cell cycle, they kill any cell that is multiplying, and they are therefore relatively nonspecific.

In order to create more precise drugs that target the cell cycle, scientists have been investigating exactly what parts of the cell cycle have gone wrong in cancer. And they have focused much of their attention on CDKs (cyclin-dependent kinases). The CDKs are **a group of kinases that control the progression of the cell from one phase of the cell cycle to the next**. The focus of scientists on CDKs is for a couple of reasons: (1) because several CDKs are overactive in many different cancer types, and (2) because, being kinases, they have a binding site for ATP that can be blocked with a kinase inhibitor.

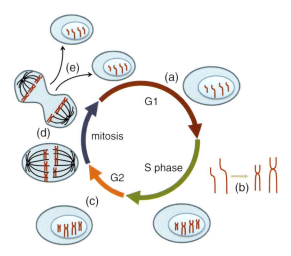

Figure 4.17 The cell cycle of a human cell. (a) The first stage in the cell cycle is G1, when the cell grows bigger and duplicates many of its proteins and other contents. **(b)** In S phase, the cell copies all 46 of its chromosomes so that it now has a duplicate set. **(c)** In G2, the cell checks its new chromosomes for mistakes and prepares for mitosis. **(d)** In mitosis, the cell separates its duplicate sets of chromosomes using a protein structure called the spindle. **(e)** The cell finally splits to create two identical cells, each with a full set of chromosomes.

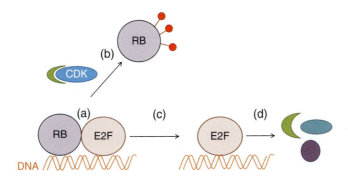

Figure 4.18 CDKs phosphorylate RB. **(a)** In a cell that is not multiplying, RB and E2F sit together on the cell's DNA. **(b)** When the cell receives a signal to enter the cell cycle, this activates its CDKs, which then phosphorylate RB (phosphates are depicted as red circles on stalks). **(c)** Once phosphorylated, RB can no longer hold onto E2F proteins, and it lets go. **(d)** Without RB, E2F proteins (which are transcription factors) activate the transcription of numerous genes, causing the cell to make proteins that force it to enter the cell cycle.
Abbreviations: RB – retinoblastoma associated protein; CDK – cyclin-dependent kinase

Scientists have been working on CDK inhibitors for over 20 years. However, it's only recently that they've been able to make highly selective CDK inhibitors that can block just one or two CDK family members [100]. These drugs are producing some exciting results in clinical trials, and two of them, palbociclib (Ibrance) and ribociclib (Kisqali), were licensed as breast cancer treatments in Europe and the United States as of December 2017. A third drug, abemaciclib (Verzenio), is licensed in the United States only.

4.5.1 CDKs Control the Cell Cycle

CDKs control the cell cycle by phosphorylating[22] an important tumor suppressor protein called **RB (retinoblastoma protein)**. When it doesn't have any phosphates attached to it, RB clings to a group of transcription factors called the E2F proteins, and this blocks the cell from entering the cell cycle. But **when RB is phosphorylated by CDKs, it lets go of E2F proteins** (Figure 4.18). When E2F proteins are free of RB, they trigger the production of

numerous proteins that force the cell into the cell cycle. And, as the cell moves through the cell cycle, more CDKs attach more phosphates to RB, making sure that the E2F proteins are free to drive the cell cycle through each of its stages [100].

The cell cycle is a vital process that enables us to grow, to replace dead cells, to heal wounds, and to replace cells sloughed off from the surface of our skin and the lining of our gut. It is also vital that our white blood cells multiply when fighting off infections. However, it's also vital that our cells only enter the cell cycle under strict conditions so that they don't become cancer cells. And, if something goes wrong during the cell cycle, it's essential that our cells can stop the process and put right whatever is awry. As a result, the cell cycle is very tightly regulated: our CDKs are subject to numerous controls, and there are many additional checks and balances.

Some of the proteins that control CDKs are the cyclins and the CDK inhibitors. The cyclins

---

[22] As you might remember from earlier chapters, kinases (such as the CDKs) are enzymes that modify the function of other proteins by attaching phosphate groups to them. Phosphate is a phosphorous atom surrounded by oxygen atoms.

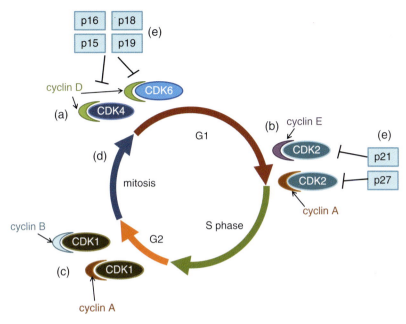

Figure 4.19 CDKs are controlled by cyclins and CDK inhibitors. (a) When a cell receives a signal to enter the cell cycle (such as activation of the MAPK and PI3K/AKT/mTOR pathways by growth factors), this causes the cell to produce cyclin D. Cyclin D activates two CDKs: CDK4 and CDK6, which phosphorylate RB and cause the cell to enter the G1 phase of the cell cycle. (b) One of the consequences of RB phosphorylation (and the resulting activity of E2F) is that the cell produces two more cyclins, cyclin E and cyclin A, which activate CDK2. CDK2 adds further phosphates to RB, triggering the cell to enter S phase and duplicate its chromosomes. (c) When all the cell's chromosomes have been copied and checked for mistakes, CDK1 becomes active due to the actions of cyclin A and cyclin B, and the cell enters mitosis. (d) Finally, once cyclin B has been destroyed, the cell can split in two. (e) If something goes wrong with the cell cycle, CDKs can be blocked by CDK inhibitors such as p16, p15, p18, p19, p21, and p27. **Abbreviations:** RB – retinoblastoma protein; CDK – cyclin-dependent kinase

are a group of proteins that are produced and then destroyed at set moments during the cell cycle. They activate each CDK in turn, allowing the cell to pass through each stage of the cell cycle (see Figure 4.19a, b, c, and d). CDK inhibitors are a separate group of proteins produced by our cells when they need to halt, or prevent, the cell cycle. They include proteins such as p16, p15, p18, p19, p21, and p27 (these proteins also get called $p16^{INK4a}$, $p15^{INK4b}$, $p18^{INK4c}$, $p19^{INK4d}$, $p21^{CIP1}$, and $p27^{KIP1}$) (see Figure 4.19e). Scientists have also discovered how to make drugs that block CDKs, and these are also referred to as CDK inhibitors.

4.5.2 Other CDKs

Human cells produce around 20 different CDK proteins [101]. Many of these proteins control the cell cycle, such as CDK4, CDK6, CDK1, and CDK2. However, some of them have completely different functions. For example, CDK8, CDK7, CDK9, and CDK11 are part of the general transcription machinery that our cells use to read the information in our genes and make mRNA (which is then used to make proteins) [100]. Thus, blocking CDKs can have various impacts on human cells depending on which CDKs are blocked.

4.5.3 How Cell Cycle CDKs Become Overactive in Cancer Cells

Various CDKs involved in the cell cycle are known to be overactive in cancer cells for a variety of reasons [100, 102, 103]:

1. **Because growth factor signaling pathways are overactive**, such as the MAPK pathway and the PI3K/AKT/mTOR pathway (Figure 4.20a). Strong activation of either pathway triggers the production of cyclin D and causes the cell to enter the cell cycle. (There are actually three different versions of cyclin D, called cyclin D1, D2, and D3.)

2. **Amplification[23] of cyclin D genes is very common in many cancers,** causing the cells to produce high levels of cyclin D (Figure 4.20b). Cancers in which this has been found include head and neck cancer, breast cancer, NSCLC, esophageal cancer, malignant melanoma, endometrial cancer, pancreatic cancer, and glioblastoma.

3. **Because of overproduction of CDK4, CDK6, cyclin E1, or cyclin E2** (Figure 4.20b). The genes for these proteins are amplified in many cancers, leading to high levels of the corresponding protein. Cancers in which this has been found include sarcomas, malignant melanoma, esophageal cancer, head and neck cancer, uterine cancer, ovarian cancer, liver cancer, breast cancer, and bladder cancer.

4. **Because p16 is missing due to its gene (called *CDKN2A*) being either deleted or mutated.** Loss of p16 leads to uncontrolled CDK4 and CDK6 activity (Figure 4.20d). Cancers in which this has been found include those of the pancreas, bladder, breast, prostate, stomach, head and neck, and in glioblastoma and malignant melanoma.

5. **Because the activity of estrogen receptors is causing overproduction of cyclin D1.** The majority of breast cancers contain estrogen receptors (ERs). ER is a transcription factor; when estrogen is present, it attaches to the cyclin D1 gene and triggers overproduction of cyclin D1 protein (Figure 4.20c). In return, cyclin D1 boosts the activity of ERs, reinforcing the link between ERs and cyclin D.

6. **Because a chromosome translocation is forcing the cells to produce high levels of cyclin D1.** A translocation between chromosomes 11 and 14[24] is found in the vast majority of mantle cell lymphomas (a type of non-Hodgkin lymphoma). The translocation forces the cell to produce high levels of cyclin D1. The same translocation, and other translocations that force overproduction of cyclin D1, are found in many multiple myelomas.

In addition, **many cancers lack RB,** which means that the E2F proteins become overactive irrespective of what the cell's CDKs are doing (Figure 4.20e). Cancers in which this has been found include lung cancer, ovarian cancer, prostate cancer, uterine cancer, and bladder cancer.

4.5.4 CDK4/6 Inhibitors as Cancer Treatments

The first CDK inhibitors created were pan-CDK inhibitors. That is, they blocked multiple CDK proteins. For example, flavopiridol (alvocidib) blocks CDKs 1, 2, 4, 6, 7, and 9. And another inhibitor called roscovitine (seliciclib) blocks CDKs 1, 2, 5, 7, and 9. Neither of these drugs gave particularly promising results in clinical trials, and both cause lots of side effects [100].

More recently, scientists have been focusing their efforts on creating drugs that are much

---

[23] Amplification is when a cell has accidentally made extra copies of a gene.
[24] The precise translocation is t(11;14)(q13;q32).

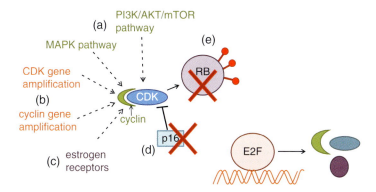

Figure 4.20 **Reasons why CDKs are overactive and E2F proteins are therefore uncontrolled in cancer cells**. **(a)** Signaling pathways such as the MAPK and PI3K/AKT/mTOR pathways are overactive in the majority of cancers, leading to increased production of cyclin D. **(b)** Many cancers contain extra copies of the genes for cyclins or CDKs, leading to increased production of these proteins. **(c)** The majority of breast cancers contain estrogen receptors, which force the cell to produce high levels of cyclin D1. **(d)** Many cancers lack important CDK inhibitors such as p16. **(e)** In some cancers, RB is missing, meaning that there is nothing to block E2F activity.
Abbreviations: MAPK – mitogen-activated protein kinase; PI3K – phosphatidylinositol 3-kinase; mTOR – mammalian target of rapamycin; RB – retinoblastoma protein; CDK – cyclin-dependent kinase

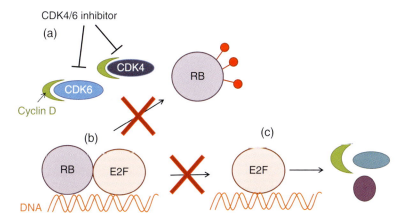

Figure 4.21 **Mechanism of action of CDK 4/6 inhibitors**. **(a)** Drugs that block CDK4 and CDK6 can prevent phosphorylation of RB. **(b)** In the absence of phosphorylation, E2F and RB stay together, and E2F is unable to trigger entry into the cell cycle. **(c)** However, if RB protein is missing from the cell, then a CDK4/6 inhibitor will have no impact. This is because there is no RB to prevent E2F activity.
Abbreviations: RB – retinoblastoma protein; CDK – cyclin-dependent kinase

more selective and that will **only block one or two CDKs,** and they are particularly interested in drugs that **block CDK4 and CDK6** (Figure 4.21). Three CDK4/6 inhibitors have so far reached phase 3 clinical trials, and three of them, palbociclib (Ibrance), ribociclib (Kisquali) and abemaciclib (Verzenio) are licensed treatments (see Chapter 6, Section 6.2.2). All three drugs work by competing with ATP for the CDKs' ATP-binding site [102].

Table 4.7   Summary of CDK4/6 inhibitors in phase 3 trials.

Stage of development (as of December 2017)	Completed and ongoing phase 3 clinical trials (as of December 2017)*
Palbociclib (Ibrance)	
• FDA and EMA: Licensed as a first-or second-line treatment for metastatic or advanced ER-positive, HER2-negative breast cancer in combination with hormone therapy (an aromatase inhibitor or fulvestrant)	• ER-positive, HER2-negative breast cancer (NCT02600923, NCT01864746, NCT02513394, NCT02297438, NCT02028507, NCT01740427, NCT01942135, and NCT02692755) • ER-positive, HER2-positive breast cancer (NCT02947685) • Squamous cell non-small cell lung cancer (NSCLC) with mutations in CDK4, CDK6, or Cyclin D1 genes, or amplification of the CDK4 gene (NCT02947685) [104] • Squamous cell or adenocarcinomas NSCLC with intact RB and a mutation that leads to overactive CDK4/6 (NCT02664935) [105]**
Ribociclib (Kisquali)	
• FDA and EMA: Licensed as a first-line treatment for ER-positive, HER2-negative metastatic breast cancer in combination with any aromatase inhibitor	• ER-positive, HER2-negative breast cancer (NCT03078751, NCT03078751, NCT02941926, NCT03096847, NCT02422615, NCT01958021, and NCT02278120)
Abemaciclib (LY2835219)	
• FDA: Licensed as a first-line treatment for ER-positive, HER2-negative metastatic breast cancer in combination fulvestrant or used alone after hormone therapy and chemotherapy	• ER-positive, HER2-negative breast cancer (NCT03155997, NCT02107703, NCT02763566, and NCT02246621) • *KRAS*-mutated NSCLC (NCT02152631)

*This information is taken from ClinicalTrials.gov.
**This trial is technically a phase 2 trial, but as it a large and ambitious trial (there are eight treatment arms) I have included it in this table.
Abbreviations and terminology: FDA – US Food & Drug Administration; EMA – European Medicines Agency; ER-positive – cancers that contain estrogen receptors; HER2-negative – cancers in which the gene for HER2 is normal; HER2-positive – cancers in which the gene for HER2 is amplified and/or the HER2 protein is present in high levels; hormone therapy – refers to treatments that either block the actions of estrogen receptors or that block the production of estrogen in the body

Because of the link between the ER and cyclin D1, most of the trials with CDK4/6 inhibitors have involved people with estrogen receptor positive (ER-positive) breast cancer. However, a handful of other phase 3 trials are investigating these drugs as treatments for NSCLC (see Table 4.7 for a summary of phase 3 trials with these drugs).

Reflecting the fact that a wide variety of tumors contain genetic defects that affect CDK4/6 activity, CDK4/6 inhibitors are also being investigated in people with a wide range of other cancer types such as, acute myeloid leukemia, pancreatic cancer, head and neck cancer, bladder cancer, mantle cell lymphoma, childhood brain tumors, prostate cancer, multiple myeloma, and glioblastoma.

4.5.5 Resistance to CDK4/6 Inhibitors

Because very few large trials with CDK4/6 inhibitors have been completed, it's a bit too soon to say what resistance mechanisms are going to be the most common or important. However, scientists have been studying cells grown in a laboratory that are resistant to CDK4/6 inhibitors, and they have discovered a number of ways that these cells are resistant (summarized in Figure 4.22). That's

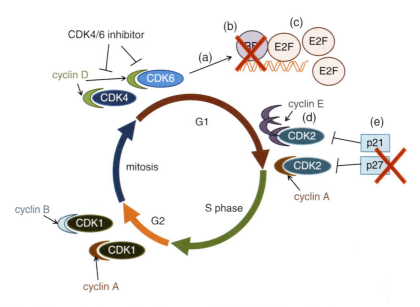

Figure 4.22 Possible mechanisms of resistance to CDK4/6 inhibitors. (a) CDK4/6 inhibitors work by preventing CDK4 and CDK6 from phosphorylating RB. **(b)** However, if RB is not present, perhaps because both of the cell's copies of the *RB1* gene are deleted or suppressed, then an CDK4/6 inhibitor will have no impact on the cell. **(c)** Equally, overproduction of E2F might overwhelm the available RB. **(d)** Resistance can also take place if the cell overproduces cyclin E or **(e)** if it lacks p21 or p27. **Abbreviations:** RB – retinoblastoma protein; CDK – cyclin-dependent kinase

why, in some ongoing trials, scientists are analyzing patients' tumor samples for RB levels and various other defects. In future, these studies might help doctors decide which patients should be given this new group of treatments.

4.6 FINAL THOUGHTS

In this chapter, I have discussed treatments that have various different targets and mechanisms of action.

First, we looked at angiogenesis inhibitors that block VEGF signaling. These drugs were first developed in the late 1990s, and the optimism surrounding them has waxed and waned. Since their creation, hundreds of clinical trials with angiogenesis inhibitors have taken place around the world. And some of them, particularly those in kidney cancer,

bowel cancer, ovarian cancer, and cervical cancer, have proven that the drug is beneficial. However, it seems these drugs can cause a wide variety of different effects on tumors, and we still lack biomarkers that would enable doctors to predict which patients are going to benefit from them.

Second, we looked at treatments that target fusion proteins such as those involving ALK, ROS1, and RET. With these treatments, we often have a very clear biomarker test: if the fusion protein is present, the person is likely to benefit from treatment. Gene rearrangements affecting ALK and ROS1 are found in a small proportion of NSCLCs. People with these tumors often benefit from ALK1 and ROS1 inhibitors. The current challenges are to overcome resistance mechanisms and to have testing procedures in place so that we can quickly identify patients whose tumors contain the relevant mutations.

The situation regarding biomarkers for PARP inhibitors is less clear and is still evolving. These treatments were created with one particular group of patients in mind: women with an inherited defect in a *BRCA* gene and who have developed breast or ovarian cancer. However, it now seems that PARP inhibitors might benefit a much wider group of patients: those whose tumors contain defects in homologous recombination. Ovarian cancers, at least 50% of which contain such defects, are therefore the focus of current trials. Scientists and doctors are also excited about the potential of PARP inhibitors as treatments for prostate cancer and other cancer types [106].

I then turned to Hedgehog pathway inhibitors. In a couple of cancer types – BCC and medulloblastoma – there are genetic defects that activate this pathway. These defects have given scientists a strong rationale for including patients with these cancers in trials. Some of the results from these trials have been very positive. However, BCC is generally cured very easily with surgery, and medulloblastoma is very rare. Because of this, some trial results have been unclear, and toxicity and drug resistance have been a problem. And, although there is reason to believe that Hedgehog inhibitors might be useful in other cancers in which Hedgehog signaling is active, this hasn't yet led to other positive trial results.

Lastly, I looked at CDK inhibitors, and specifically the drugs that block CDK4 and CDK6. Optimism around these drugs is currently sky-high [107]; the first drugs have been licensed, and others are likely to follow. However, it will be several years before we know what these drugs can do, how they should be used with other treatments, and who they should be given to. But, because so many cancers contain defects that lead to overactivity of CDK4 and CDK6, hopefully they will ultimately benefit people with many different cancer types.

REFERENCES

1 The idea of angiogenesis inhibitors as cancer treatments was first written about in 1971: Folkman J (1971). Tumour angiogenesis: Therapeutic implications. *N Engl J Med* **285**: 1182–1186.

2 NCI Drug Dictionary: https://www.cancer.gov/publications/dictionaries/cancer-drug [Accessed December 13, 2017].

3 European Medicines Agency (Europe only): http://www.ema.europa.eu/ema/ [Accessed December 13, 2017].

4 National Cancer Institute (USA only): https://www.cancer.gov/about-cancer/treatment/drugs [Accessed December 13, 2017].

5 Jayson GC et al. (2016). Antiangiogenic therapy in oncology: Current status and future directions. *Lancet* **388**: 518–529.

6 Vasudev NS, Reynolds AR (2014). Antiangiogenic therapy for cancer: Current progress, unresolved questions and future directions. *Angiogenesis* **17**(3): 471–494.

7 Escudier B, Eisen T, Porta C et al. (2012). Renal cell carcinoma: ESMO clinical practice guidelines for diagnosis, treatment and follow-up. *Ann Oncol* **23**(Suppl 7): vii65–71.

8 For a fuller list of the growth factors and other signaling molecules involved, see: Harris A, Generali D. (2008). Inhibitors of Tumour Angiogenesis. In Neidle S (ed.) Cancer Drug Design and Discovery. 2nd ed. London, UK. Elsevier Inc. pp. 275–306.

9 For a more detailed description of the process, see: Bergers G, Benjamin LE (2003). Angiogenesis: Tumorigenesis and the angiogenic switch. *Nat Rev Cancer* **3**: 401–410.

10 Jin Y, Jakobsson L (2012). The Dynamics of Developmental and Tumor Angiogenesis—A Comparison. *Cancers (Basel)* **4**(2): 400–419.

11 For a detailed description of tumor blood vessels, see: Dudley AC (2012). Tumor endothelial cells. *Cold Spring Harb Perspect Med* **2**(3): a006536.

12 For a fuller description, see: Niu G, Chen X (2010). Vascular endothelial growth factor as an anti-angiogenic target for cancer therapy. *Curr Drug Targets* **11**(8): 1000–1017.

13 Jain RK (2014). Antiangiogenesis strategies revisited: From Starving tumors to alleviating hypoxia. *Cancer Cell* **26**(5): 605–622.

14 For a summary of VEGF's actions, see: Byrne AM et al. (2005). Angiogenic and cell survival functions of vascular endothelial growth factor (VEGF). *J Cell Mol Med* **9**(4): 777–794.

15 Ellis LM, Hicklin DJ (2008). VEGF-targeted therapy: Mechanisms of anti-tumour activity. *Nat Rev Cancer* **8**: 579–591.

16 Ferrara N et al. (2004). Discovery and development of bevacizumab, an anti-VEGF antibody for treating cancer. *Nat Rev Drug Discov* **3**: 391–400.

17 Holash J et al. (2002). VEGF-Trap: A VEGF blocker with potent antitumor effects. *Proc Natl Acad Sci USA* **99**(17): 11393–11398.

18 For an example, see: Chiron M et al. (2014). Differential antitumor activity of aflibercept and bevacizumab in patient-derived xenograft models of colorectal cancer. *Mol Cancer Ther* **13**: 1636.

19 Zhang J et al. (2015). Bevacizumab, Aflibercept or Ramucirmab combined with chemotherapy as second-line treatment for metastatic colorectal cancer following progression with Bevacizumab in first-line therapy: A systematic review and indirect comparison. *J Clin Oncol* **33** (suppl; abstr e14601).

20 For a discussion of the relative usefulness of bevacizumab and aflibercept in bowel cancer, see: London S. *Evidence Is Changing Colorectal Cancer Treatment Landscape*. September 15, 2012, Volume **3**, Issue 14, Best of ASCO Supplement, The ASCO Post http://www.ascopost.com/issues/september-15-2012-boa-supplement/evidence-is-changing-colorectal-cancer-treatment-landscape.aspx [Accessed December 13, 2017].

21 Aprile G et al. (2014). Ramucirumab: Preclinical research and clinical development. *Onco Targets Ther* **7**: 1997–2006.

22 Qian CN et al. (2009). Complexity of tumor vasculature in clear cell renal cell carcinoma. *Cancer* **115**(10 Suppl): 2282–2289.

23 Stjepanovic N, Capdevila J (2014). Multikinase inhibitors in the treatment of thyroid cancer: Specific role of lenvatinib. *Biologics* **8**: 129–139.

24 Viola D et al. (2016). Treatment of advanced thyroid cancer with targeted therapies: Ten years of experience. *Endocr Relat Cancer* **23**: R185–R205.

25 Gotnik K, Verheul HMW (2010). Anti-angiogenic tyrosine kinase inhibitors: What is their mechanism of action? *Angiogenesis* **13**(1): 1–14.

26 van Geel RM, Beijnen JH, Schellens JH (2012). *The Oncologist* **17**(8): 1081–1089.

27 Yakes FM, Chen J, Tan J (2011). Cabozantinib (XL184), a Novel MET and VEGFR2 Inhibitor, Simultaneously Suppresses Metastasis, Angiogenesis, and Tumor Growth. *Mol Cancer Ther* **10**: 2298.

28 Wilhelm SM, Dumas J, Adnane L et al. (2011). Regorafenib (BAY 73-4506): A new oral multikinase inhibitor of angiogenic, stromal and oncogenic receptor tyrosine kinases with potent preclinical antitumor activity. *Int J Cancer* **129**(1): 245–255.

29 Okamoto K, Ikemori-Kawada M, Jestel A et al. (2015). Distinct binding mode of multikinase inhibitor Lenvatinib revealed by biochemical characterization. *ACS Med. Chem Lett* **6**(1): 89–94.

30 Tan Q, Wang W, Long Y et al. (2015). Therapeutic effects and associated adverse events of multikinase inhibitors in metastatic renal cell carcinoma: A meta-analysis. *Exp Ther Med* **9**(6): 2275–2280.

31 McLellan B, Kerr H (2011). Cutaneous toxicities of the multikinase inhibitors sorafenib and sunitinib. *Dermatol Ther* **24**(4):396–400.

32 Del Bufalo D, Ciuffreda L, Trisciuoglio D et al. (2006). Antiangiogenic Potential of the Mammalian Target of Rapamycin Inhibitor Temsirolimus. *Cancer Res* June 1, 2006 **66**: 5549.

33 Lin T et al. (2016). Mammalian target of rapamycin (mTOR) inhibitors in solid tumours. *Clin Pharmacist* **8**(3), online DOI: 10.1211/CP.2016.20200813

34 Limaverde-Sousa G, Sternberg C, Ferreira CG (2014). Antiangiogenesis beyond VEGF inhibition: A journey from antiangiogenic single-target to broad-spectrum agents. *Cancer Treatment Rev* **40**(4): 548–557.

35 Clarke JM, Hurwitz HI (2013). Understanding and targeting resistance to anti-angiogenic therapies. *J Gastrointest Oncol* **4**(3): 253–263.

36 For a pretty illustration of this, see Figure 1 in: Bergers G, Hanahan D (2008). Modes of resistance to anti-angiogenic Therapy. *Nat Rev Cancer* **8**: 592–603.

37 For more details, see: Sennino B, McDonald DM (2012). Controlling escape from angiogenesis inhibitors. *Nat Rev Cancer* **12**: 699–709.

38 Druker BJ (2008). Translation of the Philadelphia chromosome into therapy for CML. *Blood* **112**: 4808–4817.

39 If you are really keen, you can find a database of all known translocations found in cancers here: Mitelman F, Johansson B, Mertens, Mitelman F. Database of Chromosome Aberrations in Cancer. https://cgap.nci.nih.gov/Chromosomes/Mitelman [Accessed December 13, 2017].

40 For a review, see: Mitelman F, Johansson B, Mertens F (2007). The impact of translocations and gene fusions on cancer causation. *Nat Rev Cancer* **7**: 233–245.

41 Martens JHA, Stunnberg HG (2010). The molecular signature of oncofusion proteins in acute myeloid leukemia. *FEBS Lett* **584**(12): 2662–2669.

42 Wang Z-Y, Chen Z (2008). Acute promyelocytic leukemia: From highly fatal to highly curable. *Blood* **111**: 2505–2515.

43 Hirsch FR et al. (2016). New and emerging targeted treatments in advanced non-small-cell lung cancer. *Lancet* **388**: 1012–1024.

44 Grande E, Bolos MV, Arriola E (2011). Targeting oncogenic ALK: A promising strategy for cancer treatment. *Mol Cancer Ther* **10**: 569.

45 Other fusion partners of ALK exist in anaplastic large cell lymphoma. For a more complete list, see: Cools J, Wlodarska I, Somers R et al. (2002). Identification of novel fusion partners of ALK, the anaplastic lymphoma kinase, in anaplastic large-cell lymphoma and inflammatory myofibroblastic tumor. *Genes, Chromosomes Cancer* **34**(4): 354–362.

46 Kohno T, Nakaoku T, Tsuta K (2015). Beyond *ALK-RET, ROS1* and other oncogene fusions in lung cancer. *Transl Lung Cancer Res* **4**(2): 156–164.

47 Shaw AT et al. (2013). Tyrosine kinase gene rearrangements in epithelial malignancies. *Nat Rev Cancer* **13**(11): 772–787.

48 Viola D et al. (2016). Treatment of advanced thyroid cancer with targeted therapies: Ten years of experience. *Endocr Relat Cancer* **23**: R185–R205.

49 El Fakih R et al. (2018). Current paradigms in the management of Philadelphia chromosome positive acute lymphoblastic leukemia in adults. *Am J Hematal* **93**(2): 286–295.

50 Giles F J et al. (2009). Class effects of tyrosine kinase inhibitors in the treatment of chronic myeloid leukemia. *Leukemia* **23**: 1698–1707.

51 Ye M et al. (2016). ALK and ROS1 as targeted therapy paradigms and clinical implications to overcome crizotinib resistance. *Oncotarget* **7**(11): 12289–12304.

52 Hallberg B, Palmer RH (2016). The role of the ALK receptor in cancer biology. *Ann Oncol* **27** Suppl 3: iii4–iii15.

53 Puig de la Bellacasa R et al. (2013). ALK and ROS1 as a joint target for the treatment of lung cancer: A review. *Transl Lung Cancer Res* **2**(2): 72–86.

54 Soda M. et al. (2007). Identification of the transforming EML4-ALK fusion gene in non-small-cell lung cancer. *Nature* **448**(7153): 561–566.

55 Davies KD et al. (2012). Identifying and targeting ROS1 gene fusions in non-small cell lung cancer. *Clin Cancer Res* **18**(17): 4570–4579.

56 Summarized in: Grande E, Bolos MV, Arriola E (2011). Targeting oncogenic ALK: A promising strategy for cancer treatment. *Mol Cancer Ther* **10**(4): 569–579.

57 Heigener DF, Reck M (2014). Crizotinib. *Recent Results Cancer Res* **201**: 197–205.

58 Solomon BJ, Mok T, Kim D-W et al. (2014). First-line Crizotinib versus chemotherapy in *ALK*-positive lung cancer. *N Engl J Med* **371**: 2167–2177.

59 Goodman A (2012). Role of Crizotinib in Previously Treated ALK-positive Advanced NSCLC. *The ASCO Post*. Published online, November 1, volume 3, Issue 16. http://www.ascopost.com/issues/november-1-2012/role-of-crizotinib-in-previously-treated-alk-positive-advanced-nsclc.aspx [Accessed February 27, 2018].

60 For an overview, see: Wu J et al. (2016). Second- and third-generation ALK inhibitors for non-small cell lung cancer. *J Hematol Oncol* **9**: 19.

61 Camidge DR, Doebele RC (2012). Treating ALK positive lung cancer: Early successes and coming challenges. *Nat Rev Clin Oncol*. **9**(5): 268–277.

62 Friboulet L et al. (2014). The ALK inhibitor ceritinib overcomes crizotinib resistance in non-small cell lung cancer. *Cancer Discov* **4**(6): 662–673.

63 Awad MM, Shaw AT (2014). ALK inhibitors in non–small cell lung cancer: Crizotinib and beyond. *Clin Adv Hematol Oncol* **12**(7): 429–439.

64 For a list of ALK and ROS1 targeted treatments, see: Shaw AT et al. (2013). Tyrosine kinase gene rearrangements in epithelial malignancies. *Nat Rev Cancer* **13**(11): 772–787.

65 For an overview, see: Wu S et al. (2015). linico-pathological characteristics and outcomes of ROS1-rearranged patients with lung adenocarcinoma without EGFR, KRAS mutations and ALK rearrangements. *Thoracic Cancer* **6**(4): 413–420.

66 Mulligan LM (2014). RET revisited: Expanding the oncogenic portfolio. *Nat Rev Cancer* **14**: 173–186.

67 Espinosa A, Gilbert J (2015). *RET in Thyroid Cancer*. My Cancer Genome http://www.mycancergenome.org/content/disease/thyroid-cancer/ret/ [Accessed December 13, 2017].

68 Prescott JD, Zeiger MA (2015). The RET oncogene in papillary thyroid carcinoma. *Cancer* **121**(13): 2137–2146.

69 For more information on RET mutations, see: Espinosa A, Gilbert J, Fagin J (2014). *RET M918T Mutations in Thyroid Cancer*. My Cancer Genome http://www.mycancergenome.org/content/disease/thyroid-cancer/ret/128/ [Accessed February 27, 2018].

70 Drilon A, Wang L, Hasanovic A *et al.* (2013). Response to cabozantinib in patients with RET fusion-positive lung adenocarcinomas. *Cancer Discov* **3**: 630–635.

71 Konecny GE, Kristeleit RS (2016). PARP inhibitors for BRCA1/2-mutated and sporadic ovarian cancer: Current practice and future directions. *Br J Cancer* **115**(10): 1157–1173.

72 For a review of the creation and effects of oxygen free radicals, see: Sullivan LB, Chandel NS (2014). Mitochondrial reactive oxygen species and cancer. *Cancer Metab* **2**: 17.

73 There is much more about BRCA genes on the Cancer Research UK website: Cancer Research UK. Breast cancer genes. http://www.cancerresearchuk.org/about-cancer/causes-of-cancer/inherited-cancer-genes-and-increased-cancer-risk/inherited-genes-and-cancer-types [Accessed December 13, 2017].

74 Roy R et al. (2012). BRCA1 and BRCA2: Different roles in a common pathway of genome protection. *Nat Rev Cancer* **12**: 68–78.

75 Narod SA, Foulkes WD (2004). BRCA1 and BRCA2: 1994 and beyond. *Nat Rev Cancer* **4**: 665–676.

76 Cancer Research UK wrote about this in their Science Blog in 2013: Scowcroft H. Angelina Jolie, inherited breast cancer and the BRCA1 gene. Cancer Research UK Science blog. First published May 14, 2013. http://scienceblog.cancerresearchuk.org/2013/05/14/angelina-jolie-inherited-breast-cancer-and-the-brca1-gene/ [Accessed December 13, 2017].

77 This is Angelina Jolie Pitt's account of her cancer risk and decision to have a double mastectomy: Jolie Pitt, A. Angelina Jolie Pitt: My Medical Choice. *The New York Times*. First published March 14, 2013 http://www.nytimes.com/2013/05/14/opinion/my-medical-choice.html [Accessed December 13, 2017].

78 Some scientists argue that even a single mutation in a BRCA gene is enough to make a cell genetically unstable; see: Konishi H, Mohseni M, Tamaki A et al. (2011). Mutation of a single allele of the cancer susceptibility gene BRCA1 leads to genomic instability in human breast epithelial cells. *Proc Natl Acad Sci USA* **108**(43): 17773–17778.

79 For more about different DNA repair pathways and their importance in cancer, see: Lord CJ, Ashworth A (2012). The DNA damage response and cancer therapy. *Nature* **481**: 287–294.

80 Deng C-X, Scott F (2000). Role of the tumor suppressor gene Brca1 in genetic stability and mammary gland tumor formation. *Oncogene* **19**: 1059–1064.

81 Paul A, Paul S (2014). The breast cancer susceptibility genes (BRCA) in breast and ovarian cancers. *Front Biosci (Landmark Ed)*. **19**: 605–618.

82 Summarized in: Rouleau M, Patel A, Hendzel MJ (2010). PARP inhibition: PARP1 and beyond. *Nat Rev Cancer* **10**(4): 293–301.

83 Murai J, Huang SY, Das BB et al. (2012). Trapping of PARP1 and PARP2 by Clinical PARP Inhibitors. *Cancer Res* **72**(21): 5588–5599.

84 For a review of possible uses of PARP inhibitors see: O'Sullivan CC, Moon DH, Kohn EC et al. (2014). Beyond Breast and Ovarian Cancers: PARP Inhibitors for BRCA Mutation-Associated and BRCA-Like Solid Tumors. *Front Oncol* **4**: 42.

85 Mullane SA, Van Allen EM (2016). Precision medicine for advanced prostate cancer. *Curr Op Urol* **26**(3): 231–239.

86 Konstantinopoulos PA et al. (2015). Homologous recombination deficiency: Exploiting the fundamental vulnerability of ovarian cancer. *Cancer Discov* **5**(11): 1137–1154.

87 Brown JS et al. (2016). PARP inhibitors: The race is on. *Br J Cancer* **114**: 713–715.

88 Varjosalo M, Taipale J (2008). Hedgehog: Functions and mechanisms. *Genes Dev* **22**: 2454–2472.

89 Petrova R, Joyner AL (2014). Roles for Hedgehog signaling in adult organ homeostasis and repair. *Development* **141**: 3445–3457.

90 For an overview, see: Amakye D, Jagani Z, Dorsch M (2013). Unraveling the therapeutic potential of the Hedgehog pathway in cancer. *Nat Med* **19**: 1410–1422.

91 For a more detailed illustration of the Hedgehog pathway, I recommend: Sharpe HJ, Wang E, Hannoush RN et al. (2015). Regulation of the oncoprotein Smoothened by small molecules. *Nat Chem Biol* **11**: 246–255.

92 For a run-through of the discovery of cyclopamine, see: Heretsch P, Tzagkaroulaki L, Giannis A (2010). Cyclopamine and hedgehog signaling: Chemistry, biology, medical perspectives. *Angew Chem Int Ed Engl.* **49**(20): 3418–3427.

93 Lear JT, Corner C, Dziewulski P et al. (2014). Challenges and new horizons in the management of advanced basal cell carcinoma: A UK perspective. *Br J Cancer* **111**: 1476–1481.

94 For a review, see: McMillan R, Matsui W (2012). Molecular pathways: The Hedgehog signaling pathway in cancer. *Clin Cancer Res* **18**: 4883.

95 For a summary of clinical trial results with both vismodegib and sonidegib, see: Castellino AM. New Drug Treatments for Basal Cell Carcinoma. *Medscape* website, first published 25 May 2015: http://www.medscape.com/viewarticle/845314 [Accessed December 13, 2017].

96 For a review, see: Gajjar AJ, Robinson GW (2014). Medulloblastoma—translating discoveries from the bench to the bedside. *Nat Rev Clin Oncol* **11**: 714–722.

97 Shou Y, Robinson DM, Amakye DD et al. (2015). A five-gene hedgehog signature developed as a patient preselection tool for hedgehog inhibitor therapy in medulloblastoma. *Clin Cancer Res* **21**(3): 585–593.

98 Yauch RL, Gould SE, Scales SJ et al. (2008). A paracrine requirement for hedgehog signaling in cancer. *Nature* **455**: 406–410.

99 For a short summary of what cancer stems might be, see: The Stem Cell Theory of Cancer. Ludwig Center, Stanford Medicine website: http://med.stanford.edu/ludwigcenter/overview/theory.html [Accessed December 13, 2017].

100 Asghar U et al. (2015). The history and future of targeting cyclin-dependent kinases in cancer therapy. *Nat Rev Drug Disc* **14**: 130–146.

101 Malumbres M (2014). Cyclin-dependent kinases. *Genome Biol* **15**: 122.

102 Reviewed in: O'Leary B et al. (2016). Treating cancer with selective CDK4/6 inhibitors. *Nat Rev Clin Oncol* **13**: 417–430.

103 Musgrove EA et al. (2011). Cyclin D as a therapeutic target in cancer. *Nat Rev Cancer* **11**: 558–572.

104 Herbst RS et al. (2015). Lung Master Protocol (Lung-MAP) – A Biomarker-Driven Protocol for Accelerating Development of Therapies for Squamous Cell Lung Cancer: SWOG S1400. *Clin Cancer Res* **21**(7): 1514–1524.

105 Middleton G et al. (2015). The National Lung Matrix Trial: Translating the biology of stratification in advanced non-small-cell lung cancer. *Ann Oncol* **26**(12): 2464–2469.

106 Sartor O (2017). Biomarkers in Prostate Cancer: PARP Inhibitors and Defects in DNA Repair – The ASCO Post. [online] Ascopost.com. Available at: http://www.ascopost.com/issues/march-25-2016/biomarkers-in-prostate-cancer-parp-inhibitors-and-defects-in-dna-repair/ [Accessed December 13, 2017].

107 Bankhead C (2017). CDK4/6 Inhibitors Live Up To Predictions – MedPage Today. [online] medpagetoday.com. Available at: http://www.medpagetoday.com/hematologyoncology/BreastCancer/62306 [Accessed December 13, 2017].

CHAPTER 5

Immunotherapies for Cancer

IN BRIEF

Immunotherapies – treatments that use the immune system to destroy cancer – have been around for over a century. But only in the last ten years or so have they become really exciting. Most of the current buzz around immunotherapies is around a group of monoclonal antibody treatments called checkpoint inhibitors, which stop cancer-fighting white blood cells from being suppressed.

The first checkpoint inhibitor to become a licensed cancer treatment was ipilimumab (Yervoy) in 2011, which targets a checkpoint protein found on T cells called CTLA-4. Since that time, many more checkpoint inhibitors have come on the scene. For example, nivolumab (Opdivo), pembrolizumab (Keytruda), atezolizumab (Tecentriq), durvalumab (Imfinzi), and avelumab (Bavencio) are licensed for various solid tumors and for Hodgkin lymphoma. These antibodies target either a checkpoint protein called PD-1 or one of its ligands, PD-L1. Antibodies that target CTLA-4, PD-1, and PD-L1 reverse the suppression of T cells, and in some patients they create a strong anti-cancer immune response.

As well as checkpoint inhibitors, two other immunotherapy approaches have produced exciting clinical trials results: CAR-modified T cell therapy and TILs (tumor infiltrating lymphocytes). Both these methods rely on reprogramming, or precisely selecting, the patient's own white blood cells. At the current time, CAR-modified T cells are looking most exciting for hematological cancers, and TILs are looking most exciting for malignant melanoma. In the years to come, no doubt their use will extend to other cancer types.

Scientists are also making steady progress in creating cancer treatment vaccines – treatments that increase the visibility of the patient's cancer to their immune system. These vaccines come in many forms, but their collective goal is to activate dendritic cells – the patrolmen of our immune system, which then alert T cells to the cancer's presence.

In this chapter, I shall attempt to explain all the immunotherapy approaches described above. In order to do this, I will also need to teach you about (or at least refresh and expand your knowledge of) our immune system.

A Beginner's Guide to Targeted Cancer Treatments, First Edition. Elaine Vickers.
© 2018 John Wiley & Sons Ltd. Published 2018 by John Wiley & Sons Ltd.

5.1 INTRODUCTION

The fact that someone has cancer indicates that at least two important things have happened:

1. **One of their cells has sustained damage in the form of DNA mutations** that have caused it to become a cancer cell. This cell has then multiplied many times to become a detectable tumor or blood cancer.
2. For some reason, **their immune system has failed to recognize and destroy the cancer cells**.

So far in this book, I have focused on the DNA mutations inside cancer cells, and I have introduced you to lots of treatments that target the consequences of these mutations.

It's now time to shift our attention away from DNA mutations and look at the interaction between cancer cells and our immune system. It might feel like treatments that use a patient's immune system against cancer (the so-called immunotherapies) are a new invention, but in fact they've been around for over 100 years.[1] However, the current explosion of interest and optimism began in 2011 with the approval of ipilimumab (Yervoy) as a treatment for malignant melanoma. Since then, cancer immunotherapy has been named Breakthrough of the Year for 2013 by the prestigious Science magazine [1], and it's generated thousands of column inches in newspapers and websites around the world.

Currently there are five main groups of immunotherapies:

1. **Treatments that boost the immune system** in a relatively nonspecific way. Examples include interferon-alpha and interleukin-2.
2. **Antibodies that attach to proteins** (such as CD antigens or growth factor receptors) **on the surface of cancer cells** and that attract complement proteins and white blood cells which attack and destroy the cancer cells. Examples include many of the monoclonal antibodies I describe in Chapters 3, 4, and 7, as well as genetically modified, **bi-specific antibodies** (also called **bi-specific T cell engagers – BiTE**) that tether together cancer cells with white blood cells.
3. Treatments that **encourage the body's white blood cells to attack and destroy cancer cells** and that **overcome cancer cells' ability to suppress white blood cells**. Examples include thalidomide and its derivatives lenalidomide and pomalidomide (discussed in Chapter 7, Section 7.7); the BCG vaccine for bladder cancer (described in Chapter 6, Section 6.10); **checkpoint inhibitors** such as antibodies that target-CTLA-4, PD-1, and PD-L1.
4. Approaches in which the patient's own white blood cells are removed from their blood, modified in the laboratory, and put back into their bloodstream (this is called **adoptive cell transfer**). Examples include CAR (chimeric antigen receptor)-modified T cells, tumor-infiltrating lymphocytes (TILs), and modified dendritic cells.
5. Treatments that are injected into the patient (usually into skin or muscle) and that "educate" their white blood cells and teach them to recognize and destroy cancer cells. Examples include **peptide and DNA vaccines and oncolytic viruses**.[2]

In this chapter, I will tell you about some, but not all, of the approaches I've just listed.

---

[1] In the late 1800s and early 1900s, an American doctor called William Coley experimented with injecting bacteria into patients with various sarcomas to trigger cancer-fighting immune reactions; by the end of his career, he had treated almost 900 patients (Parish CR (2003). *Immunol & Cell Biol.* 81: 106–113).

[2] It's important to note that the word *vaccine* is used to mean different things. I am using the term to refer to **treatments** that are put into the patient's body and that activate their white blood cells *in situ* to attack and destroy cancer cells. I'm not going to talk at all about vaccines that are used to prevent cancer.

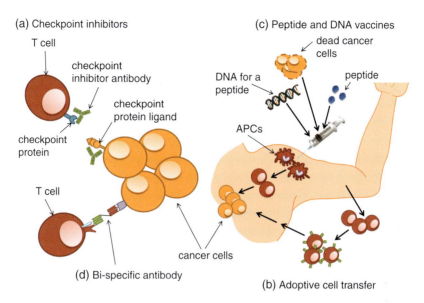

Figure 5.1 **Mechanism of action of various cancer immunotherapies. (a)** The majority of checkpoint inhibitors are monoclonal antibodies that attach to checkpoint proteins, or their ligands, on the surface of white blood cells (such as T cells) or cancer cells. By disrupting the interaction between the checkpoint protein and its ligand, the antibody increases the white blood cells' activity. **(b)** Adoptive cell transfer requires T cells (or other white blood cells) to be purified from the patient's blood. These are then modified in the laboratory and infused back into the patient, where they attack cancer cells. **(c)** Peptide and DNA vaccines are either small fragments (peptides) of proteins found on the surface of cancer cells, or the DNA for such a peptide. The DNA or peptide is injected into the skin or muscle, where it is picked up by an antigen-presenting cell (APC). The APC (usually a dendritic cell) displays the peptide on its surface (it may first need to make the peptide from the injected DNA) and presents it to T cells in lymph nodes. After receiving instructions from APCs, T cells move into the tumor and attack cancer cells. Vaccines can also be made from dead cancer cells. These are again injected into the body, where APCs digest them and display peptides from them on their surface. **(d)** Bi-specific antibodies are modified antibodies that create a physical link between cancer cells and T cells, triggering the cell-killing activity of the T cell. *Source:* Syringe image: https://upload. wikimedia.org/wikipedia/commons/3/3b/Needle_syringe.png DNA image: https://commons.wikimedia. org/wiki/File:Difference_DNA_RNA-EN.svg Arm: https://pixabay.com/en/hand-arm-man-strong-muscle-159326/ **Abbreviations:** APC – antigen-presenting cell

Treatments I cover in detail are **checkpoint inhibitors** (Figure 5.1a) and **adoptive cell transfer** (particularly CAR-modified T cells) (Figure 5.1b). I also describe **cell-based, peptide, and DNA vaccines** (Figure 5.1c) and **bi-specific antibodies** (Figure 5.1d). I'll discuss bi-specific antibodies immediately after I describe adoptive cell transfer, as there are similarities between them.

However, there are some immunotherapies that I *won't* be mentioning further in this chapter. For example, I'm not going to talk about general boosters of the immune system, as they're not targeted. And I won't talk further about antibodies that attach to cancer cell surface proteins because I've already covered many of them in other chapters. Also, I describe thalidomide and the BCG vaccine elsewhere, so there's no need to cover them here.

We'll start with some general information about how cancer and our immune system interact, as this should help you understand the various treatments I describe later in the chapter.

5.2 A BIT ABOUT CANCER AND THE IMMUNE SYSTEM

If you'd like to learn a bit about the immune system before we start, then you might want to get hold of an immunology textbook, such as *How the Immune System Works* by Lauren Sompayrac [2] or, for more detail, the classic undergraduate textbook is Janeway's *Immunobiology* [3]. Or you could look on YouTube for immunology lectures. For example, a student in the United States called Armando Hasudungan has created a series of illustrated videos that introduce you to many immunology concepts (http://armandoh. org/subjects/immunology). As he says himself, his videos don't cover everything, but they're a great starting point if you've not learned any immunology before.

Also, before I get into the nuts and bolts of how various types of immunotherapy work, it's helpful if you understand how cancer cells manage to avoid destruction by the immune system (this follows on from Section 1.3.1 in Chapter 1).

Probably the first thing to remind you of is that most cancers contain millions of white blood cells [4] (see Box 5.1 for a description of various types of white blood cells). Some of

---

Box 5.1 Descriptions of some of the white blood cells mentioned in this chapter

Antigen-presenting cells (APCs) – These include dendritic cells and macrophages. These cells display protein fragments (**peptides**) to T cells using their major histocompatibility complex (MHC) proteins. Any peptide (or other molecule) that triggers an immune response is called an **antigen**.

B cells – Specialized lymphocytes that have B cell receptors (BCRs) on their surface. When they are mature, they move to lymph nodes and other lymphoid organs (like the spleen). If their BCRs attach to an antigen (such as a protein from a bacterium or virus), the B cell may become fully active. When active, B cells move back to the bone marrow, where they become antibody-producing **plasma cells**.

Dendritic cells – Starfish-shaped APCs that shuttle between tissues and lymphoid organs (such as lymph nodes, spleen, and tonsils). In the tissues they pick up antigens. They then move to lymph nodes and other lymphoid organs, where they display peptides from these antigens to T cells. A different set of dendritic cells – the follicular dendritic cells – spend their whole life in lymph nodes and other lymph tissues. They capture antigens delivered to them by the flow of lymph fluid, and display them via MHC proteins to B cells.

Macrophages – The most versatile, jack-of-all-trades cells of the immune system. They are myeloid cells found in the skin, lungs, and other tissues. They have the capacity to ingest and destroy invaders, act as **APCs** and activate T cells, and rid the body of cell debris. However, whereas dendritic cells can shuttle to lymph nodes and other lymphoid organs, macrophages stay put in our organs and tissues.

Mast cells – Myeloid cells with histamine-containing granules inside them. Release of their histamine granules helps fight infections but also causes allergic reactions and inflammation.

Myeloid-derived suppressor cells – Scientists don't really understand these cells, but large numbers of them are found inside tumors and in the blood of cancer patients. They can suppress cytotoxic T cells and also seem to be involved in angiogenesis.

Neutrophils – Short-lived myeloid cells that enter tissues and destroy infections. They are the most numerous white blood cells in our body.

T cells (T lymphocytes):

- **Helper T cells** – T cells that respond via their T cell receptor (TCR) to peptides presented to them by APCs via **MHC class 2** proteins. They require further activation signals (called "co-stimulatory signals") from APCs to become fully active. Once active, they then activate B cells and enhance the activity of other white blood cells.

- **Cytotoxic T cells** (**CTLs**) – T cells that respond via their TCR to peptides presented to them by APCs via **MHC class 1** proteins. Once they have received the necessary co-stimulatory signals from the APC, they leave the lymph node and directly destroy virus-infected cells and cancer cells in the affected tissue by releasing cell-killing enzymes.

- **Regulatory T cells** (**Tregs**) – T cells whose job it is to suppress any T cells that might otherwise attack the body's tissues and cause autoimmune diseases; they also prevent overactivity of T cells that would otherwise cause tissue damage.

- **Natural killer (NK) cells** – Short-lived T cells that enter tissues, release cytokines, and directly destroy virus-infected cells and cancer cells.

these will be healthy white blood cells that are trying to fight cancer cells, while others will have been influenced by cancer cells and could now be helping them. In order to survive in a white-blood-cell-rich environment, cancer cells have to [5]:

1. **Live (and thrive) alongside white blood cells**
2. **Avoid being recognized** as being faulty by white blood cells that might attack them
3. Be able to **suppress any white blood cells** that do recognize them and try to destroy them

All three of these attributes are important when it comes to understanding immunotherapy, so I'll explain them in more detail below.

5.2.1 Cancer Cells Thrive alongside Millions of White Blood Cells

There are two main groups of white blood cells in our body: myeloid cells, which cause inflammation and are often involved in innate immune responses; and lymphoid cells, which mount precise attacks on invaders and are involved in adaptive immune responses (see

Box 5.2 for more on innate and adaptive immunity). Myeloid cells include macrophages, neutrophils, eosinophils, and mast cells. Lymphoid cells include B and T lymphocytes (known as B cells and T cells) and NK cells.

Cancers often contain millions of myeloid, inflammatory cells. In fact, chronic inflammation often precedes cancer and is frequently one of the reasons why the cancer came about. For example, inflammatory bowel disease puts people at risk of bowel cancer; pancreatitis can lead to pancreatic cancer; chronic liver disease often precedes liver cancer; and so on. In fact, scientists estimate that that infections and inflammatory responses are linked to 15%–20% of cancers worldwide [6].

Even when a cancer is not preceded by inflammation, it still contains inflammatory cells. This is because DNA mutations in cancer cells (such as *KRAS*, *BRAF*, and *MYC* mutations) and other faults cause cancer cells to produce signaling molecules that attract white blood cells from the bloodstream [6].

Whatever the reason for the presence of inflammatory white blood cells in a cancer,

Box 5.2   Innate and adaptive immune responses

Our body's response to infections can be split into two categories: (1) innate responses, which are almost immediate, and (2) adaptive responses, which are more precise but generally take a few days to kick in.

Innate immune responses involve lots of different types of myeloid cells such as neutrophils, macrophages, and dendritic cells. These cells ingest and destroy microbes by swallowing them up and then chemically attacking them. Innate immune responses also involve complement proteins, which circulate in the blood and attach to bacteria and other microbes. Complement proteins can clump together and directly kill some microbes, and they also help with adaptive responses. NK cells also participate in innate immune responses; they detect and destroy damaged and infected cells.

Adaptive immune responses involve two main sets of cells, the B and T lymphocytes (B and T cells). B cells can respond directly to infections via B cell receptors (BCRs) on their surface. In order to become fully active in response to an infection, they generally also need some help from specialized T cells called helper T cells and from dendritic cells. When a B cell is activated, it moves to the bone marrow and releases antibodies into the blood, or it becomes a long-lasting memory cell. T cells respond to infections through their T cell receptors (TCRs). Their TCRs bind to peptides (antigens) from bacteria and other microbes. But T cells can only recognize peptides if they are displayed to them by antigen-presenting cells (APCs) such as dendritic cells and macrophages. The initial activation of T cells is dependent on dendritic cells, but their continued activation depends on macrophages. It generally takes B and T cells a couple of days to become active, multiply, and participate in the immune response.

For more information on each cell type, see Box 5.1.

once there, they come into contact with lots of growth factors and other molecules released by cancer cells. In response to these signals, the inflammatory white blood cells release yet more signaling molecules that help cancer cells survive and thrive [6]. For example, inflammatory white blood cells produce a wide range of growth factors and cytokines[3] that trigger signaling pathways, protect cancer cells against apoptosis,[4] and facilitate metastasis and angiogenesis. A good example of their actions is in pancreatic cancer – see Figure 5.2 for some extra detail.

5.2.2 Cancer Cells Avoid Being Recognized and Destroyed by White Blood Cells

One of the functions of our white blood cells is to patrol the body looking for infections and for signs that cells have become damaged or faulty. This process is possible because all our cells constantly display their inner workings on their surface, so that passing white blood cells can see what's going on inside them. Cells do this by chopping up some of the proteins they make and putting fragments (peptides) of these proteins on their surface along with a protein called

---

[3] Cytokines are small proteins involved in cell-to-cell communication in immune responses; they can also guide white blood cells toward sites of inflammation, infection, and injury.
[4] Apoptosis is an orderly process our cells go through in which they die neatly and cleanly and without causing inflammation; it's also called "programmed cell death."

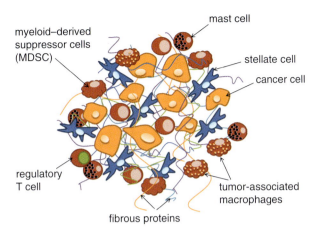

Figure 5.2 The role of white blood cells in promoting pancreatic cancer. **Mast cells** secrete growth factors that promote angiogenesis and invasion. They also produce cytokines that prevent other white blood cells from attacking cancer cells. **Tumor-associated macrophages** facilitate tumor growth and metastasis (particularly into lymph nodes). **Myeloid-derived suppressor cells (MDSC)** are immature white blood cells that actively suppress any anti-cancer immune cells (e.g., cytotoxic T cells). **Regulatory T cells** suppress cytotoxic T cells. Their presence is associated with increased aggressiveness of the cancer. Other cells in the pancreatic cancer microenvironment include **stellate cells** and **fibroblasts**, which produce and secrete a wide range of fibrous proteins such as collagen and fribronectin [7].
Abbreviations: MDSC – myeloid-derived suppressor cell

MHC[5] class 1 (Figure 5.3a). Special T cells (called cytotoxic T cells) that are passing by take a look at the peptides presented to them and decide whether they are normal peptides or faulty ones. If the peptides indicate that the cell is infected by a virus or has become faulty, the T cell immediately releases toxic, cell-killing enzymes that destroy the faulty cell.

Cancer cells often contain hundreds, if not thousands, of DNA mutations. They therefore also contain lots of damaged proteins. Cancer cells that display peptides made from damaged proteins are in danger of being spotted and destroyed by passing T cells.[6] As a result, those cancer cells that survive are the ones that for some reason (such as due to a fault in their MHC class 1 proteins) are not putting

tell-tale peptides on their surface, or that have become invulnerable to the cell-killing attempts of white blood cells [8] (Figure 5.3b).

Even when cancer cells don't present mutated peptides on their surface, it is still possible for them to alert our immune system to their presence. This is primarily because tumors generally contain lots of dead and dying cancer cells (this could be because the cells are multiplying too quickly and/or chaotically to have an adequate blood supply, or because of the effects of a treatment). Peptides from these dead and dying cells can be picked up by dendritic cells (see Box 5.1), which display them on their surface with MHC class 1 and MHC class 2 proteins[7] (Figure 5.3c) (for more on MHC proteins, see Box 5.3). The dendritic cells then move to nearby

---

[5] MHC stands for major histocompatibility complex.
[6] The fact that our immune system destroys cancer cells with tell-tale cancer peptides on their surface is known as "immune surveillance."
[7] Only APCs have both MHC class 1 and class 2 proteins. I wouldn't get too hung up on understanding the reasons why, but if it's bugging you, I suggest reading the chapter called "The Magic of Antigen Presentation" in Lauren Sompayrac's book *How the Immune System Works*.

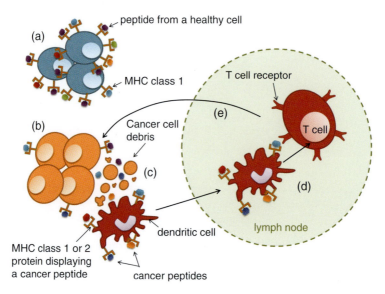

Figure 5.3 **Even cancer cells with few peptides on their surface can trigger an immune response.**
(a) Healthy cells display a wide range of peptides on the surface in conjunction with MHC class 1 proteins. These peptides are representative of the proteins the cell is making. **(b)** Cancer cells hide from the immune system by displaying a limited number of peptides on their surface. **(c)** Debris from dead and dying cancer cells includes peptides from mutated proteins. These peptides are picked up by antigen-presenting cells (APCs) known as dendritic cells, which ingest the peptides and then display them on their surface in conjunction with MHC class 1 and class 2 proteins. **(d)** Dendritic cells displaying cancer peptides move to lymph nodes, where they display the peptides to T cells. **(e)** Some T cells recognize the peptides displayed to them with their T cell receptors and mount an anti-cancer immune response.
Abbreviations: MHC – major histocompatibility complex

Box 5.3   MHC proteins [12, 13]

MHC (major histocompatibility complex) proteins come in two flavors: MHC class 1 and MHC class 2. Whereas all our cells have MHC class 1 proteins on their surface, only specialized cells called antigen-presenting cells (APCs) have MHC class 2 proteins on their surface. MHC proteins allow our cells to present small protein fragments (peptides) to one another.

MHC class 1 proteins are used by our cells to display peptides that they have manufactured themselves. Our cells use their MHC class 1 proteins to tell our immune system what they're making. So if a cell is infected by a virus, it will display peptides from the virus on its MHC class 1 proteins. In this way, the infected cell is notifying the immune system that it has been infected. The white blood cells that monitor and respond to what peptides our cells display on their MHC class 1 proteins are the cytotoxic T cells.

MHC class 2 proteins are found on APCs such as dendritic cells, which use them to display peptides that they have picked up from their environment. For example, if a dendritic cell is in an infected tissue, or in a tumor, it will pick up lots of protein fragments from its environment and display them via its MHC class 2 proteins. The dendritic cell then travels to a lymph node, where it displays these peptides to helper T cells in order to find those that recognize the peptide and can mount a response. Through a process called cross-presentation, dendritic cells can also display peptides from cancer proteins to cytotoxic T cells via MHC class 1.

lymph nodes and show their peptides to helper T cells and cytotoxic T cells. If a dendritic cell finds a T cell whose T cell receptor (TCR) matches the damaged peptide, the dendritic cell will activate it. If the dendritic cell has activated a helper T cell, the T cell will then activate B cells and enhance the activities of other white blood cells. If the dendritic cell has activated a cytotoxic T cell, the T cell will move to the tumor and destroy cancer cells [9–11] (Figures 5.3d and e).

In order to survive, cancer cells must avoid having mutated peptides on their surface. And they must also avoid leaking mutated peptides into their surroundings. Or, if they can't avoid having mutated peptides on their surface or leaking them into their surroundings, they must find a way to suppress white blood cells that try to destroy them — which brings us to our next section.

5.2.3 Cancer Cells Suppress White Blood Cells That Try to Destroy Them

Cancer cells use a variety of methods to suppress any white blood cells that try to destroy them. For example [9, 11]:

- Cancer cells secrete growth factors and other signaling molecules (e.g., prostaglandin E2, TGF-β, and IL-10) that **directly suppress cancer-fighting white blood cells** such as cytotoxic T cells.
- Signaling molecules released by cancer cells **attract and activate immune-suppressing white blood cells** such as regulatory T cells (Tregs), myeloid-derived suppressor cells (MDSCs), and certain types of B cells. These white blood cells suppress any cancer-fighting cytotoxic T cells or NK cells in their vicinity. (See Box 5.4 for more about immune-suppressing white blood cells.)
- Cancer cells (and white blood cells) sometimes **manufacture and release IDO** (indoleamine 2,3-dioxygenase), which suppresses the activity of T cells [14]

- Tumor blood vessels and growth factors that cause angiogenesis (such as VEGF[8]) act as a **barrier against the passage of cytotoxic T cells** into the tumor.
- Cancer cells display **proteins on their surface that directly kill T cells**. They also display proteins that **suppress the actions of T cells**. These proteins, known as inhibitory checkpoint proteins, include PD-L1 and PD-L2.
- The continued presence of cancer cells in a tissue can gradually lead to a phenomenon called **immune tolerance** (see Box 5.5), in which white blood cells' activity is suppressed in response to continued interaction with the same antigen.[9]
- Cancer cells seem able to **suppress the activities of dendritic cells** and limit their capacity to display cancer peptides on their surface to activate T cells. In addition, in many tumors, dendritic cells in the tumor (as well as cancer cells) have PD-L1 on their surface, which suppresses T cell activity [9].

Box 5.4 Why do we have immune-suppressing white blood cells?

Our immune system fights off infections and keeps us healthy. However, it's important that immune responses don't outlive their usefulness. If immune responses last too long, the activated white blood cells will start doing damage to otherwise healthy tissues and organs. Hence, we have white blood cells such as regulatory T cells that exist to suppress and restrain other white blood cells. In addition, these restraining white blood cells prevent our immune system from destroying helpful bacteria in our gut, and they help prevent a pregnant woman from destroying the growing embryo in her womb.

---

[8] VEGF – vascular endothelial growth factor; for more about this, see Chapter 4, Section 4.1.
[9] "Antigen" is a general term for anything (generally a peptide) that a B cell or T cell can respond to via their T cell or B cell receptors. Cancer cells have many antigens on their surface.

Box 5.5   Immune tolerance

Immune tolerance is essential to life. It describes the fact that our immune system is able to ignore (and therefore doesn't attack) the normal proteins and other molecules that make up our body. If our immune system can't ignore our own healthy proteins, then we develop autoimmune diseases. However, cancers often hide from the immune system by inducing immune tolerance. If the immune system is tolerant to cancer cells and believes that they're normal, it will no longer try to attack them.

However, despite all these mechanisms of immune suppression, **some patients' cancers do contain active, cancer-fighting cytotoxic T cells**. And the presence of cytotoxic T cells in a patient's cancer is generally a good sign and is associated with longer survival times [9]. The presence of these cells in some cancers has encouraged scientists to develop immunotherapies – treatments that use the immune system to attack cancer.

The overarching goal of most cancer immunotherapies is to activate cancer-fighting cytotoxic T cells, as these cells that have the ability to directly kill cancer cells. Each immunotherapy approach achieves this goal through a different mechanism, outlined in Table 5.1.

Having set the scene, I'll now go into more detail about these four groups of treatments.

5.3 CHECKPOINT INHIBITORS

When a doctor prescribes a checkpoint inhibitor for a patient, their hope is that it will activate any cancer-fighting T cells in the patient's body that are being suppressed via the checkpoint proteins on their surface.

At the time of writing this book in 2017, the only checkpoint inhibitors that are licensed cancer treatments are those that target checkpoint proteins called **CTLA-4, PD-1, and PD-L1**. I'm therefore going to focus on these three proteins in this chapter.

However, there are many other checkpoint proteins on human white blood cells (see Figure 5.4). And many of these proteins are being investigated by scientists and pharmaceutical companies as potential cancer drug targets. So, in future, there are likely to be a wide range of checkpoint inhibitors licensed for use that have other targets [10, 15].

Table 5.1   Mechanisms of different cancer immunotherapies.

Approach	Goal	Examples
Checkpoint inhibitors	To block inhibitory checkpoint proteins on the surface of cancer cells and on white blood cells and thereby activate pre-existing, cancer-fighting cytotoxic T cells (Figure 5.1a)	Nivolumab (Opdivo), pembrolizumab (Keytruda), atezolizumab (Tecentriq), durvalumab (Imfinzi), avelumab (Bavencio), ipilimumab (Yervoy) and tremelimumab
Adoptive cell transfer	To infuse into the body an army of cancer-fighting white blood cells (Figure 5.1b)	CD19-directed CAR T cell therapy, Provenge (dendritic cells modified with prostatic acid phosphatase), tumor-infiltrating lymphocytes
Cell-based, DNA, and peptide vaccines	To increase the number of dendritic cells that display cancer peptides on their surface and that activate cytotoxic T cells and helper T cells (Figure 5.1c)	Neuvax, L-BLP25, Allostim, OncoVAX, GV1001
Bi-specific antibodies	To physically tether together cancer cells with T cells in such a way that the T cell destroys the cancer cell (Figure 5.1d)	Blinatumomab (Blincyto)

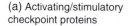

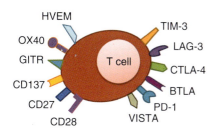

Figure 5.4 Some of the checkpoint proteins on the surface of T cells. As well as having the T cell receptor (TCR) on their surface, T cells also produce a wide range of **(a)** activating and **(b)** inhibitory checkpoint proteins that fine-tune their activity [11]. **Abbreviations:** TCR – T cell receptor

5.3.1 Introducing Checkpoint Proteins

Cytotoxic T cells (also called cytotoxic T lymphocytes – CTLs) have the capacity to directly destroy our body's cells. Their purpose is to move to sites of infection or disease and kill virus-infected cells and other faulty cells such as cancer cells. However, their activities must be tightly controlled so that they only become active under the right circumstances. And, once they are active, the body needs a mechanism to suppress them (otherwise they would start destroying the body's healthy tissues). Thus, CTLs have a range of proteins on their surface, known as checkpoint proteins, through which the body can control their activity [11, 15].

Some checkpoint proteins on CTLs help them become fully active. These are the **activating checkpoint proteins** (Figure 5.4a). For example, in order for a CTL to become fully active, two things need to happen. First, the CTL's T cell receptor (TCR) has to recognize and connect to an antigen presented to it by a dendritic cell. Second, an activating checkpoint protein on the T cell called CD28 has to interact with a protein on the dendritic cell called B7. If these two interactions take place, then the CTL will become active (Figure 5.5a).

CTLs also display on their surface a range of **inhibitory checkpoint proteins** (Figure 5.4b). These proteins limit the activity of T cells and make sure they do not remain active after a threat has passed. For example, soon after (i.e., within 24-48 hours) a CTL becomes active, and while it is still in a lymph node, it starts to display an inhibitory checkpoint protein called CTLA-4 (cytotoxic T lymphocyte-associated molecule-4) [16]. CTLA-4 binds much more tightly to B7 than CD28, and thus it displaces CD28 (Figure 5.5b). When CTLA-4 connects with B7, the T cell's activity is suppressed [15].

5.3.2 CTLA-4

As you've just heard, when CTLA-4 on the surface of CTL connects with CD28, the CTL's activity is suppressed. Other T cells, such as helper T cells and regulatory T cells, also have CTLA-4 on their surface. Helper T cells (like CTLs) are suppressed when CTLA-4 connects with B7. However, the opposite is true for regulatory T cells (Tregs). When a Treg's CTLA-4 connects with B7, the Treg's activity increases [15] (Figure 5.5c).

Thus, **CTLA-4 activation suppresses the actions of CTLs and helper T cells but enhances the activity of Tregs**. If this happens after an infection has been cleared up, it's a good thing, as it means that infection-fighting T cells are suppressed, which prevents wasteful immune responses. Also, if the helper T cells or CTLs being blocked recognize proteins on healthy tissues, then suppressing them avoids tissue damage. However, if the T cells in question recognize a protein found only on the surface of cancer cells, then by blocking them the body is unintentionally allowing the cancer to thrive.

5.3.3 Monoclonal Antibodies That Block CTLA-4

Hopefully, from the information above, you get the idea that blocking CTLA-4 might be a helpful way of treating people with cancer.

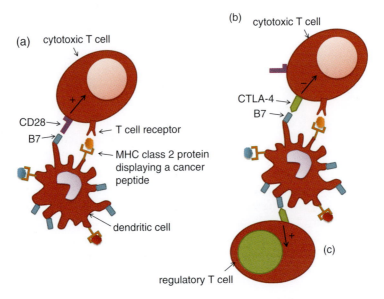

Figure 5.5 Activation and suppression of T cell activity via CD28 and CTLA-4. **(a)** Activation (+) of a cytotoxic T cell by a dendritic cell requires two signals: (1) the T cell receptor must interact with an antigen displayed to it by an antigen-presenting cell such as a dendritic cell, and (2) the CD28 protein on the T cell must engage with B7. **(b)** The activity of cytotoxic T cells is suppressed (–) when inhibitory checkpoint proteins on its surface are triggered. In this instance, suppression is mediated by CTLA-4, an inhibitory checkpoint protein found on active T cells, which, like CD28, interacts with B7. **(c)** CTLA-4 is also found on the surface of regulatory T cells (Tregs). Interaction between B7 and CTLA-4 on Tregs increases (+) their activity. **Abbreviations:** MHC – major histocompatibility complex; Treg – regulatory T cell; CTLA-4 - Cytotoxic T lymphocyte-associated molecule-4

This is because **a CTLA-4-blocking antibody would (1) increase the activity of CTLs and helper T cells and (2) suppress the activity of Tregs**. However, this will only benefit the patient if some of the CTLs and helper T cells in their body know how to recognize and fight cancer cells, and if these same T cells are being suppressed via CTLA-4 on their surface.

It's also important to remember that CTLA-4 is used by the body to **prevent any unwanted immune responses by T cells**. And it plays an important role in protecting us from protracted immune responses and tissue damage [17]. As a result, when CTLA-4 is blocked, this increases the activity of any T cells in the body that are being suppressed via

CTLA-4, often causing severe inflammatory reactions that cause diarrhea, rashes, hepatitis, and pituitary inflammation [18].

The most well-known and widely used anti-CTLA-4 antibody is ipilimumab (Yervoy). This antibody was approved as a treatment for malignant melanoma in the United States and Europe in 2011. A second CTLA-4-targeted antibody in many phase 3 trials is tremelimumab.

Response rates in trials with ipilimumab tend to be around 10%–30% [19, 20] (the wide range is partly because it depends on what you define as a response[10]). And some of the people who respond are still alive many years later [21, 22]. That is, ipilimumab can create an

---

[10] Some people who benefit from ipilimumab wouldn't be counted using standard criteria because the response is very delayed or the cancer doesn't shrink but remains stable for many months or years.

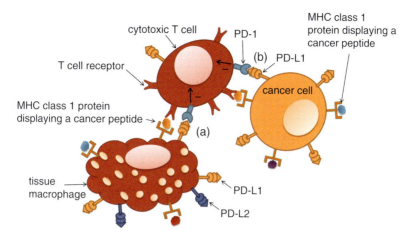

Figure 5.6 Suppression of T cells via PD-1 ligands. Once a cytotoxic T cell has been activated by dendritic cells in a lymph node, it moves out into the tissues. **(a)** In the body's tissues (e.g., in a cancer or at the site of an infection), the T cell's activity can be maintained by tissue macrophages that display peptides via their MHC class 1 and class 2 proteins. However, tissue macrophages also display PD-L1 and PD-L1, which attach to PD-1 and shut down the T cell's activity. **(b)** Cancer cells in solid tumors frequently have PD-L1 on their surface, through which they can suppress T cells with PD-1 on their surface.
Abbreviations: PD-1 – programmed cell death protein-1; MHC – major histocompatibility complex

immune response that keeps people alive for many years and potentially cures some people – something that you don't see with a B-Raf inhibitor. One unusual feature of treatment with ipilimumab is that tumors sometimes become bigger before they shrink. This is called "**pseudoprogression**," and it's thought to be a consequence of millions of white blood cells entering the tumor. It can also occur with other checkpoint inhibitors [15, 23].

5.3.4 PD-1 and PD-L1

PD-1[11] (programmed cell death protein-1), like CTLA-4, is an inhibitory checkpoint protein. However, whereas CTLA-4 controls the initial response of T cells to an infection, PD-1 is found on activated T cells out in the body's tissues.[12] The normal, healthy purpose of PD-1

is to prevent T cells from being active for too long, and to prevent autoimmune diseases [15]. As well as being found on cytotoxic T cells (CTLs) and helper T cells, PD-1 is also found on mature B cells, NK cells, dendritic cells, and Tregs [24].

There are two ligands[13] for PD-1, known as PD-L1 and PD-L2, both of which are found on the surface of tissue macrophages (Figure 5.6a). These white blood cells live permanently in our tissues. They act as a first line of defense against pathogens,[14] and they also control how long immune responses last. As well as being found on tissue macrophages, PD-1 ligands are also found on dendritic cells and, crucially, on cancer cells. In fact, cancer cells from a wide range of solid tumors (such as melanomas, ovarian cancers, bowel cancers, and lung cancers) and some hematological

---

[11] PD-1 is also called B7-H1.
[12] T cells that have CTLA-4 on their surface are generally still in the lymph node where they became active.
[13] A ligand is anything (e.g., a hormone, peptide, protein, or drug) that can attach to a receptor.
[14] Pathogen is a general term for anything (e.g., bacteria and viruses) that can cause disease.

cancers (such as Hodgkin lymphoma) have PD-L1 on their surface [25]. And a handful of cancers are known to produce PD-L2, such as Hodgkin lymphoma and some non-Hodgkin lymphomas [26].

As with CTLA-4, the activation of PD-1 has different effects on different cells. **When PD-1 on CTLs, helper T cells or B cells is activated, the T cell or B cell's activity decreases. However, activation of PD-1 on Tregs increases their activity and causes them to multiply** [15]. Cancer cells with PD-L1 on their surface can therefore use this protein to actively suppress CTLs that try to destroy them (Figure 5.6b), and to increase the activity of Tregs.

So, as with anti-CTLA-4 antibodies, **the purpose of antibodies targeted against PD-1 and PD-L1 is to increase the activity of CTLs, helper T cells, and B cells** (it's mostly the CTLs that scientists are interested in) **and decrease the activity of Tregs**. PD-1 antibodies and PD-L1 antibodies will hopefully predominantly activate T cells inside the patient's tumor. This is in contrast to CTLA-4 antibodies, which will potentially activate all suppressed T cells throughout the body.

5.3.5 Monoclonal Antibodies That Block PD-1 and PD-L1

PD-1 and PD-L1 targeted antibodies, like CTLA-4 targeted antibodies, are **designed to avoid or reverse the suppression of cancer-fighting T cells**. But these antibodies are subtly different from one another in their effects. Antibodies that target PD-1 prevent PD-1 on the surface of T cells from interacting with either of its ligands (PD-L1 and PD-L2), which might be on the surface of cancer cells or other white blood cells in the cancer microenvironment; whereas antibodies that target PD-L1 prevent PD-1 from interacting with PD-L1, but still allow PD-1 to interact with PD-L2. Because of this difference, some scientists thought that PD-L1-targeted antibodies would

be less likely to cause side effects than PD-1-targeted antibodies [27]. However, in reality, it seems their effects are very similar [28].

Various anti-PD-1 and anti-PD-L1 antibodies have been licensed as cancer treatments (see Table 5.2), but there are no PD-L2 antibodies licensed [26]. Most clinical trials so far have involved people with solid tumors such as malignant melanoma, kidney cancer, non-small cell lung cancer (NSCLC), bladder cancer, and head and neck cancer, but this is just the tip of the iceberg. Anti-PD-1 and anti-PD-L1 antibodies have so far proved useful in more than 15 different types of cancer [29, 30]. And many thousands of people with various cancers are currently being recruited into clinical trials. So I expect we'll see these antibodies licensed for numerous other cancer types in the next few years.

I've listed in Table 5.2 just the PD-1 and PD-L1 antibodies that are licensed as cancer treatments. But do be aware that there are far more antibodies being developed than the handful that I've listed, and some of them are being investigated in trials involving many hundreds of people. It's therefore likely that by the time you read this book, there will be more PD-1 and PD-L1 antibodies licensed as cancer treatments.

In trials that have investigated PD-1 and PD-L1 antibodies for people with advanced melanoma, generally around 30%–40% of them have benefited from this treatment [30] (if you remember, the response rate with ipilimumab is often about 10%–30%). Melanoma trials have also shown that antibodies targeting PD-1 and PD-L1 are more effective, and cause milder side effects, than anti-CTLA4 antibodies [30]. Trials have also shown that **two antibodies** (an anti-CTLA-4 antibody plus an anti-PD1 antibody) **can work better in combination than either of them alone** [34], and the combination of nivolumab plus ipilimumab is licensed in Europe as a treatment for melanoma. However, when you combine a

Table 5.2 PD-1 and PD-L1 targeted antibodies licensed in the United States and Europe as of December 2017.

Antibody	Target	Stage of development[a] in the United States and Europe [31–33]
Nivolumab (Opdivo; BMS-936558)	PD-1	• Licensed in the United States and Europe for malignant melanoma, alone or in combination with ipilimumab (Yervoy) • Licensed in the United States and Europe for NSCLC • Licensed in the United States and Europe for head and neck cancer • Licensed in the United States and Europe for kidney cancer • Licensed in the United States and Europe for Hodgkin lymphoma • Licensed in the United States for bladder cancer • Licensed in the United States for primary liver cancer • Licensed in the United States for MSI-high or MMR-deficient colorectal cancer[*]
Pembrolizumab (Keytruda; MK-3475)	PD-1	• Licensed in the United States and Europe for malignant melanoma • Licensed in the United States and Europe for NSCLC • Licensed in the United States and Europe for Hodgkin lymphoma • Licensed in the United States and Europe for bladder cancer • Licensed in the United States for head and neck cancer • Licensed in the United States for stomach cancer • Licensed in the United States for MSI-high or MMR-deficient solid tumors[*]
Atezolizumab (Tecentriq; MPDL3280A)	PD-L1	• Licensed in the United States and Europe for bladder cancer • Licensed in the United States and Europe for NSCLC
Avelumab (Bavencio; MSB0010718C)	PD-L1	• Licensed in the United States and Europe for Merkel cell carcinoma[**]
Durvalumab (Imfinzi; MEDI4736)	PD-L1	• Licensed in the United States for bladder cancer

*These tumors have an exceptionally high number of mutations because the cells cannot perform a type of DNA repair called mismatch repair. They account for about 5% of metastatic bowel cancers and for a small percentage of various other tumor types.
Abbreviations: NSCLC – non-small cell lung cancer; MSI – microsatellite instability; MMR – mismatch repair; PD-1 – programmed death-1; PD-L1 – programmed death ligand-1.
**Merkel cell carcinoma is a rare and aggressive form of skin cancer.

CTLA-4 antibody with a PD-1 or PD-L1 antibody, this significantly increases the proportion of patients who experience severe side effects [34]. So it won't be possible to give everyone the combination.

As I write this in December 2017, there is a huge amount of optimism for the future of PD-1 and PD-L1 targeted antibodies. For example, eminent scientists say things like: "In terms of lives saved and person-years restored, immunotherapy promises to be more significant than any other form of treatment for patients whose tumours have already metastasized" [35].

However, it will be a few years before we understand who can potentially benefit from them and how best to use them. These antibodies will crop up again in Chapters 6 and 7 when I discuss targeted treatment approaches relevant to particular cancer types.

5.3.6 Biomarkers of Response to PD-1 and PD-L1 Antibodies

Because the majority of clinical trials with PD-1 and PD-L1-targeted antibodies give response rates of 10%–30% (the response rate varies greatly depending on the type of cancer), it's **essential that we find biomarkers** that can be used to pick out those patients most likely to benefit from them.

Not surprisingly, scientists think that anti-PD-1 and anti-PD-L1 antibodies will work

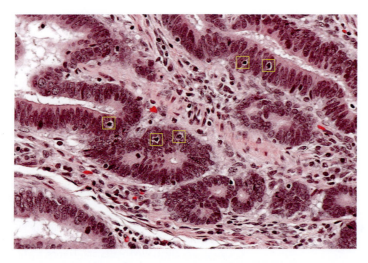

Figure 5.7 **An image taken through a microscope of a sample from a bowel cancer.** Some of the tumor-infiltrating lymphocytes have been highlighted in yellow boxes. The cells have been stained to make them show up more clearly. *Source:* https://commons.wikimedia.org/wiki/File:Tumour-infiltrating_lymphocytes_-_1_--_high_mag.jpg

best when there are CTLs in the cancer microenvironment that are being suppressed via PD-L1 (see Figure 5.7 to see what T cells infiltrating a tumor look like). But, this is not clear-cut; although PD-1 and PD-L1 antibodies often do seem to work best when you can detect the presence of PD-L1, some people benefit from these antibodies even when no PD-L1 can be found [29].

Another possible way to predict whether a patient will benefit from an anti-PD1 or anti-PD-L1 antibody is to look for CTLs in the outer margin of the tumor, as their presence appears to correlate with patient benefit [36].

In addition, people whose cancer cells have an extremely high number of mutations inside them (such as a lung cancer in a smoker) seem the most likely to have infiltrating T cells in them and to benefit from checkpoint inhibitors [37–39]. Therefore, measuring the number of mutations in a cancer might be another way of predicting response.

In an attempt to predict which patients will respond to a checkpoint inhibitor, and which won't, scientists have come up with a way of assessing tumors according to various different parameters. Called the "cancer immunogram," it brings together information such as: Has the patient's immune system recognized their cancer as something that needs destroying? Have T cells entered the tumor in order to fight it? Is their immune system generally healthy? And, are there factors other than checkpoint proteins that are blocking an effective cancer-fighting immune response? [40]

A cancer immunogram could be an accurate and sensitive way of predicting which patients will benefit from a checkpoint inhibitor. However, at the moment it is an unproven, expensive, and time-consuming way of predicting response. As a result, measuring PD-L1 in tumors is still the most common biomarker test, even though a lack of PD-L1 doesn't rule out the possibility that a person will benefit.

5.3.7 Resistance to Checkpoint Inhibitors

As with all cancer treatments, checkpoint inhibitors don't work for everyone. And even when a patient's cancer is responding (i.e., it's shrinking or remaining the same size rather than growing), the cancer can become resistant later on.

Scientists haven't had the chance to do much research to unpick the causes of resistance to checkpoint inhibitors yet. But I've listed below some of the reasons for resistance they've uncovered so far.

Reasons why some cancers, and some patients, **don't benefit at all** from checkpoint inhibitors [35]:

1. Patients who are **severely immune-suppressed** (e.g., people with HIV/AIDS and some very elderly patients) don't have enough active white blood cells in their body to mount an effective immune response against their cancer cells.

2. Checkpoint inhibitors rely on there being CTLs in the patient's body that can recognize and respond to cancer cells but that are being suppressed. They also rely on the ability of these T cells to enter and move through the tumor. Checkpoint inhibitors work by removing the suppression and triggering these cells into action. However, **some cancers don't seem to be very visible to the immune system and don't provoke any reaction from CTLs**. If this is the case, then there will be no CTLs in the cancer for the checkpoint inhibitors to work with.

3. There are **many other inhibitory checkpoint proteins** aside from CTLA-4 and PD-1. If a patient's CTLs are being suppressed by alternative inhibitory checkpoint proteins, or other mechanisms that don't involve CTLA-4 or PD-1, then they won't benefit from an anti-CTLA4, anti-PD-1 or anti-PD-L1 antibody.

Some reasons why some patients might only **partially benefit** from a checkpoint inhibitor, or only for a short time [35]:

1. Many cancers contain a high degree of **intratumoral heterogeneity**.[15] The diversity in the cancer might mean that CTLs activated by a checkpoint inhibitor kill some, but not all, cancer cells. Those cells left behind later cause the cancer to regrow.

2. **Physical and/or chemical barriers** might exist within a tumor that prevent CTLs from entering that part of the tumor. This protected region of the tumor is therefore unaffected by the presence of cancer-fighting CTLs in the body and is able to keep growing.

3. The checkpoint inhibitor may **not have activated sufficient CTLs** to keep the cancer completely under control.

5.3.8 Overcoming Resistance to Checkpoint Inhibitors

Many strategies are being explored to increase response rates to checkpoint inhibitors and to overcome resistance. Most of these strategies involve combining existing checkpoint inhibitors with other treatments. The purpose of the second treatment is often to [41]:

- Overcome the suppression mediated by a different checkpoint protein (e.g., by using combinations of multiple checkpoint inhibitors)
- Overcome the effects of CTL-suppressing chemicals in the tumor microenvironment (e.g., through the use of IDO inhibitors)
- Improve the visibility of the cancer cells to immune cells by creating lots of destruction and debris within the tumor (e.g., through the use of chemotherapy, radiotherapy, targeted therapy)
- Increase the movement of T cells into the tumor (e.g., through the use of angiogenesis inhibitors)
- Increase the variety and number of protein fragments that the immune system responds to (e.g., with vaccine strategies)
- Overcome the effects of immune-suppressing cells such as Tregs or MDSCs (e.g., by using chemokine receptor inhibitors)

---

[15] This means that the cancer contains multiple populations of cancer cells, and each population of cells contains a unique mixture of mutations and also displays a different set of peptides on its surface.

One treatment approach generating excitement is the IDO inhibitors. As I mentioned back in Section 5.2.3, IDO is an enzyme that suppresses the activity of T cells, and it is often produced by cancer cells and white blood cells in the tumor microenvironment [14]. IDO suppresses T cells by breaking down an amino acid called tryptophan, which is needed by T cells. When tryptophan levels drop due to IDO, T cells shut down and self-destruct. High IDO levels inside a tumor can also prevent T cells from gaining access [42]. In recent years, scientists have created various IDO inhibitors, and one to watch out for is epacadostat. This drug is in phase 3 trials for NSCLC, bladder cancer, malignant melanoma, kidney cancer, and head and neck cancer, and it's generating lots of interest.

5.4 ADOPTIVE CELL TRANSFER

Adoptive cell transfer (ACT[16]) refers to treatments in which some of the patient's own white blood cells are removed from their bloodstream, deliberately modified (or carefully selected) in the laboratory, allowed to multiply, and then infused back into their blood.

One advantage of this approach is that millions of cancer-fighting white blood cells are created in the laboratory in a highly efficient manner. This is a much more reliable way of activating T cells than using checkpoint inhibitors. (With checkpoint inhibitors, you just have to hope that there are already cancer-fighting T cells in the patient's body that are being suppressed but that can be provoked into action).

Another advantage with ACT is that you can prepare the way for the introduction of the laboratory-grown cells by depleting the patient's immune system beforehand (usually with chemotherapy) [43]. Then, when you introduce the new cells into the body, they aren't blocked or destroyed by regulatory T cells or the patient's other white blood cells.[17]

The types of ACT that I am going to describe in this part of the chapter are TILs and CAR-modified T cells. I'm also going to tell you about treatments that use modified dendritic cells. However, because modified dendritic cells have a lot in common with cancer vaccine approaches, I'm going to discuss them alongside vaccines in Section 5.6.

5.4.1 Tumor-Infiltrating Lymphocytes

TILs are naturally occurring lymphocytes found inside tumors. They are almost exclusively helper T cells and cytotoxic T cells (CTLs) [43]. The first evidence that TILs could be helpful as a treatment for malignant melanoma came in 1988. Since that time, the way that TILs are grown and put back into patients has slowly been improved (see Figure 5.8 for the series of steps necessary to create an active TIL treatment). However, this isn't yet a licensed treatment approach.

The goal of the TIL approach, as with checkpoint inhibitors, is to remove the suppressive forces that prevent cancer-fighting lymphocytes from destroying a tumor. Checkpoint inhibitors do this in the tumor by disrupting the interaction between lymphocytes and their suppressive neighbors. With the TIL approach, however, the lymphocytes are physically removed from the suppressive environment, encouraged to grow and multiply in the laboratory, and then returned to the patient's body [43–45]. Hopefully, the TILs then migrate into the tumor and mount an attack.

---

[16] This abbreviation is also used to mean "adoptive T cell therapy," which is essentially the same thing.
[17] You can't perform this depletion prior to using checkpoint inhibitors or vaccine approaches because you would destroy the very white blood cells you want to activate.

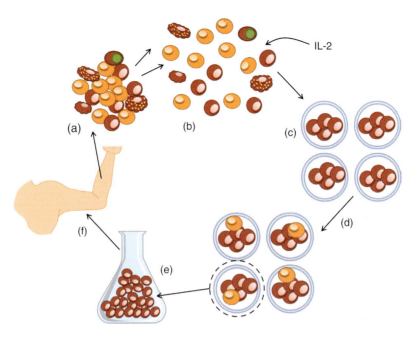

Figure 5.8 Using TILs for cancer immunotherapy. (a) A tumor (malignant melanoma) is surgically removed. It contains many different cell types including cancer cells, T cells, macrophages, and myeloid-derived suppressor cells. **(b)** The tumor is split up into single cells or small fragments. **(c)** The cells or fragments are grown in separate containers in the presence of a cytokine called IL-2 (interleukin 2), which encourages T cells to grow and multiply. Gradually, the T cells outgrow and outlast all other cell types. **(d)** Each population of T cells is tested for its ability to respond to peptides present on the patient's cancer cells. **(e)** T cells that recognize and destroy cancer cells are encouraged to multiply. **(f)** The patient's immune system is depleted with chemotherapy or radiotherapy. The T cells are then infused back into their bloodstream. Flask from: https://pixabay.com/en/flask-beaker-chemistry-container-309923/
Abbreviations: IL-2 – interleukin-2

Despite gradual improvements in the TIL approach, it is still almost exclusively being investigated as a treatment for malignant melanoma. It seems that although TILs exist in many other tumors, it's much more difficult to get them to recognize and destroy other tumors in the same way as melanomas [43].

The response rate for TIL therapy in malignant melanoma is reported to be around 40%–55%. Excitingly, some patients with advanced (i.e., metastatic) malignant melanoma treated with TILs are still alive ten years later [43].

But although TIL therapy for malignant melanoma has produced exciting results, there are some important limitations to this treatment [45]:

1. In order to select TILs that recognize cancer cells (Figure 5.8d), scientists need a supply of melanoma cells that can grow in the laboratory; these are often not available.

2. It generally takes several weeks for cancer-specific TILs to multiply to the point where there are enough of them to infuse back into the patient. Many people with advanced melanoma are extremely unwell and cannot afford to wait weeks for treatment.

3. TILs that are grown in the laboratory for several weeks are likely to lose some of their activity and capacity to survive long term when infused back into the patient.

4. Not all malignant melanomas contain TILs that recognize proteins on cancer cells.

Therefore, a proportion of melanoma patients (perhaps a third [46]) cannot be treated with this approach.

In general, trials with TILs report a high patient drop-out rate.

5.4.2 CAR (Chimeric Antigen Receptor)-Modified T Cells

The mechanism of the CAR-modified T cell approach is slightly different from that of checkpoint inhibitors and TILs. As I've mentioned before, the goal of checkpoint inhibitors and TILs is to overcome or remove things that suppress the activity of T cells. These approaches aim to increase the number and activity of cancer-killing T cells generated naturally by the patient's immune system.

The goal of CAR-modified T cells, however, is to create a genetically modified army of millions of T cells that:

1. **Would never otherwise exist** in a patient's body
2. All **attach to one particular protein** on the surface of cancer cells
3. Are **directly and powerfully activated** when their receptor attaches to its target, without requiring any further signals from other cells

I've outlined the basic premise of this approach in Figure 5.9. However, in order to explain it properly (or at least in a bit more detail), I need to tell you a bit more about T cells and the TCR. Then I need to talk you through CAR proteins. Finally, I'll tell you what cancers it's currently being explored in and why.

T Cells and the TCR

Our T cells have on their surface the T cell receptor (TCR), which is similar in structure and function to the B cell receptor (BCR) found on B cells (Figure 5.10) (if you want to find out what the BCR is, and how it works, I'd advise reading Section 7.4 in Chapter 7 of this book).

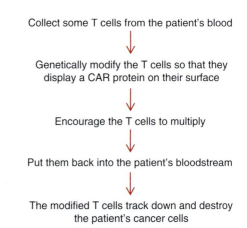

Collect some T cells from the patient's blood

↓

Genetically modify the T cells so that they display a CAR protein on their surface

↓

Encourage the T cells to multiply

↓

Put them back into the patient's bloodstream

↓

The modified T cells track down and destroy the patient's cancer cells

Figure 5.9 **The basic premise of CAR adapted T cell therapy.** The goal of CAR T cell therapy is to treat the patient with genetically modified versions of their own T cells. First, T cells are collected from their blood. The gene for a CAR protein is then introduced into the T cell's chromosomes, forcing the T cell to manufacture thousands of copies of the CAR protein and place them on its surface. The T cells are then given time to multiply. Once back in the patient's body, the CAR protein enables the modified T cells to attach to target cells (hopefully cancer cells) and destroy them. **Abbreviations:** CAR – chimeric antigen receptor

Like the BCR, the TCR has an antigen-binding site. However, unlike the BCR, the TCR can only recognise and respond to antigens if they are displayed by MHC proteins on APCs. (MHC class 1 if it's a cytotoxic T cell; MHC class 2 if it's a helper T cell). This is in contrast to the BCR, which can directly interact with antigens. (See Table 5.3 for a quick comparison between the BCR and TCR.)

So What Are CARs?

CAR proteins are **made from various bits and pieces of antibodies and other proteins** found on white blood cells (see Figure 5.11). The first CAR proteins were made back in the late 1980s. These early CAR proteins have gradually been improved to create new generations of CAR proteins with greater and greater ability to activate T cells [47, 48].

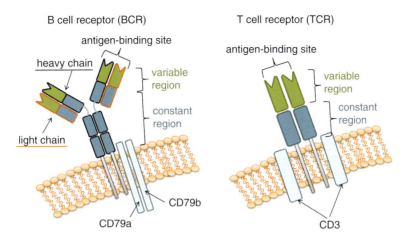

Figure 5.10 Similarities between the BCR and TCR. Both BCRs and TCRs have a constant region and a variable, antigen-binding region. Neither BCRs nor TCRs protrude far inside the cell, nor are they kinases. CD79a and CD79b are needed to transmit signals from the BCR into the cell cytoplasm. CD3 does the same for TCRs. **Abbreviations:** BCR – B cell receptor; TCR – T cell receptor

Table 5.3   Comparison between T cell receptors and B cell receptors.

	T cell receptor	B cell receptor
Contains constant and variable regions (see Chapter 2, Figure 2.4)	Yes	Yes
Has antigen-binding site(s) that attach to an antigen	Yes	Yes
Unique to each cell; constructed by mixing and matching various gene segments	Yes	Yes
Can be used by inactive T or B cells to directly attach to target antigens on the surface of pathogens and cancer cells	No – inactive T cells can only respond to their target antigen if it presented to them via MHC proteins on antigen-presenting cells such as dendritic cells	Yes
What other cells, proteins, or other signals are necessary for the cell to become active?	**Helper T cells:** require CD4 (on the T cell) and B7 (on an APC) **Cytotoxic T cells:** require CD8 (on the T cell) plus B7 and further signals from APCs; sometimes also requires helper T cells	Usually requires signals from helper T cells
Can it directly activate signaling pathways inside the cell?	No – this is done by CD3	No – this is done by CD79a and CD79b
When activated, what happens to the receptor?	It stays on the surface of the T cell	The B cell (now called a plasma cell) releases its BCRs (now called antibodies) into the blood

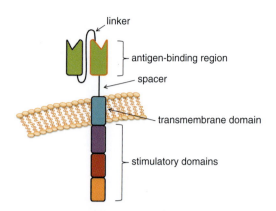

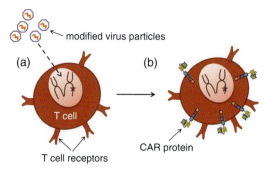

Figure 5.11 Structure of a CAR (chimeric antigen receptor) protein. CAR proteins are constructed from various pieces taken from a variety of different proteins. The extracellular, antigen-binding region is the variable region (also called the scFv) of an antibody, which is held together by a linker – a short string of amino acids. This is joined to a spacer, which provides flexibility. This in turn is connected to a protein segment known as the transmembrane domain that spans the cell membrane. Inside the cell are stimulatory domains taken from a number of proteins such as CD3, CD28, OX40, or CD247. These protein segments powerfully trigger the activity of T cells.
Abbreviations: CAR – chimeric antigen receptor

How Can a Patient's T Cells Be Persuaded to Produce and Display CAR Proteins?

T cells can be persuaded to manufacture CAR proteins and display them on their surface by inserting the instructions (i.e., the gene) to make such a protein into the T cell's chromosomes. CAR proteins are an amalgam of different protein pieces [48]. For this reason, the genetic instructions[18] telling a T cell how to make a CAR protein are in the form of a series of gene segments that correspond to each protein piece. The entire, man-made gene can

Figure 5.12 Viruses can be used to genetically modify T cells and force them to produce CAR proteins. (a) A modified virus containing the gene for a CAR protein is used to genetically modify T cells taken from the patient's blood. The CAR gene permanently integrates into the cells' chromosomes. **(b)** T cells use the instructions in the CAR gene to manufacture the desired CAR protein. They insert this protein into their outer membrane.
Abbreviation: CAR – chimeric antigen receptor

be inserted into a T cell's chromosomes using a variety of methods [49]. The most common method is to package-up the gene inside a virus capsule (see Figure 5.12). The virus (which has been emptied of all disease-causing material) infects the cell and inserts the CAR gene into the T cell's chromosomes. The T cell then uses the instructions in the CAR gene to make thousands of copies of the CAR protein, which it slots into its outer membrane.

What Do CAR Proteins Do?

CAR proteins, when present on the surface of T cells, **allow T cells to directly attach to target cells such as cancer cells.** This attachment triggers the T cells' cell-killing ability, and it directly destroys cancer cells (and any other cells with the same target on their surface). Hopefully, some of the activated T cells are

---

[18] In case you're confused or new to biology: genes are lengths of DNA that contain the instructions to make proteins. Each cell in our body contains the same DNA (our genome), which has in it the full set of instructions to make every protein in human cells. This DNA is packaged-up in the form of chromosomes. For decades now, scientists have had technology that allows them to play around with DNA and force cells to make proteins that would never otherwise exist.

memory cells, which give long-lasting protection against cancer recurrence. A vital property of CAR proteins is that they enable T cells to respond to a target without first needing to be activated by a dendritic cell.

CAR-Modified T Cells Overcome the Normal Limitations of T Cells

CAR proteins allow scientists to overcome some of the normal limitations of the immune system, such as [50–52]:

1. Cancer cells don't display peptides from every faulty protein they make. This limited display of peptides reduces the likelihood that the body will mount an anti-cancer immune response.
2. T cells need peptide fragments to be presented to them by APCs; APCs are limited in what they can present to T cells, again reducing the likelihood of the body mounting an anti-cancer response.
3. Even when T cells do recognize peptides from cancer cells displayed to them by APCs, the T cell requires further signals from other cells before it can become active; this reduces the number of T cells that are activated.
4. When activated T cells enter a tumor, they are immediately exposed to an immune-suppressing environment that can prevent them from taking action.

CAR-modified T cells overcome some of these limitations by [53]:

1. **Targeting a protein deliberatively chosen by a scientist** as being one that is consistently present in high amounts on the surface of cancer cells
2. **Attaching directly to their target** without needing it to be presented to them by APCs
3. Having **no need for signals from other cells** in order to become fully active
4. CAR-modified T cells cannot necessarily overcome immune-suppression, so this limitation remains.

What Are the CAR Proteins' Targets?

The target of CAR-modified T cells needs to:

1. Be **reliably found on a significant proportion of cells of a particular cancer**. When this is the case, the treatment will destroy enough cancer cells to bring a meaningful benefit to the patient.
2. Be **absent from healthy cells** in vital organs and tissues.

So far, most CAR proteins target a protein called CD19. Scientists think this protein best fulfills the above criteria because [54, 55]:

• There's lots of it on cancer cells of B cell leukemias (acute lymphoblastic leukemia (ALL) and chronic lymphocytic leukemia (CLL)) and on most B cell non-Hodgkin lymphomas (NHLs).

• It is also present on healthy B cells, and these cells are killed by the CAR-modified T cells. As a result, the person loses the ability to produce antibodies in response to infections. However, this can be treated with infusions of antibodies and is therefore manageable.

Other targets being explored for hematological cancers include [56–58]:

• BCMA (B cell maturation antigen), CD138 (also called SLAMF7 – signaling lymphocyte –activating molecule-7), and Kappa light chain, for the treatment of multiple myeloma

• CD123, NKG2D (Natural Killer Group 2D), CD33, CD44v6, FLT3 (FMS-like tyrosine kinase-3), CD34, and Lewis Y antigen, for the treatment of acute myeloid leukemia

• CD20, Kappa light chain, CD22, CD30, and many other targets for NHL and Hodgkin lymphoma; CD22 is also being explored as a target for ALL

Trials with CD19-Targeted CAR-Modified T Cells

No doubt, by the time you read this there will be a lot more data published, and we'll have a clearer idea of this approach's strengths and limitations. In fact, two CAR T cell therapies (called tisagenlecleucel (Kymriah) and axi-cabtagene ciloleucel (Yescarta)), were licensed by the FDA in the United States during 2017 [59], and the first one has also been put forward to the EMA in Europe for their consideration.

Although this a fast-moving field of research, I have summarized below some of the results obtained from the clinical trials that have taken place so far:

- A trial (called the ELIANA trial) of tisagenlecleucel, involving 63 children and young adults with B-cell ALL, produced a remission rate of 83%. Of the patients who responded, 64% were predicted to be free of their disease six months later [60]. Tisagenlecleucel was licensed as a treatment for children and young adults with relapsed ALL in August 2017.

- A second CAR T cell therapy, called axi-cabtagene ciloleucel, was licensed in the United States in October 2017 for patients with some aggressive types of NHL. This approval was as a result of the ZUMA-1 clinical trial, in which 101 people with relapsed, chemotherapy-resistant NHL received treatment. 82% of the people in the trial responded to the treatment, including 54% who went into complete remission. However, when the results were published, the patients involved in the trial had only been followed up for around 9 months, so it's not clear how many of these patients will later relapse [61].

- All trials with CAR-modified T cells report that patients often experience severe side effects from this therapy. These effects are generally caused by (1) the destruction of healthy cells which have the CAR's target on their surface and (2) the rapid proliferation of modified T cells in the body, and their cell-killing actions. The most dangerous side effect of anti-CD19 CAR T cells is "cytokine release syndrome" (CRS), which is a consequence of the rapid proliferation

and activity of T cells. Symptoms of CRS range from mild, flu-like symptoms to organ failure [62].

Can CAR-Modified T Cells Be Used to Treat Solid Tumors?

Making viable CAR-modified T cell treatments for solid tumors is very difficult because [63]:

- Many of the attempts to use T cells modified to attack targets on solid tumors have caused life-threatening side effects that render them unsafe to use [43]. The main reason for these toxicities is that proteins found on the surface of cancer cells in solid tumors are often the same, or very similar, to proteins found on vitally important healthy cells. That's why it's virtually impossible to create CAR-modified T cells that don't cause life-threatening side effects.

- In other trials, T cells modified to attack solid tumors have been unable to kill enough cancer cells to benefit patients. Scientists think this is because the target protein isn't present on sufficient cells in the tumor, and because the modified T cells struggle to reach their target.

- In addition, solid tumors contain more immune-suppressing cells (such as MDSCs and Tregs) than hematological cancers [64]. This makes it more difficult for the modified T cells to do their work.

Despite these obstacles, CAR-modified T cells are starting to look promising for some solid tumors. For example, HER2-targeted CAR-modified T cells have been trialled in people with sarcoma, GD2-targeted CAR-modified T cells have been trialled for neuroblastoma [63], and interleukin-13 receptor alpha 2 (IL13Rα2)-targeted T cells have been tested against glioblastoma [65]. A similar approach has also been used to create T cells that target NY-ESO-1 for the treatment of multiple myeloma [66], synovial cell sarcoma, and malignant melanoma [67].

Final Comments on CAR-Modified T Cells

Despite their limitations, the approach of using CAR-modified T cells is generating a huge amount of excitement. The reasons for this are (1) high response rates and (2) the possibility of long remissions or even cures for people for whom all other treatments have failed.

However, before we get seriously excited, we need:

- More data from more trials involving more patients with long follow-up periods proving that they really do work long-term
- Better understanding of how to treat side effects and avoid treatment-related deaths
- CAR treatments that target proteins other than CD19 and that can be used against a wider range of cancers

In addition, scientists' enthusiasm for CAR T cell therapy is tempered by various concerns, including the cost of this treatment, both in terms of the amount demanded by the creator (for example, tisagenlecleucel costs $475,000 per patient) and the costs involved in delivering the therapy and managing side effects. There is also concern that in the real world (by which I mean outside of clinical trials), the benefits will be much less than those reported in trials, because many patients will be too ill to wait for CAR T cells to be created. For example, in the ELIANA trial, an additional 16 patients who agreed to take part in the trial never received treatment [68].

5.5 MODIFIED BI-SPECIFIC ANTIBODIES

Another way of persuading T cells to attack cancer cells is to create modified antibody-based proteins that physically connect the two cell types [69] (Figure 5.13a). Scientists can create these modified antibodies using genetic engineering techniques to splice together segments from genes for two antibodies with different targets. When the modified

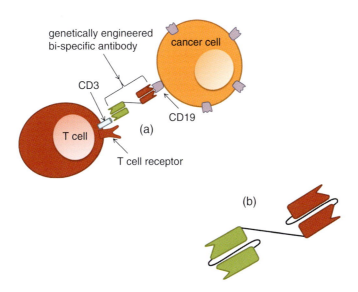

Figure 5.13 **Bi-specific antibodies**. **(a)** A genetically engineered, bi-specific antibody tethers together a T cell with a cancer cell. One part of the bi-specific antibody anchors it to CD19, while the other part attaches to CD3, which is part of the T cell receptor complex. **(b)** Bi-specific antibodies are made from the antigen-binding regions (scFvs) of two different antibodies. Three linkers (shown as black lines) hold the protein together. **Abbreviations:** scFv – single-chain variable region

gene is put into living cells, the cells create a protein that comprises the antigen-binding regions (known as scFvs) of the two antibodies. The scFvs are held together by linkers, just like in CAR proteins. The two scFvs are then fused back to back by a third linker (Figure 5.13b). These proteins are sometimes called Bi-specific T cell engagers (BiTEs) or Tandem scFvs (TaFvs).

5.5.1 Blinatumomab (Blincyto)

The first and most well-studied BiTE, and the only one licensed in the EU,[19] is a treatment for adults with ALL called blinatumomab (Blincyto). Because this treatment is only used for ALL, I mention it further in Chapter 7, Section 7.3.6.

5.6 THERAPEUTIC CANCER VACCINES

Therapeutic cancer vaccines pretty much all rely on their ability to **activate the patient's dendritic cells**.

Back in Section 5.2.2 (and Figure 5.3), I described how dendritic cells can pick up and display peptides from cancer cells on their surface. If these dendritic cells receive the correct signals, they will then travel to lymph nodes and show these peptides to helper T cells and cytotoxic T cells. If a T cell recognizes the peptide with its TCR (and receives some other signals too), it will become fully active. When active, helper T cells support the activation of other white blood cells. Active cytotoxic T cells (CTLs) leave the lymph node, enter the tumor, and (hopefully) destroy cancer cells [70]. For the activation of CTLs to happen naturally in a patient's tumor, there need to be plenty of cancer peptides floating around for the dendritic cells to pick up. The dendritic cells also have to process the peptides and present them in a way that CTLs can recognize. And, CTLs that recognize cancer peptides presented to them also need to receive further signals. Finally, cancer-fighting CTLs have to avoid being suppressed via checkpoint proteins or suppressive white blood cells such as Tregs. Perhaps not surprisingly, in many patients, their immune system fails to generate sufficient cancer-fighting CTLs to keep their cancer controlled.

Scientists have developed two methods of overcoming this problem by increasing the number of active, cancer-fighting CTLs produced:

Method 1: Using a form of **ACT.** The scientists isolate dendritic cells from the patient's blood, modify them in the laboratory, and then transfuse them back into the patient's bloodstream. The modification often involves genetically modifying or otherwise treating the dendritic cells so that they display lots of a cancer peptide[20] on their surface.

Method 2: To leave the dendritic cells where they are (i.e., in the patient's body) and deliberately inject an antigen[21] such as a peptide (or multiple peptides) from cancer cells into the patient. Or, instead of injecting a peptide, they inject the DNA instructions for making the peptide, or even just inject mushed-up dead cancer cells. The hope with these so-called **cancer vaccines** is that dendritic cells in the body that encounter the vaccine will internalize it, place cancer peptides on their surface, and display them to T cells (see Figures 5.1c and 5.14).

---

[19] It received its EU license in November 2015.

[20] Other names given to cancer peptides are tumor-associated antigens (TAAs) or tumor-associated peptides (TUMAPs).

[21] In case you don't remember, "antigen" is a general term for anything that can provoke the immune system into action; it's generally a protein, or a protein fragment (a peptide) that activates B cells and/or that can be presented to T cells by APCs like dendritic cells.

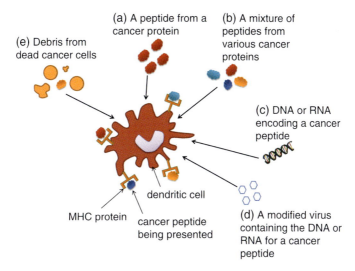

(e) Debris from dead cancer cells

(a) A peptide from a cancer protein

(b) A mixture of peptides from various cancer proteins

(c) DNA or RNA encoding a cancer peptide

dendritic cell

MHC protein

cancer peptide being presented

(d) A modified virus containing the DNA or RNA for a cancer peptide

Figure 5.14 Therapeutic cancer vaccines cause dendritic cells to display peptides from cancer proteins. **(a)** Cancer vaccines generally take the form of a fragment (peptide) from a protein found on cancer cells, which is injected into the patient. Hopefully, dendritic cells passing through the tissue pick up the peptide, internalize it, and then display it on their surface in conjunction with MHC proteins. Other vaccine strategies involve the use of **(b)** a mixture of different peptides, **(c)** the DNA or RNA instructions for making one or more peptides, **(d)** modified viruses that contain the DNA or RNA instructions for one or more cancer peptides, or **(e)** dead cancer cells taken from the patient being treated (an autologous vaccine) or from a different patient (an allogeneic vaccine).
Abbreviation: MHC – major histocompatibility complex

There's more detail about both methods below.

5.6.1 Method 1: Adoptive Cell Transfer using Dendritic Cells

Modified dendritic cells have been tested as treatments for various cancer types. One of the most well-known and well-studied applications of this technology is a treatment for prostate cancer known as sipileucel-T (also known as Provenge). Sipileucel-T involves purifying dendritic cells from the patient's blood and exposing them to a modified protein made from prostatic acid phosphatase (PAP – found on prostate cancer cells) and GM-CSF[22] (a growth factor known to trigger dendritic cells into action). The dendritic cells pick up and internalize the modified protein

and subsequently put PAP on their surface [71]. **When infused back into the patient's bloodstream, the modified dendritic cells activate CTLs, which then attack the patient's cancer cells.** Sipileucel-T has met some success in clinical trials and is approved for use in the United States [72]. However, its cost and the creation of other new prostate cancer treatments (such as abiraterone (Zytiga), enzalutamide (Xtandi), and radium-223(Xofigo)) have resulted in it being little used in Europe, and in 2015 the manufacturer of Provenge (Dendreon) asked for the marketing authorization to be withdrawn

Laboratory-grown, modified dendritic cells have also been used to treat other cancers [73], and the technology continues to evolve. However, as with other ACT methods, the creation of laboratory-grown, cancer

---

[22] GM-CSF stands for granulocyte-macrophage colony-stimulating factor.

peptide-presenting dendritic cells is both expensive and technically demanding.

5.6.2 Method 2: Antigen Vaccines and Oncolytic Viruses

The idea of creating an off-the-shelf vaccine to treat cancer isn't new [74]. In common with vaccines to prevent polio or measles, the basic idea is to introduce into the body an antigen that provokes the person's immune system into action. However, with cancer treatment vaccines, the goal is to provoke sufficient cancer-fighting white blood cells into action that they destroy an existing tumor. This is in contrast to a preventative vaccine that only needs to activate some memory cells (enough that the immune system is primed to fight off the potential invader). For a cancer treatment vaccine to work you need to generate an army of cancer-fighting white blood cells. And, these white blood cells[23] need to be so active that they can overcome the immune-suppressive cancer microenvironment.[24] So far, vaccines have struggled to do this.

Instead, where treatment vaccines have been more effective (although it's still early days) is in the destruction of cancer cells that remain in a person's body after they have received other treatments (e.g., surgery, radiotherapy, chemotherapy, or hormone therapy). Also looking promising are treatment vaccines used for pre-cancerous conditions such as: ductal carcinoma in situ (often a precursor of breast cancer); vulvar intraepithelial neoplasia (which sometimes leads to vulval cancer); and pre-malignant changes in the cervix, which can lead to cervical cancer. In these situations (post-treatment and pre-cancer), there is no immune-suppressing cancer microenvironment to have to overcome, so any T cells

that become active are more likely to destroy the cancer cells they meet [75].

When it comes to destroying an established, metastatic cancer, treatment vaccines have so far been less successful. But scientists are determined to get this approach to work, and they're making progress all the time.

Three areas they're focusing on are:

1. Choosing the right antigen for the job
2. Creating powerful adjuvants
3. Developing effective treatment combinations
4. Using oncolytic viruses to burst open cancer cells and release peptides for dendritic cells to pick up

Choosing the Right Antigen for the Job

Most antigens used in treatment vaccines are peptides (small fragments) from cancer proteins. However, if the cancer peptide used in the vaccine is very similar to (or the same as) a peptide found on healthy cells, then it's unlikely that the body will have many T cells that can recognize it.[25] Currently, peptides used in cancer vaccines include [74, 76]:

• Peptides from proteins that are overexpressed (i.e. overproduced) by cancer cells, but that are also present on a significant number of healthy cells, for example, HER2 on breast cancer cells (as mentioned above, it is not always possible to elicit an immune response against these proteins).

• Peptides from mutated cancer proteins, or those that result from chromosome translocations. The immune system is unlikely to have come across these peptides before, and it is therefore theoretically easier to target T cells against them. However, because every cancer contains a unique combination of mutated proteins, it's difficult to

---

[23] As with other immunotherapies, we're mostly talking about T cells.
[24] If you want to refresh your memory on the "immune-suppressive cancer microenvironment," I would suggest looking back at Section 5.2.
[25] This is because in the early stages of life, the body goes to great lengths to destroy any B cells or T cells that recognize the body's own proteins and could therefore lead to auto-immune diseases if allowed to survive.

translate this approach into a "one-size-fits-all" treatment.

- Peptides from **embryonic proteins** – these are proteins (such as CEA – carcinoembryonic antigen) that aren't normally found on adult cells, but that do crop up on the surface of a number of cancers.
- Peptides from "**cancer testis antigens**" and "**differentiation antigens**" – these are proteins often found on cancer cells and at low levels on other cell types.
- Peptides from **virus proteins** that are commonly found in cancer cells of certain cancer types linked to viral infections, for example, HPV (human papilloma virus) proteins in cervical cancer, vulval cancer and head and neck cancer cells; EBV (Epstein Barr virus) proteins in the cancer cells of some lymphomas and nasopharyngeal carcinoma; and HBV (hepatitis B virus) in liver cancer cells.
- Peptides that are fused together to create "**supramolecular peptide conjugates**" that are designed to be better at triggering precise, anti-cancer immune responses than standard peptides [75].

Non-peptide Vaccines

When scientists don't know what peptides to use, they sometimes take the blunt approach of using **dead cancer cells**. Their hope is that dendritic cells will pick up some of the cell debris, chop up the proteins, and display peptides on their surface. However, this is an inefficient process, and most efforts are focused on identifying suitable cancer peptides.

Another vaccine method is to inject into the body the **DNA or RNA instructions** for making a cancer peptide (or to place these instructions inside a modified virus). Again, you're hoping that passing dendritic cells pick up the instructions, use them to make the peptide, and then display this peptide to T cells. This approach has had some positive results, such as in a trial for women with pre-cancerous cells in their cervix [76].

Creating Powerful Adjuvants

Most cancer vaccines are given in the form of an injection into the skin or muscle [77]. Dendritic cells passing through the tissue pick up the vaccine and hopefully start displaying cancer peptides on their surface along with MHC class 1 and MHC class 2 proteins. When the peptide-presenting dendritic cells reach a lymph node (or other lymph tissue), they display these peptides to T cells.

This whole process is very inefficient. In addition, T cells need more than just exposure to peptides in order to become fully active. That's why **vaccine treatments rely heavily on adjuvants** – mixtures of chemicals, growth factors, or other proteins – that powerfully boost the activities of white blood cells [74, 75, 77].

Companies often keep the precise composition of their vaccine treatment adjuvants a closely guarded secret. Popular adjuvants include the growth factor GM-CSF, interleukin-2, and bacterial proteins (or fragments of them). Another way to include an adjuvant into a vaccine is to use the adjuvant as a delivery device. For example, some DNA or RNA vaccines are delivered inside modified virus particles [78]. The virus particle not only helps with vaccine delivery, but also sends activation signals to the immune system.

Developing Effective Treatment Combinations

Despite scientists' best efforts, treatment vaccines have generally been ineffective for people with established, metastatic cancers [74, 78]. And there is a growing realization that these treatments, if they are to help people with metastatic cancer, need to be given in combination with other treatments [75]. For example:

1. **In combination with checkpoint inhibitors:** The idea being that the vaccine will alert the patient's immune system to the presence of cancer, and the checkpoint inhibitor will prevent any resulting cancer-fighting T cells that are created from being suppressed.

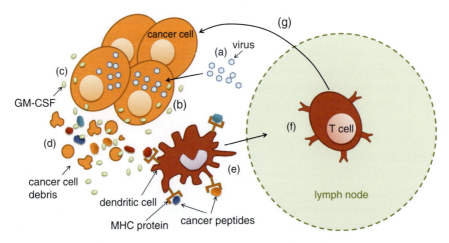

Figure 5.15 Mechanism of action of an oncolytic virus cancer treatment. **(a)** A modified virus is injected into the patient. **(b)** The virus multiplies easily in cancer cells because they contain many mutations and are less able to defend themselves from the virus than healthy cells. **(c)** The virus forces infected cells to produce GM-CSF, a growth factor that helps to activate white blood cells such as dendritic cells. **(d)** Some infected cancer cells burst open (they lyse), releasing all their inner proteins and other molecules into their surroundings. **(e)** Dendritic cells pick up some of the debris and display cancer peptides on their surface with MHC proteins. **(f)** Dendritic cells displaying cancer peptides leave the tumor and enter lymph nodes, where they activate T cells. **(g)** Activated T cells leave the lymph node, enter the tumor, and attack cancer cells. **Abbreviations:** MHC – major histocompatibility complex; GM-CSF – granulocyte-macrophage colony-stimulating factor

2. **In combination with chemotherapy**: As a result of killing lots of cancer cells, chemotherapy causes changes in the cancer microenvironment and the release of lots of cancer cell debris. Both these things can help the immune system do its work and could synergize with a cancer vaccine.

3. **In combination with ACT**: Scientists are exploring approaches such as exposing purified T cells to vaccines in the laboratory, or administering vaccines alongside T cells that are being returned to the patient's blood.

Using Oncolytic Viruses

An oncolytic virus is one that can **burst open cancer cells**. This method doesn't sit very easily in any category of cancer treatments, but it does rely on antigens and dendritic cells, which is why I'm including it here. The premise of this virus-based treatment is explained Figure 5.15.

The oncolytic viruses used in this way first of all have to be modified so that they:
- **No longer cause disease**
- **Multiply quickly in cancer cells**, causing the cells to burst open and release proteins into their surroundings
- **Contain the gene for an adjuvant** such as GM-CSF, which helps activate any dendritic cells that pick up cancer cell debris and increases the likelihood that they will travel to lymph nodes and activate T cells

The first oncolytic virus to become a licensed cancer treatment is called talimogene laherparepvec (T-VEC; Imlygic) [79]; it was given an EU license to treat malignant melanoma in December 2015. T-VEC uses a modified genetically engineered herpes simplex virus. Many other viruses, methods of delivery, and treatment combinations are being explored [80].

5.6.3 Final Thoughts on Cancer Treatment Vaccines

Cancer vaccines constantly make it into the news. However, this isn't necessarily because they work. Instead, they get coverage because they sound clever and sophisticated; because there are endless iterations of them; because they're new; or because they come under the general label of immunotherapy, which is currently generating lots of exciting trial results.

However, despite their current lack of success (particularly against established, metastatic cancers), therapeutic cancer vaccines do hold a lot of promise for the future. Hopefully they will ultimately improve survival rates in many cancer types.

5.7 THE FUTURE OF IMMUNOTHERAPY

In this chapter, I've described many different immunotherapy approaches. No doubt, by the time this book is published, more of these treatments will have been approved for use.

This rapid progress is testament to a number of factors:

1. Immunotherapy has been proven to work; therefore, there is massive optimism and massive appetite from doctors to enter patients into immunotherapy trials.
2. The optimism around immunotherapy expressed in our newspapers and cancer conferences means that cancer patients are willing to enter such trials.
3. The successes so far have whetted the appetite of pharmaceutical companies, and are driving massive investment in drug development and clinical trials.
4. Immunotherapies are potentially applicable to many, if not all, types of cancer, meaning that trials are recruiting people with tens of different cancer types.
5. Some of the cancers in which immunotherapy seems to work best (e.g., metastatic malignant melanoma and metastatic lung cancer) are relatively common and incredibly difficult to cure using other treatments.

However, future progress in immunotherapy will depend on scientists and doctors being able to overcome some of the current obstacles, such as:

- **Biomarkers** – In order to use treatments such as checkpoint inhibitors really effectively, and avoid treating patients who don't benefit, we need reliable, specific (and relatively cheap) biomarkers that tell us when the treatment is likely to work, and when it isn't.
- **Side effects** – Some of the side effects caused by immunotherapies (such as CRS and the unwanted immune reactions caused by checkpoint inhibitors) are potentially life-threatening, and we need better ways of managing them or reducing their severity.
- **Lack of efficacy** – The immune-suppressing environment in which cancer cells live (especially in solid tumors) is an enormous obstacle to the effective use of approaches such as cancer treatment vaccines.
- **Effectiveness for only some cancers** – For example, CAR-modified T cell therapy is currently only useful for hematological cancers. Many barriers need to be overcome before they can be used safely and effectively in other cancers.
- **Cost** – Some immunotherapies, such as ACT methods, rely on harvesting and modifying the patient's white blood cells. This is incredibly costly and requires specialist resources and highly trained scientists. At the time of writing, this can only be done at specialist hospitals and research institutes.
- **Effectiveness only when the body is already trying to fight** – Approaches such as checkpoint inhibitors rely on the presence of pre-existing cancer-fighting T cells. If the person's immune system isn't trying to attack the cancer, then the checkpoint inhibitor has nothing to work with.

Some of these obstacles are gradually being overcome, particularly through the use of immunotherapy combinations. For example, when immunotherapies are combined with one another or with other treatments, the response rates often rise. We've already seen a combination of two checkpoint inhibitors (nivolumab plus ipilimumab) licensed for malignant melanoma after it gave a response rate of 58% in the Checkmate 067 trial [34](for more on this, see Chapter 6, Section 6.6.3), which is more than double that reported in most other checkpoint inhibitor trials. And we'll no doubt see other combinations licensed in the near future.

I have no doubt that scientists, doctors, and drug companies will continue to make rapid progress, and develop many more effective immunotherapies and immunotherapy combinations. And, because immunotherapies are relatively insensitive to issues such as intratumoral heterogeneity that often thwart other targeted treatments, hopefully many people with metastatic cancer will be granted extra years of life because of these treatments.

REFERENCES

1 Couzin-Frankel J (2013). Breakthrough of the year 2013: Cancer immunotherapy. *Science* **342**(6165): 1432–1433.

2 Sompayrac LM (2015). How the Immune System Works (The How it Works Series) Paperback – October **23**, 2015. https://www.amazon.co.uk/How-Immune-System-Works/dp/1118997778/ref=dp_ob_title_bk (Accessed December 14, 2017).

3 Murphy K. Janeway's Immunobiology. http://www.garlandscience.com/product/isbn/9780815342434 (Accessed December 14, 2017).

4 Hanahan D, Weinberg RA (2011). Hallmarks of cancer: The next generation. *Cell* **144**: 646–674.

5 Cavallo F et al. (2011). 2011: The immune hallmarks of cancer. *Cancer Immunol Immunother* **60**: 319–326.

6 Mantovani A et al. (2008). Cancer-related inflammation. *Nature* **454**: 436–444.

7 Evans A, Costello E (2012). The role of inflammatory cells in fostering pancreatic cancer cell growth and invasion. *Front Physiol* **3**: 270.

8 Schreiber RD, Old LJ, Smyth MJ (2011). Cancer immunoediting: Integrating immunity's roles in cancer suppression and promotion. *Science* **331**(6024): 1565–1570.

9 Motz GT, Coukos G (2013). Deciphering and reversing tumor immune suppression. *Immunity* **39**: 61–73.

10 Melero I et al. (2014). Therapeutic vaccines for cancer: An overview of clinical trials. *Nat Rev Clin Oncol* **11**: 509–524.

11 For a nice illustration of this process, see: Mellman I, Coukos G, Dranoff G (2011). Cancer immunotherapy comes of age. *Nature* **480**: 480–489.

12 Sompayrac L (2012). The magic of antigen presentation. In *How the Immune System Works*. 4th ed. Chichester: Wiley, pp. 38–49.

13 Trombetta ES, Mellman I (2005). Cell biology of antigen processing in vitro and in vivo. *Annu Rev Immunol* **23**: 975–1028.

14 Brochez L et al. (2017). The rationale of indoleamine 2,3-dioxygenase inhibition for cancer therapy. *Eur J Cancer* **76**: 167–182.

15 Pardoll D (2012). The blockade of immune checkpoints in cancer immunotherapy. *Nat Rev Cancer* **12**: 252–264.

16 Jago CB et al. (2004). Differential expression of CTLA-4 among T cell subsets. *Clin Exp Immunol* **136**(3): 463–471.

17 Fife BT, Bluestone JA (2008). Control of peripheral T-cell tolerance and autoimmunity via the CTLA-4 and PD-1 pathways. *Immunol Rev* **224**: 166–182.

18 Horvat TZ et al. (2015). Immune-related adverse events, need for systemic immunosuppression, and effects on survival and time to treatment failure in patients with melanoma treated with ipilimumab at Memorial Sloan Kettering Cancer Center. *J Clin Oncol* **33**(28): 3193–3198.

19 Flaherty KT (2015). Gauging the long-term benefits of Ipilimumab in Melanoma. *J Clin Oncol* **33**(17): 1865–1866.

20 Hoos A (2016). Development of immuno-oncology drugs — from CTLA4 to PD1 to the next

generations. *Nat Rev Drug Discov* **15**(4): 235–247.

21 Schadendorf D et al. (2015) Pooled analysis of long-term survival data from phase II and phase III trials of ipilimumab in unresectable or metastatic melanoma. *J Clin Oncol* **33**(17): 1889–1894.

22 For a useful discussion of the Schadendorf paper, see: NHS Choices (September 2013). More data on survival with new skin cancer drug. [Online]. Retrieved from http://www.nhs.uk/news/2013/09September/Pages/More-data-on-survival-with-new-skin-cancer-drug.aspx [Accessed December 14, 2017].

23 Chiou VL, Burotto M (2015). Pseudoprogression and immune-related response in solid tumors. *J Clin Oncol* **33**(31): 3541–3543.

24 Ohaegbulam KC et al. (2015). Human cancer immunotherapy with antibodies to the PD-1 and PD-L1 pathway. *Trends Mol Med* **21**(1): 24–33.

25 Dong H et al. (2002). Tumor-associated B7-H1 promotes T-cell apoptosis: A potential mechanism of immune evasion. *Nat Med* **8**: 793–800.

26 Goodman A et al. (2017). PD-1 – PD-L1 immune-checkpoint blockade in B-cell lymphomas. *Nat Rev Clin Oncol* **14**: 203–220.

27 Reviewed in: Buchbinder EI, Desai A (2016). CTLA-4 and PD-1 pathways: Similarities, differences, and implications of their inhibition. *Am J Clin Oncol* **39**(1): 98–106.

28 Pillai RN et al. (2018). Comparison of the toxicity profile of PD-1 versus PD-L1 inhibitors in non-small cell lung cancer: A systematic analysis of the literature. *Cancer* **124**(2): 271–277.

29 Sharma P, Allison JP (2015). The future of immune checkpoint therapy. *Science* **348**(6230): 56–61.

30 Smyth MJ et al. (2016). Combination cancer immunotherapies tailored to the tumour microenvironment. *Nat Rev Clin Oncol* **13**(3):143–158.

31 European Medicines Agency website: http://www.ema.europa.eu (Accessed December 18, 2017).

32 National Cancer Institute: A to Z list of Cancer Drugs: http://www.cancer.gov/about-cancer/treatment/drugs (Accessed December 18, 2017)

33 ClinicalTrials.gov website: https://clinicaltrials.gov/ (Accessed December 18, 2017).

34 Larkin J et al. (2015) Combined nivolumab and ipilimumab or monotherapy in untreated melanoma. *N Engl J Med* **373**: 23–34.

35 Restifo NP, Smyth MJ, Snyder A (2016). Acquired resistance to immunotherapy and future challenges. *Nat Rev Cancer* **16**(2): 121–126.

36 Tumeh PC et al. (2014). PD-1 blockade induces responses by inhibiting adaptive immune resistance. *Nature* **515**: 568–571.

37 Rizvi NA et al. (2015). Mutational landscape determines sensitivity to PD-1 blockade in non-small cell lung cancer. *Science* **348**(6230): 124–128.

38 Le DT at al. (2015). PD-1 blockade in tumors with mismatch-repair deficiency. *N Engl J Med* **372**(26): 2509–2520.

39 Van Allen EM et al. (2015). Genomic correlates of response to CTLA-4 blockade in metastatic melanoma. *Science* **350**(6257): 207–211.

40 Blank CU et al. (2016). The "cancer immunogram." *Science* **352**(6286): 658–660.

41 Swart M et al. (2016). Combination approaches with immune-checkpoint blockade in cancer therapy. *Front Oncol* **6**: 233.

42 Brochez L et al. (2017). The rationale of indoleamine 2,3-dioxygenase inhibition for cancer therapy. *Eur J Cancer* **76**: 167–182.

43 For a review of ACT, see: Rosenberg SA, Restifo NP (2015). Adoptive cell transfer as personalized immunotherapy for human cancer. *Science* **348**(6230): 62–68.

44 Restifo NP, Dudley ME, Rosenberg SA (2012). Adoptive immunotherapy for cancer: Harnessing the T cell response. *Nat Rev Immunol* **2**: 269–281.

45 Geukes Foppen MH at al. (2015). Tumor-infiltrating lymphocytes for the treatment of metastatic cancer. *Mol Oncol* **9**: 1918–1935.

46 Goff SL et al. (2010). Tumor infiltrating lymphocyte therapy for metastatic melanoma: Analysis of tumors resected for TIL. *J Immunotherapy* **33**(8): 840–847.

47 Tasian SK, Gardner RA (2015). CD19-redirected chimeric antigen receptor-modified T cells: A promising immunotherapy for children and adults with B-cell acute lymphoblastic leukemia (ALL). *Ther Adv Hematol* **6**(5): 228–241.

48 Maher J (2012). Immunotherapy of malignant disease using chimeric antigen receptor engrafted T cells. *ISRN Oncology* 2012: 278093.

49 For an overview of different methods, see: Ghorashian S, Pule M, Amrolia P (2015). CD19 chimeric antigen receptor T cell therapy for

haematological malignancies. *Br J Haematol* **169**: 463–478.

50 Vinay DS et al. (2015). Immune evasion and cancer: Mechanistic basis and therapeutic strategies. *Sem Cancer Biol* **35**: S185–S198.

51 Spranger S, Gajewski TF (2018). Mechanisms of tumor cell-intrinsic immune evasion. *Ann Rev Cancer Biol* **2**: 213–228.

52 Muenst S et al. (2016). The immune system and cancer evasion strategies: Therapeutic concepts. *J Intern Med* **279**: 541–562.

53 Newick K et al. (2016). Chimeric antigen T-cell therapy for solid tumors. *Mol Ther-Oncolytics* **3**: 16006.

54 Maude SL et al. (2015). CD19-targeted chimeric antigen receptor T-cell therapy for acute lymphoblastic leukemia. *Blood* **125**(26): 4017–4023.

55 Sadelain M et al. (2015). CD19 CAR therapy for acute lymphoblastic leukemia. *Am Soc Clin Oncol Educ Book*. 2015: e360–3.

56 Mikkilineni L, Kochenderfer J (2017). Chimeric antigen receptor T-cell therapies for multiple myeloma. *Blood* **130**(24): 2594–2602.

57 Gill S (2016). Chimeric antigen receptor T-cell therapy in AML: How close are we? *Best Pract Res Clin Haematol* **29**(4): 329–333.

58 Brudno JN, Kochenderfer JN (2018). Chimeric antigen receptor T-cell therapies for lymphoma. *Nat Rev Clin Oncol* **15**: 31–46.

59 National Cancer Institute. With FDA Approval for Advanced Lymphoma, Second CAR T-Cell Therapy Moves to the Clinic. [Online] https://www.cancer.gov/news-events/cancer-currents-blog/2017/yescarta-fda-lymphoma (Accessed December 18, 2017).

60 Novartis. Novartis pivotal CTL019 6-month follow-up data show durable remission rates in children, young adults with r/r B-cell ALL. [Online] https://www.novartis.com/news/media-releases/novartis-pivotal-ctl019-6-month-follow-data-show-durable-remission-rates (Accessed December 18, 2017).

61 Locke FL et al. (2017). Clinical and biologic covariates of outcomes in ZUMA-1: A pivotal trial of axicabtagene ciloleucel (axi-cel; KTE-C19) in patients with refractory aggressive non-Hodgkin lymphoma (r-NHL). Abstract #7512.

Presented at the 2017 ASCO Annual Meeting, June 5, 2017; Chicago, Illinois.

62 For a wide-ranging and helpful review of CAR T cell therapy, including its side effects, see: National Cancer Institute. CAR T Cells: Engineering Patients' Immune Cells to Treat Their Cancers. [Online] https://www.cancer.gov/about-cancer/treatment/research/car-t-cells (Accessed December 18, 2017).

63 Summarized from: Dai H et al. (2016). Chimeric antigen receptors modified T-cells for cancer therapy. *J Natl Cancer Inst* **108**(7): pii:djv439.

64 Brentjens RJ (2016). Are chimeric antigen receptor T cells ready for prime time? *Clin Adv Hematol Oncol* **14**(1): 17–19.

65 Brown CE et al. (2016). Regression of glioblastoma after chimeric antigen receptor T-cell therapy. *New Engl J Med* **375**: 2561–2569.

66 Rapoport AP et al. (2015). NY-ESO-1–specific TCR–engineered T cells mediate sustained antigen-specific antitumor effects in myeloma. *Nat Med* **21**: 914–921.

67 Robbins PF et al. (2011). Tumor regression in patients with metastatic synovial cell sarcoma and melanoma using genetically engineered lymphocytes reactive with NY-ESO-1. *J Clin Oncol* **29**(7): 917–924.

68 Prasad V (2018). Immunotherapy: Tisagenlecleucel — the first approved CAR-T-cell therapy: Implications for payers and policy makers. *Nat Rev Clin Oncol* **15**: 11–12.

69 Huehls AM et al. (2016). Bispecific T cell engagers for cancer immunotherapy. *Immunol Cell Biol* **93**(3): 290–296.

70 Chen DS, Mellman I (2013). Oncology meets immunology: The cancer-immunity cycle. *Immunity* **39**(1): 1–10.

71 Reviewed in: Di Lorenzo G, Buonerba C, Kantoff PW (2011). Immunotherapy for the treatment of prostate cancer. *Nat Rev Clin Oncol* **8**: 551–561.

72 Gerritsen WR (2012). The evolving role of immunotherapy in prostate cancer. *Ann Oncol*. **23** Suppl 8: viii22–7.

73 Reviewed in Palucka K, Banchereau J (2012). Cancer immunotherapy via dendritic cells. *Nat Rev Cancer* **12**: 265–277.

74 For a timeline of progress, see: Melero I et al. (2014). Therapeutic vaccines for cancer: An overview of clinical trials. *Nat Rev Clin Oncol* **11**: 509–524.

75 For a review, see: van der Burg SH et al. (2016). Vaccines for established cancer: Overcoming the challenges posed by immune evasion. *Nat Rev Cancer* **16**(4): 219–33.

76 Trimble CL et al.(2015). Safety, efficacy, and immunogenicity of VGX-3100, a therapeutic synthetic DNA vaccine targeting human papillomavirus 16 and 18 E6 and E7 proteins for cervical intraepithelial neoplasia 2/3: A randomised, double-blind, placebo-controlled phase 2b trial. *Lancet* **386**: 2078–2088.

77 Also reviewed in: Melief CJM et al. (2015). Therapeutic cancer vaccines. *J Clin Investigation* **125**(9): 3401–3412.

78 For more information on this, see: Drake CG, Lipson EJ, Brahmer JR (2014). Breathing new life into immunotherapy: Review of melanoma, lung and kidney cancer. *Nat Rev Clin Oncol* **11**(1): 24–37.

79 Andtbacka RH et al. (2015). Talimogene laherparepvec improves durable response rate in patients with advanced melanoma. *J Clin Oncol* **33**(25): 2780–2788.

80 Turnbull S et al. (2015). Evidence for oncolytic virotherapy: Where have we got to and where are we going? *Viruses* **7**(12): 6291–6312.

CHAPTER 6

Targeted Treatments for Common Solid Tumors

IN BRIEF

In this chapter, I will summarize the progress we've made to date in developing targeted treatments for each of the top ten most common solid tumors diagnosed in the United Kingdom. Four of these cancers (breast, bowel, lung, and prostate) account for over half of all new cancers diagnosed in the United Kingdom, and almost half of all deaths.

Every cancer in every patient is driven by a unique set of DNA mutations. However, by studying thousands of samples from thousands of patients, scientists have discovered some mutations that are very common in particular cancer types, such as *HER2* amplifications in breast and stomach cancer, *EGFR* mutations in lung cancer, and *BRAF* mutations in melanoma skin cancer. Hence, treatments that block the proteins made from these genes are important treatments for people with breast, stomach, lung, and melanoma skin cancer.

In other situations, it's possible to target a faulty process rather than a faulty protein that is important for the cancer's survival. A blood supply is important to every solid tumor, and this has led to the use of angiogenesis inhibitors for various cancer types.

We're also seeing enormous numbers of trials in which treatments are being combined together in the hopes that the two treatments will synergize with one another, or that one of the treatments will overcome some of the limitations of the other. For example, combinations of HER2-targeted treatments are licensed for HER2-positive breast cancers. And B-Raf inhibitors combined with MEK inhibitors are licensed for melanoma skin cancer, as is a combination of two checkpoint inhibitors.

Since 2011, checkpoint inhibitors such as ipilimumab, nivolumab, and pembrolizumab have proved their worth in a variety of tumor types. Initially their use was limited to melanoma skin cancer, but since then they've been licensed for various other cancer types. Because checkpoint inhibitors and other immunotherapies are in a huge number of trials and there's enormous interest in them, I've included information on the possible usefulness of immunotherapy for all ten cancers.

A Beginner's Guide to Targeted Cancer Treatments, First Edition. Elaine Vickers.
© 2018 John Wiley & Sons Ltd. Published 2018 by John Wiley & Sons Ltd.

6.1 INTRODUCTION

In this chapter, I summarize the progress made in applying the treatments I have described elsewhere in this book to people with the ten most common solid tumors in the United Kingdom.

Probably rather obviously, people with early stage cancer are usually treated with surgery, and many thousands of these people are cured. **Most targeted treatments are therefore predominantly given to people with metastatic cancer**, which is generally still an incurable disease. However, some of them, such as HER2-targeted treatments, are given as adjuvant treatments to people with early-stage cancers that haven't spread.

The details of which treatments are licensed for which cancer patients is a constantly changing picture, and what is true now, in December 2017, will not be accurate when this book is published. Consequently, I have focused on the treatments themselves, rather than providing lots of detail about the licensing or availability of each treatment. And where I have included data from trials, this is just to give you a flavor of the treatment's impact. **The analysis of trial data and assessment of a treatment's worth are well beyond the scope of this book**.

The aim of this chapter is to allow you to navigate to other information in this book that is most relevant to you, and to put the information in previous chapters into context. For example, if you most commonly come into contact with lung cancer patients, hopefully by looking at the relevant section of this chapter, you will quickly learn that Chapter 3, Section 3.3 on EGFR (epidermal growth factor receptor) inhibitors, Chapter 4, Section 4.2 on ALK and ROS1 inhibitors, and Chapter 5, Section 5.3 on checkpoint inhibitors will be most relevant to you.

In this chapter, you'll find a lot more information about some cancers than others. This is simply because some cancers have more targeted treatments licensed for them than others. For example, there are now eight licensed targeted treatments and immunotherapies for malignant melanoma but only one for brain tumors (specifically glioblastoma). You'll therefore find a lot more information in this chapter about melanoma than you do about brain tumors.

Finally, if the cancer you work on isn't included in this chapter, I may have covered relevant treatments elsewhere in the book. For example, in Chapter 3 you'll find out about RET inhibitors for thyroid cancer and in Chapter 4 you'll find information about PARP inhibitors for ovarian cancer.

6.2 TARGETED TREATMENTS FOR BREAST CANCER

Breast cancer is the most common cancer in the United Kingdom, with over 55,000 cases diagnosed (including 390 in men) each year [1].[1] As with all cancers, the location of the cancer, whether it has spread, how aggressive its behavior is, and the general health of the person, are all important factors when it comes to selecting the right treatment. However, when diagnosing breast cancers, the cells are also tested for the **presence of hormone receptors and HER2**.

Hormone receptors (estrogen receptors and/or progesterone receptors) are found inside the cancer cells of about 70% of women with breast cancer and in about 90% of men with breast cancer [2]. People with hormone

---

[1] Because so few men are diagnosed with breast cancer compared to women, from here on I'll just talk about women. However, some of the treatments I mention, particularly the hormone treatments, are also relevant to men with breast cancer.

receptor positive cancers are often treated with hormone therapies alongside their other treatments. Also, about 15%–20% of breast cancers massively overproduce HER2, and women with these cancers are generally given HER2-targeted treatments.

Around 15% of breast cancers are called "triple-negative" breast cancers (TNBCs), because they don't have hormone receptors inside them or HER2 on their surface [3]. At the moment, there are no licensed targeted treatments for TNBC, but treatments such as PARP inhibitors and checkpoint inhibitors are in trials. Increasingly, TNBC is being thought of as a group of several different types of breast cancer, each of which is likely to respond to different treatments.

6.2.1 Targeting the Estrogen Receptor with Hormone Therapies

Estrogen (and progesterone) receptors are proteins found in both normal and cancer-causing breast cells. They respond to the presence of estrogen (or progesterone) by pairing up and attaching to genes in the cell's chromosomes. Once attached to genes, they act as transcription factors and trigger the production of many different proteins [4] (see Figure 6.1).

Hormone therapies for breast cancer work in one of two ways: they either block the actions of estrogen receptors, or they block the production of estrogen in the woman's body.

Treatments That Block Estrogen Receptors
Selective estrogen receptor modulators (SERMs) [5]

- **Tamoxifen** – This drug is chemically very similar to estrogen, and it can attach to estrogen receptors (ERs). But, once attached, it distorts their shape. The altered ERs can still bind to target genes, but (in the breast) they recruit co-repressors rather than co-activators and therefore suppress (rather than activate) gene transcription.

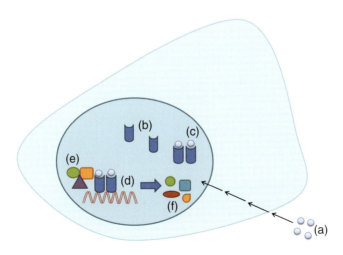

Figure 6.1 Estrogen receptors. **(a)** Estrogens are made by the ovaries, adrenal glands, and other tissues. Estrogens are tiny, lipid-soluble hormones that easily enter the cell. **(b)** Breast cells contain estrogen receptors (ERs). **(c)** In the presence of estrogen, the receptors pair up. **(d)** Paired-up receptors attach to genes in the cell's chromosomes. **(e)** Various other proteins (co-activators) join the paired-up ERs. **(f)** The cell manufactures many proteins involved in cell survival and proliferation.
Abbreviations: ER- estrogen receptor

- Because of its properties, tamoxifen is able to block the actions of estrogen in the breast, but it has estrogen-like effects (i.e., it activates ERs) in the uterus and bones.
- **Raloxifene** (Evista) – This is similar to tamoxifen but is able to block ER activity in both the breasts and uterus.
- **Toremifene** (Fareston) – This is similar to tamoxifen but is activated and metabolized differently in the body.

Fulvestrant (Faslodex) [6]

- Fulvestrant attaches to the ER and causes it to change shape, which prevents ERs from pairing up.
- It also causes destruction of the altered ERs, lowering the amount of ERs in the cell.
- Unlike other SERMs, fulvestrant does not have any estrogen-like effects; it is therefore a "pure anti-estrogen."

Treatments That Block Estrogen Production

Aromatase inhibitors (AIs) [7]

Aromatase is an enzyme (a catalyst) that creates estrogen from other hormones called androgens; it is present in ovaries and other tissues (breast, uterus, vagina, bone, brain, heart, blood vessels, and adipose (fat)).

Letrozole (Femara), anastrozole (Arimidex), and exemestane (Aromasin) block aromatase and effectively block the production of estrogen in post-menopausal women.

AIs are less effective at suppressing estrogen production in pre-menopausal women (this is because AIs cause increased aromatase production by the ovaries).

Pre-menopausal women can be given an aromatase inhibitor if they are willing to take medication to suppress their ovaries [8].

Without estrogen, ERs can't pair up or attach to genes – their activity is therefore blocked.

6.2.2 Overcoming Hormone Therapy Resistance

Hormone treatments are very effective treatments for women with hormone-sensitive breast cancer. For example, when given as adjuvant therapy following surgery, they can cut the risk of recurrence by around 40% [9]. However, they are less effective against metastatic breast cancer and can only cause around 50% of these cancers to shrink or stop growing [10]. The other 50% are resistant. Because of their limitations against metastatic breast cancer, understanding the mechanisms of resistance and overcoming them is hugely important.

Scientists who have studied hormone-therapy-resistant breast cancer have uncovered a multitude of different resistance mechanisms. These include interplay between hormone receptors and growth factor signaling pathways (including the PI3K/AKT/mTOR pathway) and overproduction of cyclin D [10] (see Figure 6.2).

Other resistance mechanisms include [9, 10]:

- Mutations that affect the ER, and that cause ERs to become independent of estrogen or hypersensitive to estrogen – occurs in 15%–40% of women
- Gradual loss of ERs in cancer cells, with corresponding increases in growth factor receptors to sustain the cells' survival and proliferation
- Overproduction of ER co-activators such as AIB1 and loss of co-repressors such as NCoR; this leads to ER activity even in the absence of estrogen
- Presence of stem cells that lack ERs; these cells will therefore be unaffected by hormone treatments and may later cause recurrence
- Protection of cancer cells by non-cancer cells in the microenvironment, such as fibroblasts

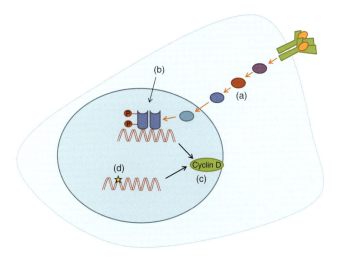

Figure 6.2 **Mechanisms of resistance to hormone therapies: growth factor signaling and cyclin D. (a)** Growth factor signaling pathways are overactive in breast cancer cells for a variety of reasons and cause resistance to hormone therapies. **(b)** Proteins involved in growth factor signaling phosphorylate ERs and cause them to attach to genes independently of estrogen. **(c)** ERs force the cell to produce many proteins involved in proliferation and survival including cyclin D, which forces the cell to enter the cell cycle and multiply. **(d)** In over 50% breast cancers, cyclin D is overproduced due to gene amplification or other mechanisms; this bypasses the cell's requirement for ERs in order to multiply.
Abbreviations: ER – estrogen receptor

Currently the only treatments that have been proved to delay resistance to hormone therapies are an mTOR inhibitor, everolimus (Afinitor), and a class of treatments known as CDK4/6 inhibitors.

Overcoming Hormone Resistance with mTOR Inhibitors

The PI3K/AKT/mTOR pathway is overactive in a large proportion of breast cancers due to mutations affecting the *PIK3CA*[2] gene and other components of the pathway [6]. When the PI3K pathway is overactive, hormone-receptor-positive breast cancers become resistant to hormone therapies [9]. This discovery led to various clinical trials investigating mTOR inhibitors (and other drugs that block the PI3K/AKT/mTOR pathway) in combination with hormone therapy. At the moment,

only everolimus, an mTOR inhibitor (see Chapter 3, Section 3.8.4 for more on mTOR inhibitors), has been licensed as a breast cancer treatment. This license was granted because of the results of the BOLERO-2 clinical trial (see Table 6.1).

Overcoming Hormone Resistance with CDK4/6 Inhibitors

Mutations that affect proteins involved in the cell cycle are very common in breast cancer. These proteins include various cyclins, CDKs, and RB (for a review of the cell cycle and CDK inhibitors, see Chapter 4, Section 4.5). When scientists conducted experiments with breast cancer cells, they discovered that cancer cells with overactive CDK4 and CDK6 were resistant to hormone therapies [9]. This led to clinical trials investigating a combination of

---

[2] The *PIK3CA* gene is the gene for making the active, catalytic part of PI3K.

Table 6.1   Results from the BOLERO-2 study of exemestane plus everolimus or placebo in 724 women with hormone treatment-resistant metastatic breast cancer.

	Exemestane + everolimus	Exemestane + placebo
Progression-free survival	7.8 months	3.2 months
Overall response rate	12.6%	1.7%
Clinical benefit rate (complete or partial response or stable disease for ≥24 weeks)	51.3%	26.4%
% of patients requiring dose interruptions or reductions due to adverse events	66.8% had the everolimus dose reduced; 23.9% had their exemestane dose reduced	11.8%

Source: Yardley DA et al. (2013). Everolimus plus exemestane in postmenopausal patients with HR(+) breast cancer: BOLERO-2 final progression-free survival analysis. *Adv Ther* **30**(10): 870–884.

Box 6.1   *Understanding the language of clinical trials*

When researchers design a clinical trial, they think long and hard about what measures of success to use. For example, if the treatment they're investigating is being used early on in the patient's treatment, then measuring overall survival won't be appropriate – by the time the patient dies, they might have received many subsequent treatments that might have all contributed to the length of time they lived. So for every trial, the researchers decide what measure will give them the greatest amount of information about the effectiveness of their treatment. Common measures include [11, 12]:

Overall survival (OS) – The length of time from when a person is entered into a trial until their death from any cause

Progression-free survival (PFS) – The length of time from when a person is entered into a trial until they die or their cancer progresses (i.e., starts growing again, spreads or gets worse)

Time to progression (TTP) – The length of time from when a person is entered into a trial until their cancer progresses (this measure doesn't include deaths)

Disease-free survival (DFS) – The length of time from when a person is entered into a trial until their cancer returns or they die due to any cause (this measure can only be used if the people entering the trial have no signs of cancer when they enter the trial; for example, they might have had an early-stage cancer which has been removed by surgery)

Event-free survival (EFS) – The length of time from when a person is entered into a trial until their cancer returns, they die, or they have to discontinue treatment for any reason

Objective response rate (ORR) – The proportion of patients whose cancer shrinks by a predefined amount and for a minimum time period

Complete response rate (CRR) – The proportion of patients in whom all detectable signs of cancer have disappeared

Partial response rate (PRR) – The proportion of patients in whom their tumor has shrunk by about 30%[3]

---

[3] The criteria for a partial response depends on how many dimensions of the tumor you measure.

Stable disease (SD) – When a patient's cancer appears to stay about the same size and hasn't got any worse

Durable response rate (DRR) – The length of time that a partial or complete response lasts for

Duration of response (DoR) – The length of time from when the cancer appears to have responded to treatment until the time when it spreads or gets worse

Many of these response measures aren't useful for assessing the effectiveness of immuno-therapies, as (1) the benefits of these treatments often take longer to become apparent, (2) cancers sometimes appear to grow before they begin to shrink, (3) durable stable disease can be a sign that the treatment is working very well, and (4) sometimes small new metastases appear that are insignificant and can safely be ignored [13]. For this reason, scientists have created a new set of criteria for measuring responses to immunotherapies. These measures emphasize measuring the total amount of tumor in the patient's body (primary tumor and metastases) and requiring repeat scans to confirm whether a cancer is indeed getting worse [14].

Finally, for most of the measures used in clinical trials the researchers will generally calculate the **median** value because this gives you a more useful and representative figure than using the mean [15].

a CDK4/6 inhibitor with hormone therapy. Three CDK4/6 inhibitors have been studied in phase 3 trials: palbociclib (Ibrance), ribociclib (Kisqali), and abemaciclib (Verzenio). The results of these trials are summarized in Table 6.2. Both palbociclib and ribociclib are licensed treatments in Europe and the United States. Abemaciclib is licensed in the United States only (as of December 2017).

6.2.3 Targeting HER2

Treatments that target HER2 (explained in Chapter 3, Section 3.4) have become extremely important as treatments for HER2-positive breast cancer (that is, breast cancers that contain extra copies of the HER2 gene and that massively overproduce HER2 protein – see Chapter 3, Figure 3.13). Five HER2-targeted treatments are licensed as breast cancer treatments (see Table 6.3). Three of them are antibodies, and each has a slightly different mechanism of action (Chapter 3, Figure 3.12).

Trastuzumab (Herceptin) was the first HER2-targeted treatment to be licensed and it has become part of standard treatment for women with early, locally advanced, or metastatic HER2-positive breast cancer [20].

Overcoming Resistance and Extending Responses to Trastuzumab

As with hormone treatment resistance, resistance to HER2-targeted treatments such as trastuzumab is almost inevitable for women with metastatic breast cancer. If and when trastuzumab stop working, this may be for a variety of different reasons (see Chapter 3, Section 3.4.1 and Figure 3.14).

That's why we have seen lots of clinical trials in which treatment combinations have been tried. These combinations include:

- Trastuzumab with another HER2-targeted treatment such as pertuzumab (Perjeta) or lapatinib (Tyverb)
- Trastuzumab with hormone therapies such as anastrozole or letrozole
- Trastuzumab with mTOR, AKT, or PI3K inhibitors
- Trastuzumab with immunotherapy

Table 6.2   Results from phase 3 trials investigating a combination of an aromatase inhibitors plus a CDK4/6 inhibitor for the treatment of post-menopausal women with hormone receptor-positive (HR-positive) breast cancer.

PALOMA-2 study [16]

A phase 3 study of letrozole plus palbociclib or placebo in 666 women with HR-positive advanced or metastatic breast cancer who had received no prior therapy for advanced disease.

	Letrozole + palbociclib	Letrozole + placebo
Progression-free survival	24.8 months	14.5 months
Incidence of grade 3 or 4 adverse events*	75.7%	24.4%

PALOMA-3 study [17]

A phase 3 study of fulvestrant plus palbociclib or placebo in 521 women with hormone treatment-resistant metastatic breast cancer

	Fulvestrant + palbociclib	Fulvestrant + placebo
Progression-free survival	9.5 months	4.6 months
Incidence of grade 3 or 4 adverse events*	73%	22%

MONALEESA 2 [18]

A phase 3 study of letrozle plus ribociclib or placebo in 668 women with HR-positive advanced or metastatic breast cancer who had received no prior therapy for advanced disease.

	Letrozole + ribociclib	Letrozole + placebo
Progression-free survival	Not yet reached	14.7 months
Incidence of grade 3 or 4 adverse events*	81.2%	32.7%

MONARCH 2 [19]

A phase 3 study of fulvestrant plus abemaciclib or placebo in 669 patients with HR-positive, HER2-negative metastatic breast cancer with disease progression following endocrine therapy who had not received chemotherapy in the metastatic setting.

Progression-free survival	16.4 months	9.3 months
Incidence of grade 3 or 4 adverse events*	60.5%	22.8%

*The most common side effects caused by these treatments are neutropenia, leukopenia and other consequences of bone marrow suppression.
Abbreviations: HR – hormone receptor

Not all the results of these trials have been positive, but we are seeing some progress. For example, the CLEOPATRA trial showed that a combination of trastuzumab with pertuzumab and chemotherapy is better than trastuzumab plus chemotherapy as the first course of treatment for women with metastatic breast cancer. In the trial, women given pertuzumab alongside their other treatments survived a median of 56.5 months versus 40.8 months for women given trastuzumab plus chemotherapy alone. This is a survival improvement of 15.7 months [21].

Various other phase 3 trials are ongoing that explore the trastuzumab/pertuzumab combination in HER2-positive breast cancer in different settings, such as:
- as an adjuvant treatment after surgery (BOLD-1 trial; NCT02625441)
- as a re-treatment in women who have already received trastuzumab/pertuzumab (PRECIOUS trial; NCT02514681)

Table 6.3   Summary of licensed HER2-targeted treatments for breast cancer.

Drug	Target	Mechanism
Monoclonal antibodies		
Trastuzumab/ Herceptin	HER2	Not completely understood; blocks paired HER2s from activating signaling pathways; recruits and activates white blood cells; prevents HER2 shedding.
Pertuzumab/ Perjeta	HER2	Prevents HER2s from pairing up with one another or with other EGF receptors (i.e., EGFR, HER3, and HER4).
Trastuzumab emtansine/ T-DM1/ Kadcyla	HER2	Made from trastuzumab fused to chemotherapy – delivers chemotherapy to HER2-positive cancer cells.
Small molecule kinase inhibitors		
Lapatinib/ Tyverb/ Tykerb	EGFR & HER2	Reversibly inhibits activation of HER2 and EGFR by competing for their ATP binding sites.
Neratinib/Nerlynx	EGFR, HER2, HER4	Similar to lapatinib, but neratinib is an irreversible inhibitor that targets EGFR, HER2, and HER4. It is classed as a "pan-HER" inhibitor.

Abbreviations: HER2 – human epidermal growth factor receptor 2; EGF – epidermal growth factor; EGFR – EGF receptor; HER3 – human epidermal growth factor receptor 3; HER4 – human epidermal growth factor receptor 4
Source: Schramm A et al. (2015). Targeted therapies in HER2-positive breast cancer – a systematic review. *Breast Care* 10(3): 173–178.

- as neoadjuvant treatment[4] (i.e., prior to surgery) (PREDIX HER2 trial; NCT02568839)
- in combination with hormone therapy or chemotherapy for HER2-positive and hormone receptor-positive metastatic breast cancer (Detect V / CHEVENDO trial; NCT02344472)
- in combination with hormone therapy and an anti-CDK4/6 inhibitor for HER2-positive and hormone receptor-positive metastatic breast cancer (PATINA trial; NCT02947685)

Trials are also investigating different doses, schedules, and routes of delivery (i.e., subcutaneous rather than intravenous delivery).

Newer HER2-Targeted Antibodies

Trastuzumab Emtansine
Trastuzumab emtansine (Kadcyla) is the **trastuzumab antibody linked to chemotherapy**

(Chapter 3, Section 3.4.1 and Figure 3.12c). Clinical trials have shown that it, combined with lapatinib, is better than lapatinib plus capecitabine against HER2-positive breast cancer that has progressed (i.e., continued to grow and spread) after treatment with trastuzumab plus capecitabine. The trial that investigated this comparison was the EMILIA trial. It reported a five- month survival advantage (30.9 months vs. 25.1 months) for the women given the trastuzumab emtansine/lapatinib combination [22].

Current phase 3 trials involving patients with HER2-positive breast cancer are investigating trastuzumab emtansine:

- For patients with metastatic breast cancer who have already received chemotherapy and other HER2-targeted treatments (NCT01702571)
- As a neoadjuvant treatment in comparison to trastuzumab/pertuzumab (PREDIX HER2 trial; NCT02568839)

---

[4] Trastuzumab, pertuzumab plus chemotherapy is already a licensed, NICE-approved neoadjuvant treatment for HER2-positive locally advanced, inflammatory or early-stage breast cancer at high risk of recurrence.

- In combination with pertuzumab as an adjuvant treatment for invasive breast cancer following chemotherapy (KAITLIN trial; NCT01966471)
- As a neoadjuvant treatment in combination with pertuzumab (NCT02131064)
- As an adjuvant treatment for patients who have residual disease following surgery (KATHERINE trial; NCT01772472)

Trastuzumab Biosimilars

The **patents on trastuzumab expired in July 2014 in Europe** and will expire in the United States in June 2019. That's why various companies are creating biosimilars of trastuzumab. These antibodies are virtually identical to trastuzumab and should be equally effective as well as cheaper.[5] They include Herzuma (CT-P6), ABP-980, Hercules (Myl-1401O), PF-05280014 and SB3 [23]. The first trastuzumab biosimilar, called Ontruzant, was licensed in Europe in November 2017 [24].

Margetuximab

Also in phase 3 trials is a HER2-targeted antibody called margetuximab. It binds to the same part of HER2 as trastuzumab, but it is designed to be better at attracting and activating white blood cells [25]. It's currently being tested in a phase 3 trial called SOPHIA (NCT02492711), which is due to report its results in 2021.

HER2-Targeted Kinase Inhibitors

Lapatinib is a reversible, competitive kinase inhibitor (see Chapter 2, Section 2.3.2) that blocks both EGFR and HER2. Results from clinical trials investigating lapatinib haven't been uniformly positive. When it was directly compared to trastuzumab in a phase 3 trial, it came out worse [26] (the trial was called NCIC CTG MA.31). However, it is licensed in three settings [27]:

- In combination with capecitabine for patients with advanced or metastatic breast cancer who have already received chemotherapy and trastuzumab
- In combination with trastuzumab for patients with advanced or metastatic breast cancer who have already received chemotherapy and trastuzumab
- In combination with an aromatase inhibitor for post-menopausal women with HER2-positive and hormone-receptor positive breast cancer

More recently, irreversible inhibitors of EGF receptors have been created and tested in trials. One of these, neratinib (Nerlynx), which blocks EGFR, HER2, and HER4, was investigated in the ExteNET study. This study investigated giving women with HER2-positive breast cancer neratinib for a year following previous adjuvant treatment with trastuzumab. Five years later, 90.2% of women given neratinib, and 87.7% women given placebo, were free of invasive breast cancer [28].

There is also some evidence from other trials that neratinib might be better than trastuzumab at preventing brain metastases in women with metastatic breast cancer [29].

6.2.4 Angiogenesis Inhibitors

There are various reasons to believe that angiogenesis inhibitors might be useful breast cancer treatments [30]:

1. Levels of HIF-1, an important controller of angiogenesis, are high in invasive breast cancers.
2. High HIF-1 levels, high VEGF levels, and high numbers of blood vessels, go hand in hand with short survival times.

---

[5] They're called "biosimilar" antibodies rather than "generic" antibodies because antibodies are large proteins, and it's impossible to create exactly the same antibody again – the cells you use to manufacture them will always add subtly different modifications to the basic antibody protein. For more on biosimilars see Chapter 2, Section 2.2.5.

3. In experiments with mice, angiogenesis inhibitors work well against triple-negative breast cancer.

Various angiogenesis inhibitors have been investigated in many different clinical trials involving thousands of women with breast cancer [30]. Treatments tested include antibodies such as bevacizumab (Avastin) and ramucirumab (Cyramza), and a variety of kinase inhibitors such as sorafenib (Nexavar), sunitinib (Sutent), and pazopanib (Votrient) (see Chapter 4, Section 4.1.5). However, despite being able to improve PFS and response rates, angiogenesis inhibitors haven't had a substantial impact on survival times. The only license awarded to an angiogenesis inhibitor is a European license for bevacizumab as a treatment for metastatic breast cancer in combination in with paclitaxel or capecitabine chemotherapy. At one point, bevacizumab held a similar license in the United States, but this was later rescinded [31].

6.2.5 Targeted Treatments for Triple-Negative Breast Cancer

Unlike for HER2-positive or hormone receptor-positive breast cancer, there are very few non-chemotherapy treatment options for women with breast cancers that produce neither HER2 nor hormone receptors – the so-called triple-negative breast cancers (TNBCs). However, there are signs that some TNBCs might respond to PARP inhibitors (see Chapter 4, Section 4.3) or immunotherapy with checkpoint inhibitors (see Chapter 5, Section 5.3).

PARP Inhibitors for TNBCs

Around 8%–16% of women with TNBC have an inherited (germline) *BRCA* gene mutation [32]. And it's likely that a far greater percentage of TNBCs have other problems with homologous recombination that might render them sensitive to treatment with a PARP inhibitor [33] (see Chapter 4, Section 4.3.6). Various phase 2 trials have investigated PARP inhibitors for TNBC, and there have been some signs of activity. Various phase 3 trials are now taking place with olaparib (Lynparza), veliparib, talazoparib, niraparib (Zejula) and rucaparib (Rubraca) (see Table 6.4).

Data from the first phase 3 trial of a PARP inhibitor in *BRCA*-mutated breast cancer (called OlympiAD) were announced in 2017. In the OlympiAD trial, 302 women were randomized to receive either olaparib or chemotherapy (capecitabine, eribulin, or vinorelbine). All the women involved in the trial had an inherited *BRCA1* or *BRCA2* mutation and had received no more than two prior chemotherapy regimens for metastatic HER2-negative breast cancer. Results from the trial showed that the median PFS was longer for women in the olaparib group (7.0 months versus 4.2 months). However, the median overall survival in the two groups of women was almost identical (19.3 months versus 19.6 months) [34].

The phase 3 EMBRACA trial also reported its results in 2017. Again, the trial involved women with inherited *BRCA* mutations. The trial included 431 women, who were randomized to receive either talazoparib or chemotherapy (capecitabine, vinorelbine, eribulin, or gemcitabine). As with the OlympiAD trial, the PARP inhibitor produced a longer PFS than chemotherapy (8.6 months versus 5.6 months) [35]. The survival data weren't yet available when the study was published.

A doctor writing about the OlympiAD trial has since pointed out some important limitations of the trial [36]. These include the suggestion that carboplatin chemotherapy might have been a better control, as it is known to be particularly effective against BRCA-mutated breast cancer [37]. The same could perhaps be said for the EMBRACA trial.

Table 6.4   Summary of randomized phase 3 trials investigating PARP inhibitors as treatments for *BRCA*-mutated breast cancer.

Treatments under investigation	Estimated study completion date	Study population and ClinicalTrials.gov Identifier
Olaparib trials		
Olaparib versus physician's choice of chemotherapy	December 2018	Women with metastatic HER2-negative breast cancer who have an inherited mutation in a *BRCA* gene (OlympiAD trial; NCT02000622)
Adjuvant olaparib versus placebo following surgery, neoadjuvant, and adjuvant chemotherapy	March 2020	Women with high-risk triple-negative breast cancer (TNBC) who have an inherited mutation in a *BRCA* gene (OlympiA; NCT02032823)
Neoadjuvant olaparib + chemotherapy (paclitaxel + carboplatin) versus chemotherapy	January 2032	Women with operable *BRCA*-mutated breast cancer and/or TNBC (PARTNER trial; NCT03150576)
Olaparib after chemotherapy versus chemotherapy	August 2029	Patients with HER2-negative breast cancer with features of defective homologous recombination (Subito trial; NCT02810743)
Veliparib trials		
Carboplatin + paclitaxel with or without veliparib	May 2018	Women with HER2-negative, *BRCA*-mutated metastatic breast cancer (BROCADE-3; NCT02163694)
Standard chemotherapy versus standard chemotherapy plus carboplatin versus standard chemotherapy + veliparib + carboplatin	November 2020	Patients with early-stage TNBC (NCT02032277)
Talazoparib trials		
Talazoparib versus physician's choice	June 2017	Women with locally advanced or metastatic breast cancer who have an inherited mutation in a *BRCA* gene (EMBRACA trial; NCT01945775)
Niraparib trials		
Niraparib versus physician's choice	February 2018	Women with HER2-negative, advanced, or metastatic breast cancer who have an inherited mutation in a *BRCA* gene (BRAVO trial; NCT01905592)
Rucaparib trials		
Adjuvant chemotherapy with or without rucaparib	August 2017	Women with triple-negative breast cancer or HER2-negative breast cancer with a *BRCA* gene mutation (NCT01074970)*

Note: Some of these trials include patients whose cancer is hormone-receptor positive as well as those with triple-negative disease.
*This is a phase 2 trial.

Table 6.5 Summary of randomized phase 3 trials investigating checkpoint inhibitors as treatments for triple-negative breast cancer.

Treatments under investigation	Number of women taking part and estimated study completion date	Study population and ClinicalTrials.gov Identifier
Pembrolizumab or chemotherapy	600; May 2019	Women with metastatic TNBC (NCT02555657)
Chemotherapy with or without pembrolizumab	858; December 2019	Women with previously untreated metastatic TNBC (NCT02819518)
Neoadjuvant chemotherapy with or without pembrolizumab, followed by adjuvant pembrolizumab or placebo	855; March 2025	Women with operable TNBC (NCT03036488)
Adjuvant pembrolizumab versus observation	1000; May 2026	Women with operable TNBC (NCT02954874)
Chemotherapy with or without atezolizumab	900; April 2020	Women with previously untreated metastatic TNBC (NCT02425891)
Chemotherapy with or without atezolizumab	540; June 2021	Women with previously-untreated locally advanced or metastatic TNBC (NCT03125902)
Neoadjuvant chemotherapy with or without atezolizumab, followed by adjuvant atezolizumab or placebo	1520; June 2024	Women with operable TNBC (NCT03281954)
Neoadjuvant chemotherapy with or without atezolizumab	272; October 2022	Women with locally advanced TNBC (NCT02620280)
Neoadjuvant chemotherapy with or without atezolizumab	204; September 2021	Women with early-stage TNBC (NCT03197935)
Chemotherapy with or without atezolizumab	350; January 2021	Women with inoperable recurrent TNBC (NCT03371017)
Adjuvant avelumab versus observation	335; June 2023	Women with high-risk, operable TNBC (NCT02926196)

Immunotherapy for TNBCs

TNBC's tend to contain more DNA mutations than other types of breast cancer,[6] and they contain higher levels of infiltrating B-cells and T-cells. There's also more PD-L1 on the surface of TNBC cells than on the cells of other breast cancers [33]. So it makes sense to test out monoclonal antibody checkpoint inhibitors that target PD-1 or PD-L1. So far, the trials have been pretty small, and the response rates have tended to be fairly low – about 18% (complete responses plus partial responses) [33]. But, when patients do benefit from checkpoint inhibitors, they often benefit for many months, or even years. For this reason, doctors are very excited about the potential of checkpoint inhibitors as treatments for TNBC. And as a result, various checkpoint inhibitors are being investigated in phase 3 trials (Table 6.5).

6.2.6 Conclusions

The survival times for women with breast cancer have improved hugely over the past few decades. For example, since the 1970s the death rate for breast cancer has dropped by

---

[6] In many clinical trials, cancers with high numbers of mutations have often been sensitive to treatment with checkpoint inhibitors.

32% [38]. However, much of this is due to improved treatments for hormone receptor-positive and HER2-positive breast cancer. The treatments available for the 15% or so of women whose cancers lack these receptors (TNBCs) have remained pretty much the same – that is, surgery, chemotherapy, and radiotherapy. Thankfully, advances made in our understanding of so-called TNBC are leading to new treatment opportunities such as PARP inhibitors and checkpoint inhibitors. Hopefully these advances will mean that the survival times for women with TNBC soon begin to climb.

6.3 TARGETED TREATMENTS FOR PROSTATE CANCER

Over 46,000 men are diagnosed with prostate cancer each year in the United Kingdom [39]. Prostate cancers depend on the hormone testosterone for their growth and survival, and hormone therapies are very important treatments. Other treatment approaches for prostate cancer include a number of treatments that are beyond the scope of this book. These include photodynamic therapy, brachytherapy, high-intensity focal ultrasound, and Radium-223 – a calcium-mimicking radiation-emitting particle that gets incorporated into bones, and targets bone metastases [40].

Apart from hormone therapies, none of the other targeted treatments mentioned in this book are yet licensed as prostate cancer treatments. Some approaches, such as angiogenesis inhibitors, have been tried but failed to improve survival times. Other treatments, such as PARP inhibitors, are looking highly promising.

6.3.1 Hormone Therapies for Prostate Cancer

As with hormone therapies for breast cancer, those used for prostate cancer work in one of two ways: they either block the actions of the receptor, which in this case is the androgen receptor,[7] or they block the production of the hormone that activates the receptor: testosterone. There are similarities between androgen receptors (ARs) and ERs:

- ARs are present in both normal and cancer-causing prostate cells.
- ARs respond to the presence of testosterone by pairing up and attaching to genes in the cell's chromosomes.
- Once attached to genes, ARs act as transcription factors and trigger the production of many different proteins [41].

Treatments That Block Testosterone Production
Testosterone is made in a man's testes and adrenal glands in response to hormones released by the brain (see Figure 6.3). Two sets of treatments can block the production of testosterone: the LHRH (GnRH)[8] agonists and the LHRH (GnRH) antagonists (again, to see what role LHRH/GnRH has in the production of testosterone, see Figure 6.3).

LHRH Agonists (Also Known as GnRH Agonists) [43]
- LHRH agonists have been used as prostate cancer treatments for over 25 years.
- Because they activate LHRH receptors, they first of all cause luteinizing hormone (LH) and follicle stimulating hormone (FSH) production by pituitary cells in the brain to increase, causing a surge in testosterone levels. But after further treatment, pituitary cells lose their LHRH receptors and shut down LH and FSH production.

---

[7] Androgen receptors are similar to estrogen receptors except that they respond to testosterone and other androgens (male sex hormones) such as dihydrotestosterone.
[8] LHRH stands for luteinizing hormone-releasing hormone; GnRH is gonadotropin-releasing hormone.

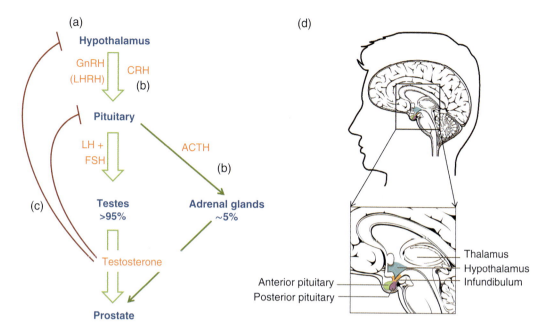

Figure 6.3 How testosterone production is controlled in men [42]. **(a)** The hypothalamus releases gonadotropin-releasing hormone (GnRH) (also called luteinizing hormone releasing hormone – LHRH). GnRH binds to cells in the pituitary gland, prompting them to secrete follicle stimulating hormone (FSH) and luteinizing hormone (LH). LH and FSH travel through the body and cause cells in the testes to produce testosterone. Testosterone binds to androgen receptors in the testes, and both testosterone and FSH are required for the creation and maturation of sperm. Testosterone also binds to androgen receptors in the prostate. **(b)** A small amount of testosterone is made by the adrenal glands that sit on top of the kidneys. They produce testosterone in response to ACTH (adrenocorticotropic hormone) released by the pituitary. ACTH release is in turn controlled by CRH (corticotropin-releasing hormone) released by the hypothalamus. **(c)** Rising levels of testosterone trigger a feedback loop that suppresses further production of GnRH, LH, or FSH. **(d)** The location of the hypothalamus and pituitary in the brain.
Abbreviations: GnRH – gonadotropin-releasing hormone; LHRH – luteinizing-hormone-releasing hormone; FSH – follicle stimulating hormone; LH – luteinizing hormone; ACTH – adrenocorticotropic hormone; CRH – a corticotropin-releasing hormone Brain image from: https://en.wikipedia.org/wiki/File:1806_The_Hypothalamus-Pituitary_Complex.jpg

- They include treatments such as goserelin (Zoladex or Novgos), leuprorelin acetate (Prostap or Lutrate), triptorelin (Decapeptyl or Gonapeptyl Depot), and buserelin acetate (Suprefact).

LHRH Antagonists (Also Known as GnRH Antagonists) [43]

- The first LHRH antagonist (abarelix) was licensed as a prostate cancer treatment in 2003.

- They reduce testosterone levels more quickly than the LHRH agonists, and don't cause any surge in LH and FSH levels.
- They include treatments such as degarelix (Firmagon), abarelix (Plenaxis),[9] and relugolix.

Treatments That Block ARs (Anti-androgens) [44]

- Anti-androgens all have a chemical structure that is similar to testosterone, and they

---

[9] Abarelix was withdrawn when it caused life-threatening allergic reactions in clinical trials.

compete with testosterone for its binding site on the AR.

- Once bound to the AR, they trigger ARs to pair up, just as testosterone does, but once the paired-up ARs reach the nucleus they can't work properly and can't activate target genes.[10]
- They include treatments such as bicalutamide (Casodex), flutamide (Drogenil), and cyproterone acetate (Cyprostat).

6.3.2 Second-Generation Hormone Therapies

Hormone therapies are standard treatments for men with advanced prostate cancer. However, although they can keep a man's cancer at bay for many months and years, the cancer inevitably becomes resistant and starts growing again. Scientists investigating hormone therapy-resistant prostate cancers (often known as castration-resistant prostate cancers) have discovered that the resistant cancer cells are generally still driven by testosterone. So their focus has been on creating drugs that lower testosterone levels still further or that block ARs more completely. This work has led them to create two new hormone therapies: abiraterone (Zytiga) and enzalutamide (Xtandi).

Enzalutamide (Xtandi) [44]

Enzalutamide has three benefits over first-generation anti-androgens:

- It has a far greater affinity for the androgen receptor than other anti-androgens, and hence it's better at preventing testosterone from binding to ARs.
- It prevents ARs from entering the nucleus, whereas other anti-androgens don't.
- It prevents paired-up ARs from activating genes. This is important, as other anti-androgens can only suppress ARs when they're present at normal levels; in cells that are producing high levels of ARs, the first-generation drugs actually activate them rather than suppress them; whereas enzalutamide always suppresses ARs.

Abiraterone (Zytiga)

One limitation of LHRH agonists and antagonists is that although they can block testosterone production by the testes, they can't prevent testosterone production by the adrenal glands. However, abiraterone gets around this problem by blocking testosterone production via an entirely different mechanism. It blocks an enzyme (a catalyst) necessary for the manufacture of testosterone anywhere in the body. The enzyme is called CYP17A. As a result, abiraterone can lower testosterone levels even further than first-generation drugs [45].

6.3.3 Overcoming Resistance to Hormone Therapies

Sadly, even with the creation of second-generation hormone therapies, prostate cancers still inevitably become resistant,[11] and scientists have discovered many different resistance mechanisms. These include [45]:

- Prostate cancer cells and adrenal glands use alternative enzymes to create androgens.
- Mutations in the AR gene cause the production of shortened versions of ARs that respond to hormones other than testosterone, or that don't need any hormones at all.
- Amplification of the AR gene and subsequent overproduction of AR protein allows cells to survive even when only tiny amounts of testosterone are present.

---

[10] Remember that ARs, like ERs, are transcription factors that, once paired up, attach to genes and trigger the production of many different proteins.
[11] Hormone therapy-resistant prostate cancer is sometimes called hormone-refractory, castrate-resistant or castration-resistant prostate cancer.

- The cancer cells produce high levels of glucocorticoid receptors, which can partly substitute for ARs.
- The cancer cells increase their production of AR co-activators (there are over 150 different AR co-regulators).
- Growth factor receptor signaling pathways become overactive, and they activate ARs in the absence of testosterone, or allow the cell to survive even when its ARs are suppressed.

Strategies to overcome resistance include using PARP inhibitors, signaling pathway blockers, angiogenesis inhibitors, and immunotherapies.

PARP Inhibitors

Around 20% of prostate cancers have defects affecting DNA repair. Scientists have also discovered that prostate cancer cells that contain a translocation that creates a fusion protein called TMPRSS2-ERG are sensitive to PARP inhibitors [46]. Phase 1 and phase 2 trials with PARP inhibitors have been very promising, with trials such as TOPARP reporting a response rate of 88% in men whose tumors contained defects in DNA repair genes [47]. Two PARP inhibitors, olaparib and rucaparib, are now being investigated in phase 3 trials. For example, the PROfound study (NCT02987543) is investigating olaparib versus enzalutamide or abiraterone in 340 men whose disease has progressed despite hormone therapy and whose cancer cells contain defects in genes involved in homologous recombination. The rucaparib trial (TRITON3; NCT02975934) is very similar and is recruiting 400 men.

Blocking Signaling Pathways

Almost 50% of hormone-therapy resistant prostate cancers contain defects in various proteins involved in the PI3K/AKT/mTOR pathway. Another discovery is that suppression of ARs automatically leads to increased PI3K/AKT/mTOR signaling, and vice versa. That's why scientists think it might be useful to suppress both pathways together [48]. Various trials are under way to find out whether a combination of an mTOR or PI3K inhibitor along with a hormone treatment will benefit men with previously-treated, hormone-therapy-resistant prostate cancer. For example, a phase 3 trial (NCT03072238) is investigating ipatasertib (an AKT inhibitor) plus abiraterone in 850 men with hormone-therapy-resistant prostate cancer.

6.3.4 Immunotherapy for Prostate Cancer

Back in Chapter 5, Section 5.6.1 I mentioned an immunotherapy approach for prostate cancer called sipileucel-T (Provenge). Although the trials with this treatment were successful, the cost and practicalities of implementing it have proved to be its downfall. After first being licensed for prostate cancer, the treatment was later withdrawn [49]. However, some prostate cancers do contain very high numbers of mutations and they might therefore respond to other immunotherapies such as checkpoint inhibitors. And, prostate cancers often contain lots of infiltrating T cells, which again is a hopeful sign for the possible usefulness of checkpoint inhibitors [50].

So far, the only completed phase 3 trial investigating a checkpoint inhibitor in prostate cancer was a trial with ipilimumab (Yervoy) (see Chapter 5, Section 5.3.3). This trial wasn't successful – the survival time wasn't improved with ipilimumab [51] – but other ipilimumab trials are in progress.

There are also trials under way investigating PD-1 and PD-L1 antibodies (see Chapter 5, Section 5.3.5), including a phase 3 trial investigating atezolizumab (NCT03016312). None of the trials completed so far have involved enough men with prostate cancer to draw any firm conclusions. However, some prostate cancers do contain PD-L1, and there is some evidence for a role of PD-L1 in causing resistance to hormone therapies [50]. And with many trials taking place, hopefully it'll soon be clear whether or not they have a future as prostate cancer treatments.

6.3.5 Conclusions

Advanced prostate cancers are dependent on ARs. And this dependence is generally still there even when available hormone therapies have failed. Scientists working on new treatments are therefore predominantly focusing their efforts on lowering testosterone levels yet further, or blocking ARs with greater and greater efficacy. However, new insights into the biology and genetics of advanced prostate cancers are leading to some new treatment approaches, such as PARP inhibitors and signaling pathway inhibitors. And, as with pretty much all cancers at the present time, there are also many trials with checkpoint inhibitors.

6.4 TARGETED TREATMENTS FOR LUNG CANCER

Each year around 25,000 men and 21,500 women are diagnosed with lung cancer in the United Kingdom [52]. Lung cancers are divided into two main types: non-small cell lung cancer (NSCLC) and small cell lung cancer (SCLC). NSCLCs are by far the most common, accounting for around 85%–90% of cases. 86% of all lung cancers are caused by smoking [53].

Within NSCLC there are subdivisions that have important implications for treatment. For example, the two most common types of NSCLC are adenocarcinomas and squamous cell carcinomas. *EGFR* mutations, *ALK* mutations, and *ROS1* mutations are all more common in adenocarcinoma NSCLC [54], and people whose cancers contain these mutations are now generally treated with EGFR and ALK (and ROS1[12]) inhibitors. In addition, the different types of lung cancer develop from different cells in the lungs (see Figure 6.4), and they also contain mutations in different genes [55] (see Table 6.6). These genetic differences are likely to become more and more important as we move into an era where lung cancers are treated according to the mutations they contain.

Another important fact is that lung cancers in people who have a history of smoking contain different DNA mutations than non-smokers.[13] For example *EGFR*, *ALK*, and *ROS1* mutations are all more common in non-smokers [54]. In addition, lung cancers in smokers contain around 10 times the amount of DNA damage compared with lung cancers in non-smokers [55]. This has important implications for immunotherapy with checkpoint inhibitors: this approach has so far been most effective against lung cancers in smokers, presumably because of their high number of mutations [55]. Checkpoint inhibitors are also looking promising against SCLC. SCLC is notoriously difficult to treat, and many different approaches have failed to improve survival times. As well as checkpoint inhibitors, other approaches for SCLC in phase 3 trials include an antibody-drug conjugate called rovalpituzumab tesirine [58] and an angiogenesis inhibitor called apatinib.

Over the past ten years or so, a wide variety of targeted cancer treatments have been approved for use against NSCLC (but none for SCLC). These are summarized in Table 6.7.

---

[12] Testing for *ROS1* mutations and treating *ROS1*-mutated lung cancer with ROS1 inhibitors are currently the subject of a scoping exercise by NICE that began in February 2017.

[13] If a non-smoker develops lung cancer, it's mostly likely to be an adenocarcinoma NSCLC.

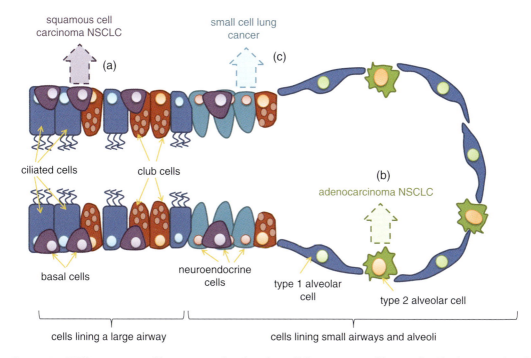

Figure 6.4 Different types of lung cancer develop from different types of lung cells. The lungs are lined by a variety of different cell types. **(a)** Squamous cell carcinoma NSCLCs tend to arise in the large airways in the lungs and develop from faulty basal cells. **(b)** Adenocarcinoma NSCLCs arise from alveolar cells in the tiny air sacs in the lungs called alveoli. **(c)** Small cell lung cancers arise from neuroendocrine cells [55]. **Abbreviations:** NSCLC – non-small cell lung cancer

Table 6.6 Common driver mutations in non-small cell lung cancers.

Pathway/process affected	Genes that are altered (% of cases) [55–57]	
	Adenocarcinoma (AC)[a]	**Squamous cell carcinoma (SqCC)[a]**
Cell-cycle control	*TP53* (63%), *CDKN2A*[b] (43%), *RB1* (7%), *CDK4* (7%), *CCNE1* (3%), *CCND1* (4%)	*TP53* (81%), *CDKN2A*[b] (72%), *RB1* (7%)
Growth factor signaling	*KRAS* (33%), *EGFR* (14%), *HER2* (3%), *BRAF* (10%), *STK11* (17%), *MET* (8%), *NF1* (11%), *PIK3CA*[c] (7%), *RIT1* (2%), *ALK* (4%), *ROS1* (2%), *RET* (1%)	*PIK3CA*[c] (16%), *PTEN* (15%), *EGFR* (9%), *HRAS* (3%), *KRAS* (3%), *NRAS* (1%), *FGFR1/2/3* (12%), *HER2* (4%), *BRAF* (4%), *TSC1/2* (6%), *NF1* (11%), *AKT 1/2/3* (20%)
Oxidative stress response	*KEAP1* (17%)	*CUL3* (6%), *KEAP1* (12%), *NFE2L2* (15%)
Aberrant splicing	*U2AF1* (3%), *RBM10* (8%)	
Squamous differentiation:		*NOTCH1* (8%), *ASCL4* (3%), *NOTCH2* (5%)

[a] Do note that this isn't a definitive list of either mutations or percentages – the mutations found, and their frequency, depend on the number of samples studied and the make-up of the study population, such as how many smokers there were, what age, what gender, and so on.
[b] *CDKN2A* is the gene for making p16, an important CDK inhibitor.
[c] *PIK3CA* is the gene for making the catalytic part of PI3K.

Table 6.7 Summary of licensed targeted treatments for lung cancer in the United States and the European Union (EU).

Drug	Licensed for [59]
EGFR inhibitors	
Gefitinib/Iressa	NSCLC with activating mutations in the *EGFR* gene
Erlotinib/Tarceva	NSCLC with activating mutations in the *EGFR* gene
Afatinib/Giotrif/Gilotrif	NSCLC with activating mutations in the *EGFR* gene
Osimertinib/Tagrisso	NSCLC with the T790M activating mutation in the *EGFR* gene (this mutation causes resistance to gefitinib, erlotinib and afatinib EGFR inhibitors)
Necitumumab/Portrazza	Squamous cell NSCLCs in which EGFR is present on the cells' surface (in combination with platinum-based chemotherapy)
ALK inhibitors	
Crizotinib/Xalkori	NSCLC with an *ALK* gene rearrangement
Alectinib/Alecensa	NSCLC with an *ALK* gene rearrangement as a first-line treatment and for patients previously treated with crizotinib
Ceritinib/Zykadia	NSCLC with an *ALK* gene rearrangement as a first-line treatment and for patients previously treated with crizotinib
Brigatinib/Alunbrig	NSCLC with an *ALK* gene rearrangement previously treated with crizotinib (United States only)
ROS1 inhibitors	
Crizotinib/Xalkori	NSCLC with a *ROS1* gene rearrangement
B-Raf inhibitors	
Dabrafenib/Tafinlar	NSCLC with the *BRAF* V600E mutation, in combination with the MEK inhibitor trametinib (Mekinist)
Angiogenesis inhibitors	
Bevacizumab/Avastin	As a first-line treatment for: • NSCLCs that are not squamous cell carcinomas (in combination with platinum-based chemotherapy) • NSCLC with activating mutations in the *EGFR* gene (for which it is given in combination with erlotinib, an EGFR-inhibitor)
Ramucirumab/Cyramza	As a second-line treatment for NSCLC, in combination with docetaxel chemotherapy
Nintedanib/Vargatef	As a second-line treatment for NSCLC, in combination with docetaxel chemotherapy (EU only)
Checkpoint inhibitors	
Nivolumab/Opdivo	NSCLCs previously treated with chemotherapy
Pembrolizumab/Keytruda	• NSCLCs previously treated with chemotherapy in which >1% of cancer cells are known to have PD-L1 on their surface • Previously untreated NSCLCs in which >50% of cancer cells are known to have PD-L1 on their surface
Atezolizumab/Tecentriq	NSCLCs previously treated with chemotherapy

Abbreviations: NSCLC – non-small cell lung cancer; EGFR – epidermal growth factor receptor; ALK – anaplastic lymphoma kinase; ROS1 – ROS proto-oncogene 1; PD-L1 – programmed death ligand-1

6.4.1 First- and Second-Generation EGFR Kinase Inhibitors

Back in Chapter 3, Section 3.3.2, I wrote about various kinase inhibitors that block EGFR. And I told you that they are highly effective against the 10% or so of NSCLCs in which the *EGFR* gene is mutated in such a way that EGFR is overactive.

Two particular mutations, called exon[14] 19 deletions and L858R (the normal lysine (L) amino acid at position 858 has become an arginine (R)), account for 85% of all *EGFR* mutations found in lung cancer patients. The mutated receptors are up to 50 times more active than normal EGFRs [60]. Generally, only one copy of the *EGFR* gene in the cancer cells is mutated,[15] but the mutated gene is generally also amplified; that is, there are lots of copies of it. Other mutations that sensitize NSCLCs to EGFR inhibitors are glycine 719 in exon 18, which accounts for about 5% of *EGFR* mutations, and rarer mutations such as G719C, G719S, G719A, L861Q and S768I. *EGFR* mutations are most common in East Asian people, in non-smokers, and in people with adenocarcinoma NSCLC rather than squamous cell NSCLC [60].

There are also some mutations that make NSCLCs insensitive to EGFR inhibitors. These include the T790M mutation in exon 20, which is present in about 5% of newly diagnosed NSCLCs, and in up to 60% of NSCLCs resistant to EGFR inhibitors [60].

The two most well-known first-generation EGFR kinase inhibitors are gefitinib (Iressa) and erlotinib (Tarceva). When these drugs were first tested in clinical trials in the late 1990s and early 2000s, scientists thought that all patients with NSCLC might benefit from them. However, clinical trials generally showed a response rate of about 10%. Then, in 2004, scientists studying biopsy samples from NSCLC patients discovered how to predict who would or wouldn't benefit. They found that patients whose NSCLC cells contained mutated, overactive versions of EGFR were those that benefited, whereas patients whose NSCLC didn't contain an *EGFR* gene mutation didn't get any better [61]. This realization led to clinical trials involving only people with sensitizing *EGFR* mutations. And these trials led to the licensing of both treatments.

First-generation EGFR inhibitors such as gefitinib and erlotinib are reversible inhibitors of EGFR. Second-generation EGFR inhibitors such as afatinib (Giotrif/Gilotrif) in contrast are irreversible inhibitors.

Many scientists have tried to compare the usefulness of erlotinib, gefitinib, or afatinib by comparing the results from many clinical trials [62–64]. There have also been a couple of clinical trials in which two EGFR kinase inhibitors have been directly compared against one another (gefitinib vs. afatinib in the LUX-Lung-7 trial [65]; gefitinib versus erlotinib in the WJOG 5108L trial [66]). The results from these analyses generally suggest that all three drugs are pretty similar in their effectiveness. Having said that, there is some evidence that second-generation inhibitors may be more effective, but cause more severe side effects, than first-generation drugs [67].

6.4.2 Third-Generation EGFR Kinase Inhibitors

Most people with *EGFR*-mutated NSCLC benefit from treatment with an EGFR inhibitor like gefitinib, erlotinib, or afatinib. However, the benefit they get from these drugs generally lasts between 9 and 13 months [68]. The most common reason why a patient's tumor starts growing again is because of cancer cells that contain the T790M mutation. This mutation changes the shape of EGFR's ATP-binding site in such a way that its affinity

---

[14] Most of our genes contain exons and introns. Exons contain the information needed to make the corresponding protein, whereas the information from introns gets discarded.
[15] Our cells have two copies of every chromosome, and hence two copies (alleles) of every gene.

for ATP increases, and drugs like gefinitib and erlotinib can no longer block it [68].

Scientists believe that in some patients a handful of T790M mutant cells are there right from the start, before the person has received any treatment. Having survived treatment with a first- or second- generation EGFR inhibitor, these cells continue to multiply and become the most dominant cells in the tumor, eventually causing the patient to relapse. In other patients, it's thought that cancer cells that somehow survive EGFR inhibitor treatment later pick up the T790M mutation by chance, and then grow and cause relapse [69].

Third-generation EGFR inhibitors like osimertinib (Tagrisso) can kill T790M-mutant cancer cells (see Chapter 3, Section 3.3.2 for more details). And they can kill cells with *EGFR* mutations that render them sensitive to first- and second-generation EGFR inhibitors – for a comparison of first-, second-, and third-generation drugs, see Chapter 3, Table 3.3. In trials, osimertinib has proved effective for lung cancers that are resistant to first- and second-generation drugs. For example, in a phase 3 trial involving people whose cancer was resistant to a first- or second-generation drug due to the T790M mutation, the response rate for osimertinib was 71% (compared to 31% with chemotherapy) [70]. The PFS from this trial was 10.1 months with osimertinib, versus 4.4 months with chemotherapy.

There have also been promising results with osimertinib as a first-line treatment. In a phase 3 trial involving 556 patients with previously untreated advanced NSCLC, osimertinib was compared to gefitinib or erlotinib. All three drugs gave similar response rates (76%–80%), but the median duration of response with osimertinib was 17.2 months, compared to 8.5 months with gefitinib or erlotinib [71].

6.4.3 EGFR-Targeted Antibodies

The only EGFR-targeted antibody licensed for lung cancer is necitumumab (Portrazza). This antibody, although very similar to the bowel cancer treatments cetuximab and panitumumab, has been investigated almost exclusively in lung cancer. The phase 3 clinical trial that led to the approval of necitumumab was the SQUIRE trial, which demonstrated that when necitumumab is added to chemotherapy, it improve survival times by about 6 or 7 weeks (11.5 months vs. 9.9 months) [72]. Perhaps the most interesting aspect of this trial was that it exclusively involved people with squamous cell NSCLC, whereas we normally talk about EGFR-targeted treatments for adenocarcinomas. In Europe, the approval of necitumumab is only for people whose cancer cells have EGFR on their surface (which is about 95% of patients with squamous cell NSCLC[16]). In this group of people, the OS result was 11.7 months versus 10.0 months [73].

Because of benefits of necitumumab are modest, as with many other treatments there has been much discussion in the medical community over what is a reasonable price to pay for it [74, 75].

6.4.4 Targeting ALK and ROS1

Around 3%–5% of NSCLCs contain an *ALK* gene rearrangement, and a further 1%–2% contain a *ROS1* gene rearrangement [76] (I wrote about both of them in Chapter 4, Section 4.2.4).

As with *EGFR* mutations, gene mutations affecting *ALK* and *ROS1* are more common in non-smokers and light smokers rather than in heavy smokers, and they're more common in adenocarcinomas than other NSCLC types [54]. *ALK* and *ROS1* mutations

---

[16] This might seem high, but most lung cancers have EGFR on their surface; but only 10% or so have mutated versions of EGFR that make them sensitive to the first-, second-, and third-generation EGFR kinase inhibitors.

are also more common in relatively young lung cancer patients [77].

ALK Inhibitors

Crizotinib (Xalkori), ceritinib (Zykadia), alectinib (Alecensa), and brigatinib (Alunbrig)[17] are all licensed treatments for *ALK*-mutated NSCLC (for their comparison with other ALK inhibitors, see Chapter 4, Table 4.4).

Crizotinib was the first ALK inhibitor to be licensed as a first-line treatment for people with *ALK*-mutated lung cancer. Ceritinib and alectinib were later licensed for people whose cancer was resistant to crizotinib. However, it looks like the second-generation drugs may eventually take over from crizotinib. Both ceritinib and alectinib were awarded approval as first-line treatments in 2017. The approval of alectinib was based on the ALEX trial, in which 303 people with *ALK*-mutated lung cancer were randomized to receive either alectinib or crizotinib. Results from this trial are shown in Table 6.8. As you can see, alectinib was superior to crizotinib, particularly in terms of PFS and its ability to prevent brain metastases [78].

ROS1 Inhibitors

As well as blocking ALK, crizotinib and some other ALK inhibitors can also block ROS1. This realization, and the discovery of *ROS1* mutations in 1%–2% of NSCLCs, led to a trial of 50 patients with *ROS1* mutations.[18] 72% of the people in the trial responded to treatment with crizotinib with a median PFS of 19.2 months (which is longer than the PFS seen with crizotinib in *ALK*-mutated NSCLC, which is generally more like 7–10 months) [76]. Crizotinib is now licensed for *ROS1*-mutated NSCLC in both the United States and Europe.

6.4.5 Targeting B-Raf

The *BRAF* gene is mutated in 1%–4% of people with NSCLC [79], and around half of these people have the *BRAF* V600E mutation commonly found in malignant melanoma.

In people with malignant melanomas that contain the V600E *BRAF* mutation, a combination of a B-Raf inhibitor with a MEK inhibitor works better than either drug alone (see Section 6.6 for more about this). Scientists have investigated the same combination in

Table 6.8 Results from ALEX trial which involved 303 people with *ALK*-mutated NSCLC who hadn't received any prior treatment with an ALK inhibitor.

	Alectinib	Crizotinib
Estimated median progression-free survival	25.7 months	10.4 months
Objective response rate	79%	72%
Incidence of brain metastases at 12 months	9.4%	41.4%
Incidence of grade 3 or 4 adverse events	41%	50%

Source: Peters S et al. (2017). Alectinib versus crizotinib in untreated ALK-positive non-small-cell lung cancer. *N Engl J Med* 377(9):829–838.

---

[17] At the time of writing, brigatinib is licensed in the United States only.
[18] This might not seem like a lot of patients, but do take a moment to think about the number of people's tumors they will have had to test to find 50 people with *ROS1* mutations.

people with V600E *BRAF*-mutated NSCLC. For example, in a trial of 57 patients, 36 of them (63%) responded to a combination of dabrafenib (Tafinlar) plus trametinib (Mekinist) [80].

The dabrafenib/trametinib combination was approved for V600E *BRAF*-mutated NSCLC in Europe and the United States in 2017 [81].

6.4.6 Targeting Other Mutations

Scientists around the world have studied hundreds of biopsy samples from people with adenocarcinoma NSCLC and squamous cell NSCLC to find out what gene mutations drive them. As well as discovering that 10%–15% of adenocarcinomas contain *EGFR* mutations, that 3%–5% contain *ALK* mutations, and that 1%–2% contain *ROS1* mutations, they have also discovered many other mutations (see Table 6.6).

These mutations include several that it might be possible to target directly or indirectly with existing targeted treatments. For example, there are trials in progress with HER2 inhibitors, RET inhibitors, and MET inhibitors for *HER2-*, *RET-*, and *MET*-mutated lung cancers. There are also trials of Trk inhibitors for the 3% or so of adenocarcinoma NSCLCs that contain *NTRK1* mutations.

Two other groups of mutations are worth mentioning: those that affect CDK activity (including *CDKN2A* mutations, *CCND1* amplification, and *CDK4* amplification), and those that affect K-Ras activity (i.e., *KRAS* mutations). There is evidence that people with either of these sets of mutations might benefit from a CDK4/6 inhibitor such as palbociclib (for more on CDK4/6 inhibitors, see Chapter 4, Section 4.5). In the National Lung Matrix Trial – a UK trial in which NSCLC patients are

being subdivided into 21 groups depending on the mutations their cancers contain – people whose tumors contain *CDKN2A*, *CCND1*, *CDK4*, or *KRAS* mutations will receive palbociclib [82]. In the same trial, the investigators are also testing out an FGFR[19] inhibitor for cancers with *FGFR* mutations; an mTOR inhibitor for cancers with *TSC1/2* mutations (see Chapter 3, Section 3.8.2); crizotinib[20] for cancers with *MET* or *ROS1* mutations; a MEK inhibitor (selumetinib) plus chemotherapy for cancers with *NF1*[21] or *NRAS* mutations; an AKT inhibitor for cancers with mutations affecting PI3K, PTEN, or AKT1; and finally immunotherapy with a checkpoint inhibitor for cancers in which none of these mutations can be detected [82].

Scientists hope that in the coming years, we will be in a position where we can test lung cancer cells for a wide variety of mutations, and be able to treat patients with appropriate, effective, targeted treatments.

6.4.7 Angiogenesis Inhibitors

Like other solid tumors, **NSCLCs depend on angiogenesis to deliver adequate oxygen and nutrient supplies**. And, again similar to other cancers, angiogenesis, and VEGF production are associated with an increased risk of tumor recurrence, metastasis and death [83]. It's therefore logical to think that treatments that block angiogenesis might be useful lung cancer treatments.

Frustratingly, **angiogenesis inhibitors have had a mixed history as treatments for lung cancer** (for lots more information on angiogenesis inhibitors, see Chapter 4, Section 4.1). And it's not for a want of trials – a quick search of clinicaltrials.gov reveals 32 phase 3 trials investigating bevacizumab (Avastin) for

---

[19] FGFR – fibroblast growth factor receptor – a growth factor receptor similar to EGFR and VEGFR.
[20] Remember that crizotinib blocks ALK, MET, and ROS1.
[21] NF1 suppresses Ras proteins; mutations in the *NF1* gene lead to loss of NF1 protein.

NSCLC, two with ramucirumab (Cyramza), and three with nintedanib (Vargatef).[22] There have been many other large trials with kinase inhibitors such as pazopanib (Votrient), cabozantinib (Cometriq), axitinib (Inlyta), sorafenib (Nexavar), lenvatinib (Lenvima), apatinib, and sunitinib (Sutent). Further trials have investigated some of these drugs as treatments for SCLC.

A common pattern with trials investigating angiogenesis inhibitors for people with lung cancer is that they are often able to improve PFS but rarely able to improve OS [84]. A problem seems to be that the predominant mechanism of action of all licensed angiogenesis inhibitors is that they block VEGF signaling. But lung tumors rapidly switch to using alternative growth factors rather than VEGF [85].

Rather than discuss every trial that has investigated an angiogenesis inhibitor for lung cancer, I'll just give a run through of the drugs that have been licensed so far, and why.

If you want to refresh your memory as to the mechanism of action of each drug, do look back at Chapter 4, Section 4.1.5.

Bevacizumab (Avastin)

In both the United States and Europe, bevacizumab is licensed as a first-line treatment for non-squamous NSCLC (it's too likely to cause bleeding in people with squamous cell NSCLC). The license was granted on the basis of two large phase 3 trials. The first trial (ECOG 4599) showed a two-month improvement in OS (12.3 months vs. 10.3 months) when bevacizumab was added to chemotherapy. But the second trial (AVAiL) showed smaller improvements in PFS and no improvement in survival times [84].

Bevacizumab is also licensed in Europe in combination with erlotinib for the treatment of NSCLC in people with activating *EGFR* mutations. This license was granted on the basis of the JO25567 phase 2 trial, which in involved 154 Japanese people with *EGFR*-mutated NSCLC. The PFS as 16.0 months with the combination, versus 9.7 months with erlotinib alone [86].

Ramucirumab (Cyramza)

A phase 3 trial (REVEL) demonstrated that ramucirumab can improve PFS from 3.0 months to 4.5 months, and OS from 9.1 months to 10.5 months, in people with NSCLC who had already received platinum-based chemotherapy [87].

Nintedanib (Vargatef)

Nintenanib is licensed in Europe, but not in the United States, as a second-line treatment for advanced adenocarcinoma NSCLC. Proof of its benefits came from the LUME-Lung 1 trial. This trial showed that the addition of nintedanib to docetaxel improved PFS from 2.8 months to 4.2 months, and OS from 10.3 months to 12.6 months [88].

6.4.8 Immunotherapy for NSCLC

Despite being the new kids on the block, as of December 2017 three checkpoint inhibitors are already licensed as NSCLC treatments: nivolumab (Opdivo), pembrolizumab (Keytruda), and atezolizumab (Tecentriq) (see Table 6.7). Nivolumab and pembrolizumab both block PD-1 (which is found on the surface of T cells, B cells, and NK cells [89]), whereas atezolizumab blocks PD-1's ligand, PD-L1 (found on T cells, B cells, macrophages, dendritic cells, and cancer cells [89]) (see Chapter 5, Section 5.3 for more about checkpoint proteins and checkpoint inhibitors).

In around 20%–65% of NSCLCs, you can find PD-L1 present at some level within the

---

[22] I used www.clinicaltrials.gov to search for trials on February 17, 2017.

tumor [89] (the percentage depends on what test you use and what cutoff you set). The presence of PD-L1, and of infiltrating T cells, is generally seen as an encouraging sign that treatment with a checkpoint inhibitor might be helpful for that patient.

Confusingly, **trials with checkpoint inhibitors have been inconsistent in terms of patient selection**. In some trials, no threshold of PD-L1 level has been set; whereas in other trials, patient inclusion has been dependent on the presence of PD-L1. Even when a PD-L1 cutoff has been used, trials with different checkpoint inhibitors have used different cutoffs and different testing methods. However, from trials conducted to date, it does seem that PD-1 and PD-L1 antibodies are more likely to benefit [90, 91]:

- Patients whose NSCLCs contains high levels of PD-L1
- Smokers and ex-smokers (rather than non-smokers), as their cancers contain a high number of DNA mutations
- People whose tumors contain high numbers of infiltrating lymphocytes and high levels of IFN-gamma (a signaling molecule produced by natural killer cells and activated T cells)

Response rates to PD-1 and PD-L1 inhibitors are generally around 15%–30% [90], but these responses are often delayed, which can produce confusing results in clinical trials. The delay appears to be because it takes a while for the activated T cells to kill enough cancer cells to start seeing an impact. Also, tumors sometimes get bigger before they get smaller – this is because so many white blood cells are entering the tumor that it initially appears to grow [92].

Perhaps one of the most impressive indicators of the impact that checkpoint inhibitors can have is "duration of response." For example, in the CheckMate 057 trial (see Table 6.9), the median duration of response was 17.1 months for nivolumab versus 5.6 months for docetaxel. This result was despite underwhelming PFS data (2.3 months for nivolumab vs. 4.2 months for docetaxel) [93]. Also, the same trial demonstrated that anti-PD-1/PD-L1 antibodies are much safer than chemotherapy, with grade 3–5 toxicities occurring in 10% of patients given nivolumab versus 54% with docetaxel. Other trials investigating pembrolizumab and atezolizumab have given similar results for people with either squamous or non-squamous NSCLC.

One of the current limitations with checkpoint inhibitors is the relatively low proportion of patients who benefit from them. Because of this, efforts are under way to select

Table 6.9 Results from the Checkmate 057 trial which involved 582 people with non-squamous NSCLC who had received prior platinum-based chemotherapy.

	Nivolumab	Docetaxel
Median OS	12.2 months	9.4 months
Median PFS	2.3 months	4.2 months
1 year survival	50.5%	39%
18 month survival	39%	23%
1 year PFS	18.5%	8.1%
Median duration of response	17.1 months	5.6 months
Objective response rate	19%	12%
Incidence of grade 3–5 adverse events	10%	54%

Abbreviations: OS – overall survival; PFS – progression-free survival

patients according to biomarkers that predict response, or to find combinations of treatments that can boost the number of people who benefit.

For example, in the KEYNOTE-024 trial, only people with tumors that contained PD-L1 on at least 50% of their tumor cells were allowed to take part. None of the 305 people in the trial had received any previous treatment for advanced NSCLC. The response rate in this trial was 44.8% for pembrolizumab, compared to 27.8% in the control group of patients given chemotherapy [94]. However, only 26% of the people screened for the trial had the required level of PD-L1 and were allowed to enroll. And in other trials, some people with no detectable PD-L1 have benefited from a checkpoint inhibitor. So by using a cutoff of 50% for KEYNOTE-024, a lot of people who might have benefited were unable to receive the new treatment. This might seem harsh, but a similar trial called Checkmate-026, which investigated nivolumab, used a PD-L1 cut-off of 1%. Partly as a result of this low cutoff, the results from the trial weren't positive enough for nivolumab to become an approved treatment for previously untreated NSCLC. In fact, the response rate with nivolumab was lower than that for chemotherapy (26% versus 33%) [95]. In contrast, because of the KEYNOTE-024 trial, pembrolizumab is a licensed treatment for people with untreated advanced NSCLC in which at least 50% of their tumor cells produce PD-L1.

Combinations of treatments under investigation include combining an anti-PD-1 or anti-PD-L1 antibody with an anti-CTLA-4 antibody, with chemotherapy or with radiotherapy. The hope with these combinations is that the non-checkpoint inhibitor treatment will increase the number of infiltrating T cells in the tumor and/or make the cancer more visible to the immune system [90]. Some data from these approaches is already being published, suggesting that these sorts of combinations might boost response rates but may add to the side

effects [96]. For example, in 2016 results were published from the Keynote-21 trial in which pembrolizumab was added to chemotherapy as the first line of treatment for 123 people with advanced NSCLC [97]. The response rate was 55% for pembrolizumab plus chemotherapy versus 29% for chemotherapy alone. The incidence of grade 3 or worse side effects (see Box 6.2 for an explanation of how side effects are graded) was 39% compared to 26%.

We are also seeing trials of checkpoint inhibitors in people with earlier-stage NSCLC, rather than just in people with advanced NSCLC. For example, the PACIFIC trial investigated durvalumab (Imfinzi) (a PD-L1 targeted checkpoint inhibitor), for people with stage 3, locally advanced NSCLC, whose disease hadn't worsened following a combination of

---

Box 6.2 Grading of toxicities in clinical trials

Toxicities (also called side-effects or adverse events) are given a grade from one to five depending on how severe they are. A commonly used scale is the National Cancer Institute Common Toxicity Criteria:

1 = Mild side-effects
2 = Moderate side-effects
3 = Severe side-effects
4 = Life Threatening or disabling side-effects
5 = Fatal

Common side effects from cancer treatments include skin reactions, diarrhea, hair loss, fatigue, and nausea and vomiting. But they also include changes in white blood cell numbers that the patient might not realize is happening. Exactly how the side effects are assessed, graded, and reported varies between clinical trials.

chemotherapy and radiotherapy. The results of the trial showed that people who received durvalumab rather than a placebo did better. For example, after 18 months of treatment, 72.8% of people in the durvalumab arm had an ongoing response to treatment, compared to 46.8% in the placebo arm. And the median PFS was 16.8 months versus 5.6 months [98].

An unanswered question with the checkpoint inhibitors is whether they can actually cure some people with NSCLC. It seems that this probably is the case with melanoma skin cancer,[23] but as yet it's impossible to tell with NSCLC. The only information on long-term survival that has been published so far comes from a phase 1b trial with nivolumab called CA209-003. The five-year survival rate for this trial is 16%, compared to a historical figure of around 4%–5% for people receiving standard treatments [99].

6.4.9 Monoclonal Antibody Checkpoint Inhibitors for SCLC

SCLC is an incredibly aggressive disease. Although it generally responds to chemotherapy, it rapidly becomes resistant, and people often only survive a few months. Because it almost always develops in smokers, the cells of SCLC have one of the highest numbers of DNA mutations of any cancer [100].

So far only a handful of trials have assessed the effectiveness of checkpoint inhibitors for people with SCLC. They have given some promising signs of activity. For example, the CheckMate 32 trial, which investigated nivolumab alone versus nivolumab plus ipilimumab, gave reasonable response rates (about 10%–20%), duration of response, and survival times [101]. A trial with pembrolizumab involving 24 people also gave a 37.5% response rate [102]. Phase 3 trials are now talking place with both anti-PD-1 and anti-PD-L1

antibodies, both alone and in combination with anti-CTLA-4 antibodies. These include the KEYNOTE-604 (NCT03066778) trial of pembrolizumab combined with chemotherapy and the CheckMate 331 (NCT02481830) and CheckMate 451 (NCT02538666) trials investigating nivolumab or nivolumab plus ipilimumab. Durvalumab and atezolizumab are also in phase 3 trials.

6.4.10 Conclusions

As you can tell from the long list of targeted treatments for advanced NSCLC, a lot of progress has been made in recent years. Some of the most exciting treatments are the first, second, and third generations of targeted kinase inhibitors that block mutated EGFR, ALK, or ROS1. These drugs are often now capable of increasing PFS by one or two years for people whose cancer contains the relevant mutations.

Also exciting are the checkpoint inhibitors. Seeing a median duration of response figure of 17.1 months in the CheckMate 057 trial shows that when these treatments work, they really can make a huge difference. But the challenge now is to increase the proportion of people who benefit from them.

Sadly, a lot less progress has been made against SCLC. It continues to be a rapidly deadly disease, although checkpoint inhibitors may perhaps be able to make a difference.

6.5 TARGETED TREATMENTS FOR BOWEL CANCER

Around 22,800 men and 18,400 women are diagnosed with bowel cancer each year in the United Kingdom [103]. The vast majority of bowel cancers have EGFRs on their surface [104]. As a result, treatments that block EGFR

---

[23] Doctors and scientists are understandably hesitant to say that anyone with advanced cancer has been cured, but when someone with metastatic melanoma is alive and free of disease 10 years after treatment with a checkpoint inhibitor, it's *probably* safe to say that their disease isn't going to come back.

have been a major focus of drug development for bowel cancer for many years. **Angiogenesis inhibitors** also seem to benefit some people with bowel cancer. Two EGFR-targeted antibodies and four angiogenesis inhibitors are licensed as bowel cancer treatments in Europe and the United States (see Table 6.10). In addition, both nivolumab and pembrolizumab are licensed in the United States for people with MSI-high/MMR-deficient bowel cancer. These bowel cancers contain thousands of DNA mutations, and are consequently particularly sensitive to treatment with checkpoint inhibitor immunotherapy.

As with many common cancers, scientists have studied hundreds of bowel cancer samples to discover what gene mutations and other defects drive their development. This work has led to a four-way classification of bowel cancer (Table 6.11), which will hopefully be helpful in guiding the treatment of future bowel cancer patients [106]. Scientists have also uncovered important differences between right-sided bowel cancers and left-sided bowel cancers. For example, right-sided cancers are more common in women [107]; these cancers tend to be more aggressive and are more likely to be hyper-mutated[24] and to contain *BRAF* mutations. They are linked to a high-fat, high-sugar diet. In contrast, left-sided bowel cancers are more common in men, carry a better prognosis, and are associated with a high-protein diet full of red meat and deficient in calcium [108].

At the current time, the various new ways of categorizing bowel cancer are not directly being used to select which treatments people are given.

Table 6.10 Summary of licensed targeted treatments for bowel cancer.

Drug	Licensed for [105]
EGFR-targeted antibodies	
Cetuximab/Erbitux	For people with metastatic bowel cancer whose cancer does not contain a mutation in the *KRAS* gene
Panitumumab/Vectibix	For people with metastatic bowel cancer whose cancer does not contain a mutation in the *KRAS* gene
Angiogenesis inhibitors	
Bevacizumab/Avastin	For people with persistent, recurrent, or metastatic bowel cancer in combination with chemotherapy
Ramucirumab/Cyramza	Licensed in combination with chemotherapy for people with metastatic bowel cancer who have already received bevacizumab + chemotherapy
Aflibercept /Zif-Aflibercept/ Zaltrap	Licensed in combination with chemotherapy for people with metastatic bowel cancer who have already received chemotherapy
Regorafenib/Stivarga	Licensed in combination with chemotherapy for people with metastatic bowel cancer who have already received chemotherapy + bevacizumab, or chemotherapy + an anti-EGFR antibody
Checkpoint inhibitors	
Nivolumab/Opdivo	Licensed in the United States for people with dMMR, MSI-high metastatic bowel cancer
Pembrolizumab/Keytruda	Licensed in the United States for people with any dMMR, MSI-high metastatic solid tumor

Abbreviations: dMMR – mismatch repair-deficient; MSI – microsatellite instability

---

[24] That is, they contain many thousands of small DNA mutations.

Table 6.11 Four-way classification of bowel cancer.

CMS1	CMS2	CMS3	CMS4
14% of cases Often right-sided bowel cancers in women	37% of cases Mainly left-sided	13% of cases Contain fewer mutations than other types	23% of cases Show strong activation of transforming-growth factor-beta
Often hyper-mutated (MSI-H) due to defective DNA repair	Have very unstable chromosomes (CIN) with lots of breaks, rearrangements, duplications, and deletions		
Often contain *BRAF* mutations	WNT/beta-catenin pathway is overactive; MYC is overactive	Contain the most *KRAS* mutations	Lots of cells are mesenchymal and have gone through the EMT; lots of angiogenesis
Often contain lots of infiltrating T cells and natural killer cells; the cancer cells are very visible to the immune system		Metabolic pathways are rewired	Many inflammatory white blood cells; the cancer cells are hidden from the immune system
Generally carry a good prognosis; but if they relapse, they carry a poor prognosis	Associated with better survival after relapse than other subtypes		Generally diagnosed late and carry a worse prognosis than other subtypes

Abbreviations: CMS – consensus molecular subtypes; MSI-H – microsatellite instability high; CIN – chromosomal instability; EMT – epithelial to mesenchymal transition
Source: Guinney J et al. (2015). The consensus molecular subtypes of colorectal cancer. *Nat Med* **21**(11): 1350–1356. Dienstmann R et al. (2017). Consensus molecular subtypes and the evolution of precision medicine in colorectal cancer. *Nat Rev Cancer* **17**(2): 79–92.

However, many new treatment approaches are in trials, which will hopefully be useful for specific groups of patients. These include:

- **Combinations of kinase inhibitors and antibodies** for the 8%–10% of bowel cancers that contain *BRAF* mutations
- **A combination of HER2-blockers** for the 7% of bowel cancers in which the *HER2* gene is mutated or amplified
- **Anti-PD-1 or anti-PD-L1 monoclonal antibodies** (checkpoint inhibitors) for the 14%–17% of bowel cancers that contain thousands of small DNA mutations **(hypermutated, MSI-high or MMR-deficient bowel cancers)**

6.5.1 Targeting EGFR

Two EGFR-targeted monoclonal antibodies are approved as bowel cancer treatments: panitumumab (Vectibix) and cetuximab (Erbitux). (I described these antibodies back in Chapter 3. Section 3.3.2). Both have been the subject of numerous trials. From these trials, we know that about 15% of all bowel cancer patients benefit from an EGFR-targeted antibody [109]. However, work still goes on to define and implement the necessary tests so that they're only given to people who have the best chance of benefiting from them.

For a long time, EGFR antibodies were given to anyone whose cancer cells didn't contain common mutations in the *KRAS*[25] gene (see Chapter 3, Section 3.3.1 and Figure 3.10). However, *KRAS* mutations are only found in around 40% of bowel cancers [110], whereas we know that the proportion of bowel cancer patients who don't benefit from cetuximab or panitumumab is far greater than that. In fact, **about 73% of bowel cancers contain gene mutations that affect EGFR signaling pathway proteins and that cause resistance to EGFR-targeted antibodies.** And

---

[25] *KRAS* is the gene for making K-Ras protein.

Table 6.12 People with left-sided bowel cancers benefit more from EGFR-targeted antibodies than people with right-sided bowel cancers; analysis of the CRYSTAL and PRIME trials.

CRYSTAL trial:	FOLFIRI chemotherapy + cetuximab		FOLFIRI chemotherapy alone	
	Left (n=142)	Right (n=33)	Left (n=138)	Right (n=51)
Progression-free survival (months)	12.0	8.1	8.9	7.1
Overall survival (months)	28.7	18.5	21.7	15
Objective response rate	72.5%	42.4%	40.6%	33.3%

PRIME trial:	FOLFOX chemotherapy + panitumumab		FOLFOX chemotherapy alone	
	Left (n=169)	Right (n=39)	Left (n=159)	Right (n=49)
Progression-free survival (months)	12.9	7.5	9.2	7.0
Overall survival (months)	30.3	11.1	23.6	15.4
Objective response rate	68%	42%	53%	35%

FOLFIRI – a chemotherapy combination of folinic acid (also called leucovorin, FA or calcium folinate), 5-fluorouracil, and irinotecan.
FOLFOX – a chemotherapy combination of folinic acid (also called leucovorin, FA or calcium folinate), 5-fluorouracil, and oxaliplatin.
Source: Holch JW et al. (2017) The relevance of primary tumour location in patients with metastatic colorectal cancer: A meta-analysis of first-line clinical trials. *Eur J Cancer* 70: 87–98.

a further 13% are resistant for other reasons [109, 111]. So, to push up response rates to EGFR antibodies further, we need to be testing for more than just *KRAS* mutations.

As part the effort to improve the use of EGFR inhibitors, an international group of scientists analyzed over a thousand tumor samples from people who had taken part in trials investigating cetuximab plus chemotherapy. They found that patients whose tumors didn't contain a mutation in *KRAS*, *NRAS*, *BRAF*, or *PIK3CA*[26] genes were the most likely to benefit from cetuximab [112]. However, in the United Kingdom at least, we don't yet test for all the various mutations in *KRAS* and *NRAS* that cause resistance, nor do we test for other mutations that cause resistance [113].

Another insight that may guide the use of cetuximab and panitumumab is that **left-sided bowel cancers are more likely to respond to these antibodies than right-sided bowel cancers** [114] (see Table 6.12). You can see from the data that left-sided bowel cancers are more common, carry a better prognosis, and are more likely to respond to EGFR-targeted antibodies. For example, the response rate of right-sided bowel cancers to a combination of chemotherapy and an EGFR antibody is about 40%, whereas in left-sided bowel cancers it's about 70%.

In conclusion, although EGFR-antibodies are important treatments for bowel cancer, **there's probably much more we can do to improve their usefulness**. There appear to be various opportunities to improve response

[26] Remember that *PIK3CA* is the gene for the enzyme part of PI3K, which is involved in the PI3K/AKT/mTOR pathway.

rates and avoid giving them unnecessarily to people who don't benefit from them.

6.5.2 Overcoming Resistance to EGFR-Targeted Antibodies

Resistance to panitumumab and cetuximab is generally **driven by mutations in genes involved in EGFR signaling pathways** and by **alternative growth factors on the cell surface** [111]. Because we have drugs that target some of the faulty proteins and growth factor receptors that cause resistance, it might someday become possible to test for the resistance-causing mechanism and then treat the patient accordingly. One promising example of this is the Heracles clinical trial conducted in Italy. This trial focused on patients whose tumors were resistant to cetuximab or panitumumab because they had extra copies of the HER2 gene. They discovered that treatment with two HER2-targeted treatments – lapatinib and trastuzumab – was helpful for some of these people [115].

Other strategies to improve response rates and delay resistance to EGFR antibodies include [112, 116]:

- Using two EGFR-targeted treatments in combination, such an EGFR antibody and an EGFR kinase inhibitor
- Using combinations of antibodies that attach to different parts of EGFR
- Combining an EGFR antibody with a treatment that blocks other growth factor receptors or proteins involved in either the MAPK pathway or the PI3K/AKT/mTOR pathway

Hopefully, the ongoing clinical trials testing out these various combinations will mean longer lives for people with metastatic bowel cancer.

6.5.3 Targeting Other Signaling Pathway Proteins

Targeting B-Raf

BRAF mutations are found in around 8%–10% of bowel cancers. People with *BRAF* mutations aren't currently excluded from receiving cetuximab or panitumumab, but the available evidence suggests that they don't benefit from these antibodies [117].

The *BRAF* gene mutation found in bowel cancers is the same as that found in malignant melanoma (i.e., the V600E mutation). However, giving people a B-Raf inhibitor on its own only gives a response rate of 5%–10%. A more promising approach for *BRAF*-mutated bowel cancer is to use a combination involving two or three treatments. For example, trials of a B-Raf inhibitor plus either an EGFR or MEK inhibitor have been conducted, as have various trials that tested a triple combination of a B-Raf inhibitor, an EGFR-targeted antibody, and a MEK inhibitor, PI3K-alpha inhibitor or chemotherapy. These trials have typically given response rates of 10%–35% [111, 117, 118].

Targeting HER2

HER2 mutations and amplifications are found a small proportion of bowel cancers before treatment with an EGFR antibody, and in a larger proportion of bowel cancers that have become resistant to an EGFR antibody [111]. A combination of trastuzumab plus lapatinib seems promising for people with metastatic, EGFR antibody-resistant bowel cancers [115], but it's unclear whether the same combination will be better than an EGFR antibody for people who haven't yet been treated for metastatic bowel cancer, as this hasn't yet been investigated in trials.

6.5.4 Angiogenesis Inhibitors for Bowel Cancer

Metastatic bowel cancer was one of the first cancers in which angiogenesis inhibitors were tried (for an introduction to angiogenesis inhibitors, see Chapter 4, Section 4.1). The first phase 3 trial of an angiogenesis inhibitor for metastatic bowel cancer reported its findings in 2004. In this first phase 3 trial, adding bevacizumab to chemotherapy improved survival times by about five months [119]. But more recently, most large phase 3 trials (those involving over 500 people) tend to show a survival improvement of one or two months [120]. For example, in the N016966 study, which involved 1,400 people, adding bevacizumab to chemotherapy improved PFS from 8.0 to 9.4 months, and OS from 19.9 months to 21.3 months [121] (the OS result wasn't deemed to be statistically significant).

Results with other licensed angiogenesis inhibitors, aflibercept, ramucirumab, and regorafenib, have been fairly similar to those with bevacizumab [120]. For example, aflibercept improved PFS from 4.7 to 6.9 months, and OS from 12.1 to 13.5 months, when added to chemotherapy in the VELOUR study [122]. Ramucirumab improved PFS from 4.5 to 5.7 months, and OS from 11.7 to 13.3 months, when added to chemotherapy in the RAISE study [123]. Regorafenib improved PFS from 1.7 to 1.9 months, and OS from 5.0 to 6.4 months, compared to placebo in the CORRECT study [124].

Two of the perpetual frustrations with angiogenesis inhibitors are (1) the variety of resistance mechanisms that tumors can use to continue growing (see Chapter 4, Section 4.1.7) and (2) our lack of biomarkers to predict who they'll be helpful for (see Chapter 4, Section 4.1.8). Because we can't predict who will benefit from them, angiogenesis inhibitors are often given to patients with KRAS mutations and who therefore wouldn't benefit from an EGFR-targeted antibody.

In many trials, EGFR-targeted antibodies and angiogenesis inhibitors seem to have given fairly similar levels of benefit. As a result, there have been trials to compare the two treatment approaches in people whose tumors don't have KRAS mutations.[27] In these head-to-head trials, the PFS data has often been almost the same, whereas there are some

signs that the EGFR-targeted antibody results in better OS. But the results haven't been terribly consistent [117]. As a result, both EGFR-targeted antibodies and angiogenesis inhibitors are prescribed to people with KRAS wild-type metastatic bowel cancer [125]. However, there do seem to be promising opportunities to refine the use of EGFR-targeted antibodies, which might gradually make treatment decisions clearer.

6.5.5 Immunotherapy for Bowel Cancer

As I've said previously, immunotherapy, and specifically checkpoint inhibitors, often work best for patients whose tumors contain lots and lots of DNA mutations. And the group of bowel cancers with the highest numbers of mutations are the so-called MSI (microsatellite instability[28])-high bowel cancers. These cancers develop from cells that have defects in a DNA repair pathway called mismatch repair. As a result, the cancer cells generally contain 10 to 100 times the number of DNA mutations compared with other bowel cancers [126].

Two groups of bowel cancer patients have MSI-high bowel cancers. The larger group, accounting for 12% of all bowel cancers, have developed MSI-high bowel cancer due to faults in mismatch repair that have occurred during their lifetime. The other group of patients, accounting for 3% of all bowel cancers, have inherited a defect in a mismatch repair gene [127]. These people have Lynch syndrome, a condition that is associated with a very high risk of bowel cancer.

There is growing evidence from clinical trials that people with MSI-high bowel cancers (or other hyper-mutated bowel cancers) benefit from checkpoint inhibitors, whereas

---

[27] The un-mutated, normal version of any gene is often referred to as the "wild-type" gene.
[28] The name MSI reflects the pattern of mutations seen in the cancer cells of people with bowel cancers that have arisen due to faults in mismatch repair DNA.

people whose tumors have normal mismatch repair don't. For example, in a series of small clinical trials with the PD-1 antibody pembrolizumab (Keytruda), the antibody gave a response rate of 36% in 90 people with mismatch repair-deficient bowel cancer [128]. In addition, the CheckMate 142 trial investigating nivolumab, another PD-1-targeted antibody, gave a response rate of 31% in 74 patients with MSI-high bowel cancer [129]. As a result of these trials, both pembrolizumab and nivolumab have both been approved in the United States as treatments for MSI-high bowel cancer. In addition, pembrolizumab is approved for any metastatic, MSI-high solid tumor. Alongside bowel cancer, MSI-high/MMR-deficiency is present in a proportion of many other cancers, such as endometrial, stomach, biliary, pancreatic, prostate, bladder, and esophageal cancer [130]. This is the first time that any cancer treatment has been approved based on a feature of the cancer cells, rather than the cancer's location in the body.

The evidence so far suggests that checkpoint inhibitors will only be useful for people with MSI-high bowel cancer. And, although around 15% of people diagnosed with bowel cancer have MSI-high bowel cancer, it generally carries a pretty good prognosis (see Table 6.11). So the proportion of metastatic bowel cancers that are MSI-high is only 4% [131]. Consequently, it's possible that checkpoint inhibitors will have a relatively small role to play in the future treatment of bowel cancer. The caveat to this is that it might be possible to find combinations of checkpoint inhibitors with other treatments that increase the infiltration of T cells and thereby increase response rates in non-MSI-high bowel cancer. The first hint that this might be possible comes from a phase 1b trial in which atezolizumab was combined with a MEK inhibitor (cobimetinib). In this small trial involving 23 patients the response rate was 17% [132].

6.5.6 Conclusions

So far, the two main targeted treatment approaches that are licensed for people with bowel cancer are EGFR-targeted antibodies and angiogenesis inhibitors. To date, these treatments have brought relatively modest benefits. However, with further refinements to patient selection, response rates to EGFR-targeted antibodies will hopefully climb. Also, we are heading toward a future in which bowel cancers will be tested for mutations and amplifications in genes such as *BRAF* and *HER2*. Sadly though, little progress has been made against bowel cancers that contain *KRAS* and *NRAS* mutations, or against the CMS4 group of bowel cancers. One current glimmer of hope for people with these cancers is trials such as the FOCUS 4 clinical trial taking place in the United Kingdom, which is testing out various different treatment combinations for people with a number of different mutations [133].

As in many other cancers, checkpoint inhibitors will likely play a future role in the treatment of bowel cancer. The people with bowel cancer most likely to benefit from these treatments are the 4% or so of people with MSI-high metastatic bowel cancer.

6.6 TARGETED TREATMENTS FOR MALIGNANT MELANOMA SKIN CANCER

6.6.1 Introduction to Melanoma Skin Cancer

Around 15,400 people are diagnosed with malignant melanoma skin cancer each year in the United Kingdom, and Cancer Research UK estimates that 86% of melanoma skin cancers are caused by UV radiation from the sun [134].

Happily, if people are diagnosed early, then they can virtually always be cured with surgery. However, only 8% of men and 25% of women diagnosed in the UK with metastatic melanoma in the years 2002–2006 (i.e., a melanoma that has spread to elsewhere in the body) were still alive five years later [135].

Around 45%–50% of melanomas contain faulty, overactive versions of the B-Raf protein [136]. In 80%–90% of these cancers, the cancer-causing mutation in *BRAF* is the V600E mutation. This mutation in the gene causes the cell to create a version of the B-Raf protein that is only one amino acid different from the normal protein: the 600th amino acid is a glutamic acid rather than the normal valine.[29] However, even this seemingly small change is enough to cause the B-Raf protein to be continually active [137]. Melanomas that aren't driven by faulty B-Raf often contain *NRAS* mutations (see Figure 6.5).

Since 2011, eight new treatments have been licensed for advanced melanoma: two

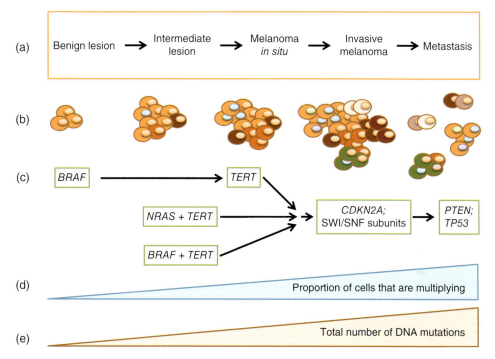

Figure 6.5 Progression from a benign skin lesion to an invasive, metastatic cancer [138, 139]. **(a)** Melanomas generally develop from benign skin lesions, which gradually evolve to become an invasive melanoma and finally spread to other locations. **(b)** During the stages of progression, the cancer gradually becomes more and more diverse as individual cells pick up mutations and multiply to create new populations of cells. **(c)** By studying samples taken from people with different stages of disease, scientists have uncovered the order in which some mutations take place. For example, *BRAF* and *NRAS* mutations commonly occur very early on, and these mutations set in motion a chain of events that finally leads to invasive melanoma. Other mutations, such as *PTEN* and *TP53* mutations, are generally found in metastases. **(d)** As the cancer progresses, the proportion of multiplying cells within the tumor gradually increases, and **(e)** the cancer cells tend to contain more and more mutations.

---

[29] If you remember, our proteins are made from 20 different amino acids which are chemically connected to one another. Each amino acid is made from a particular arrangement of carbons, oxygens, hydrogens, and nitrogens – see https://en.wikipedia.org/wiki/Amino_acid.

B-Raf inhibitors, two MEK inhibitors, three checkpoint inhibitors, and an oncolytic virus (see Table 6.13 for a summary).

6.6.2 Targeting B-Raf and MEK

The first clinical trials with a B-Raf inhibitors were conducted from 2008 to 2010, and they showed that around 50%–80% of people with *BRAF*-mutated melanoma benefit from treatment with a B-Raf inhibitor [137]. Larger trials were conducted from 2010 to 2012, and as a result of these trials, two B-Raf inhibitors, vemurafenib (Zelboraf) and dabrafenib (Tafinlar), were licensed in the United States and Europe between 2011 and 2013.

Over the past six to eight years, two main problems with B-Raf inhibitors as a standalone treatment for melanoma have emerged:

1. **The Raf-inhibitor paradox** (see Chapter 3, Figure 3.16) means that people treated with a B-Raf inhibitor are at risk of developing benign skin tumors and other cancers driven by *RAS* gene mutations [141, 142].

2. Although most patients with *BRAF*-mutated melanoma benefit from B-Raf inhibitors, **resistance develops rapidly**, and PFS is generally about 5 to 7 months [143].

As I mentioned back in Chapter 3, Section 3.7.4 (and Figure 3.17), there are many different reasons why a *BRAF* mutant cell might be resistant to a B-Raf inhibitor. And, because of the genetic diversity of melanomas, when a patient's cancer starts growing again, it's not just one cell that is driving the resistance. Instead, there will be many different populations of cancer cells that have survived for different reasons [144]. But, having said that, many of the resistance-causing mutations cause reactivation of the MAPK

Table 6.13 Licensed targeted treatments for malignant melanoma.

Treatment	Target	Licensed for [140]
Kinase inhibitors		
Vemurafenib/Zelboraf	B-Raf	For metastatic melanoma with the V600* BRAF mutation – it can be given on its own or in combination with cobimetinib.
Dabrafenib/Tafinlar	B-Raf	For metastatic melanoma with the V600* B-Raf mutation– it can be given on its own or in combination with trametinib.
Trametinib/Mekinist	MEK	For metastatic melanoma with the V600* B-Raf mutation – it can be given on its own or in combination with dabrafenib.
Cobimetinib/Cotellic	MEK	For metastatic melanoma with the V600* B-Raf mutation in combination with vemurafenib.
Immunotherapies		
Ipilimumab/Yervoy	CTLA-4	• For metastatic melanoma. • As an adjuvant therapy for people with melanoma who have already received surgery (United States only).
Nivolumab/Opdivo	PD-1	For metastatic melanoma, either on its own or in combination with ipilimumab.
Pembrolizumab/ Keytruda	PD-1	For metastatic melanoma.
T-VEC/talimogene laherparepvec; Imlygic	N/A	For metastatic melanoma in the skin and lymph nodes (but not to bone, lung, brain, and other internal organs) that cannot be removed by surgery. It is used as local treatment in patients whose disease has returned after surgery.

*The most common mutation is V600E, but other substitutions have been discovered, such as V600K; hence, the regulators simply write "V600" to encompass any substitution of the 600th amino acid in B-Raf.

pathway [142, 143]. Because of this, many resistance-causing mutations can be blocked with another drug that blocks the MAPK pathway, such as a MEK inhibitor. And we now know that when you use a combination of a B-Raf inhibitor with a MEK inhibitor, the response rate improves by around 10%–30%, and the median duration of response also improves by about 2 to 3 months [143]. On top of this, the addition of a MEK inhibitor also avoids the problem of the Raf-inhibitor paradox, and patients no longer develop Ras-driven cancers [145].[30] Two B-Raf/MEK inhibitor combinations are licensed in the United States and Europe: vemurafenib + cobimetinib (Cotellic) and dabrafenib + trametinib (Mekinist).

Sadly though, because melanomas are so genetically diverse, and because not every resistance-causing mutation works by reactivating the MAPK pathway, resistance is still almost inevitable. And because of this, further drugs and combinations are being tested in trials with the hope of extending survival times further. Approaches include [143]:

- Developing new B-Raf inhibitors that are more effective than vemurafenib and dabrafenib [146].
- Combining other targeted treatments with the B-Raf/MEK inhibitor combination. Drugs added into the combination include HSP90 inhibitors (which cause various resistance-causing proteins to be destroyed by the cell), AKT inhibitors (to shut down the PI3K/AKT/mTOR pathway), and an MDM2 inhibitor (which activates p53 and might be able to trigger cell death).
- Combining immunotherapies with the B-Raf/MEK inhibitor combination. (Because I haven't discussed immunotherapies for

melanoma yet, I'll talk about these combinations in Section 6.6.3. below.)

6.6.3 Immunotherapy for Malignant Melanoma

Immunotherapy has been used to treat melanoma skin cancer since the late 1980s. But to begin with, the only treatments available were drugs such as high-dose interleukin-2 (Aldesleukin/Proleukin) that worked very generally to boost the patient's immune system [147]. These treatments produce complete remissions in about 5%–10% of patients, but at the expense of lots of side effects.

Much more recently, scientists have created much more targeted immunotherapies such as the checkpoint inhibitors (Chapter 5, Section 5.3). Three checkpoint inhibitors are now licensed as melanoma treatments, as well as an oncolytic virus called T-VEC (Chapter 5, Section 5.6.2) (see Table 6.13 for a summary). Scientists are also making progress with using infiltrating T lymphocytes (Chapter 5, Section 5.4.1).

Monoclonal Antibody Checkpoint Inhibitors for Malignant Melanoma

Response rates with checkpoint inhibitors vary from about 10%–20% with anti-CTLA-4 antibodies [148] to 30%–40% with anti-PD-1 antibodies [149, 150]. We've also seen the results of the phase 3 CheckMate 067 trial, which investigated a combination of two antibodies (ipilimumab + nivolumab) (Table 6.14). The trial gave an impressive response rates of almost 60% for the combination [151]. However, it appears that the additional benefit with the combination over nivolumab alone is more profound in people with low or no detectable PD-L1 in their tumor. It also appears that

[30] You might have noticed in this section, I sometimes talk about *BRAF*, sometimes B-Raf, and we also have *RAS* and Ras. In general, something written in capitals and italics is a gene, where as something not in italics and lowercase is likely to be a protein.

Table 6.14 Results from the CheckMate 067 clinical trial investigating a combination of ipilimumab plus nivolumab in 945 people with previously untreated, metastatic melanoma.

	Nivolumab + ipilimumab	Nivolumab alone	Ipilimumab alone
Objective response rate across the entire patient population	58.9%	44.6%	19%
Complete response rate	17.2%	14.9%	4.4%
Grade 3-4 side effects	55%	16.3%	27.3%
Median PFS	11.5 months	6.9 months	2.9 months
2-year OS rate	64%	59%	45%
Median PFS in PD-L1–negative tumors**	11.2 months	5.3 months	2.8 months
Median PFS in PD-L1–positive tumors***	14.0 months	14.0 months	3.9 months

*PFS – progression-free survival – that is, the length of time the cancer was kept under control.
**PD-L1-negative is defined as cancers in which less than 5% of tumor cells had PD-L1 on their surface.
***PD-L1-positive is defined as cancers in which more than 5% of tumor cells had PD-L1 on their surface.
Source: Larkin J et al. (2015) Combined nivolumab and ipilimumab or monotherapy in untreated melanoma. *N Engl J Med* 373: 23–34.
OncLive website (2017). Nivolumab/Ipilimumab Combo Shows Modest OS Benefit in Advanced Melanoma in Updated Phase III Findings. Available at: http://www.onclive.com/conference-coverage/aacr-2017/nivolumabipilimumab-combo-shows-modest-os-benefit-in-advanced-melanoma-in-updated-phase-iii-findings?p=1 (accessed December 29, 2017).

people with *BRAF*-mutated melanomas gain more benefit from checkpoint inhibitor therapy than people with un-mutated (*BRAF*-wild-type) tumors [152]. Because anti-CTLA-4 antibodies often cause severe side effects, it's just as important to know who won't benefit from them as who will.

Perhaps the most exciting aspect of checkpoint inhibitors (and of other immunotherapies) is that **they sometimes keep cancer under control for many months, if not years** [154, 155]. And there's a good chance that some people with metastatic melanoma have been cured through checkpoint inhibitor treatment.[31] However, until fairly recently, response rates for immunotherapy in melanoma patients were lower than those for B-Raf inhibitors. So the doctor and patient

had to choose: do you go for a high response rate but relatively short duration of response with a B-Raf/MEK inhibitor combination, or a lower response rate but potentially a longer duration of response with a checkpoint inhibitor? However, this balance is now shifting. In fact, we're already at a stage where response rates with a combination of checkpoint inhibitors are nearing those of B-Raf/MEK inhibitor combinations.[32] Hence, the next step is to discover, for a person with *BRAF*-mutated metastatic melanoma, which treatment approach should be used first: a B-Raf/MEK inhibitor combination, or checkpoint inhibitors. In order to answer this question, various clinical trials are under way. For example, one trial (NCT02224781) is investigating whether dabrafenib + trametinib fol-

---

[31] See footnote 23.
[32] Of course, the B-Raf/MEK inhibitor combination is only relevant for people with *BRAF*-mutated melanoma.

lowed by nivolumab + ipilimumab is better or worse for patients than nivolumab + ipilimumab followed by dabrafenib + trametinib. Results are expected in 2022.

In addition, as we discover and implement biomarker tests, and try out new immunotherapy combinations, response rates and survival times will no doubt improve further.

T-VEC (Talimogene Laherparepvec; Imlygic)

The only other immunotherapy to be so far licensed as a treatment for melanoma is T-VEC, an oncolytic virus (see Chapter 5, Figure 5.15). T-VEC was approved on the basis of one phase 3 trial (called the OPTiM trial [156]). Although the trial did report positive results (see Table 6.15), this was only one trial. So it's a bit too soon to say what impact oncolytic viruses are going to have on the treatment of melanomas.

6.6.4 Conclusions

Since 2011, two B-Raf inhibitors, two MEK inhibitors, three checkpoint inhibitors, and an oncolytic virus have all proved their effectiveness against metastatic melanoma skin cancer in large clinical trials. All of these treatments are licensed for use both in Europe and the United States. **Between them they have given thousands of people with an aggressive and previously incurable cancer many additional months, if not years of life.** Scientists and

Table 6.15 Results from the OPTiM trial of T-VEC in people with metastatic melanoma.

	TVEC	GM-CSF
Durable response rate*	16.3%	2.1%
Objective response rate	26.4%	5.7%

*They defined a durable response as one lasting at least six months.
Source: Andtbacka RH et al. (2015). Talimogene Laherparepvec Improves Durable Response Rate in Patients With Advanced Melanoma. *J Clin Oncol* **33**(25): 2780–2788.

doctors are therefore understandably feeling hugely optimistic. However, important challenges remain, such as:

- How to increase the length of time that B-Raf/MEK inhibitor combinations keep melanoma under control
- How to predict exactly who is going to benefit from checkpoint inhibitors in order to avoid unnecessary treatment
- How to ensure that the majority, rather than the minority, of people given checkpoint inhibitors live for many years afterward
- How to manage all the side effects that checkpoint inhibitors cause – particularly those caused by anti-CTLA-4 antibodies like ipilimumab
- How to decide which treatment to give first

However, no doubt, perhaps even before this book gets published, we'll see more progress made.

6.7 TARGETED TREATMENTS FOR KIDNEY CANCER

Around 7,800 men and 4,700 women are diagnosed with kidney cancer each year in the United Kingdom [157]. About a quarter of cases are due to smoking, and a quarter can be attributed to being overweight [158].

The most common type of kidney cancer is renal cell carcinoma – RCC (other types of kidney cancer include transitional cell cancers and Wilm's tumor). About 75% of RCCs are clear cell renal cell carcinomas. Other types of RCC include papillary type 1 (5%), papillary type 2 (10%), and chromophobe (5%) kidney cancers [159]. Because clear cell RCCs are by far the most common type of kidney cancer, I'll only be talking about them in this section.

Two groups of targeted therapies are important treatments for metastatic RCCs: angiogenesis inhibitors (Chapter 4, Section 4.1) and checkpoint inhibitors (Chapter 5, Section 5.3), summarized in Table 6.16.

Table 6.16   Licensed targeted treatments for renal cell carcinoma (RCC).

Treatment	Targets [164, 165]
Angiogenesis inhibitors licensed as first-line treatments	
Bevacizumab/Avastin	VEGF-A
Sorafenib/Nexavar	Blocks multiple targets including Raf-1, B-Raf, VEGF receptors, PDGF receptors, RET, FLT3, and KIT
Sunitinib/Sutent	Blocks multiple targets including VEGF receptors, PDGF receptors, KIT, and FLT3
Pazopanib/Votrient	Blocks multiple targets including VEGF receptors, PDGF receptors, and KIT
Temsirolimus/Torisel	mTOR
Cabozantinib/Cabometyx/Cometriq	Blocks multiple targets including VEGF receptors, AXL, MET, RET, TIE-2, KIT, and FLT3 (approval granted in the United States only as of December 2017)
Angiogenesis inhibitors licensed as second-line treatments	
Axitinib/Inlyta	Blocks multiple targets including VEGF receptors, PDGF receptors, and KIT
Cabozantinib/Cabometyx/Cometriq	Blocks multiple targets including VEGF receptors, AXL, MET, RET, TIE-2, KIT, and FLT3
Lenvatinib/Kisplyx/Lenvima	Blocks multiple targets including VEGF receptors, PDGF receptors, FGF receptors, RET, and KIT. Given in combination with everolimus.
Everolimus/Afinitor	mTOR
Checkpoint inhibitors licensed as second-line treatments	
Nivolumab/Opdivo	PD-1

6.7.1 Angiogenesis Inhibitors for Kidney Cancer

RCC and Angiogenesis

Solid tumors need a blood supply to grow, and angiogenesis inhibitors are licensed treatments for many tumor types. But it's in the treatment of clear cell RCCs that angiogenesis inhibitors are most effective [160]. This effectiveness is because the cancer cells of clear cell RCCs have almost always lost an important tumor suppressor protein called VHL (von Hippel Lindau). In healthy cells, VHL normally suppresses angiogenesis. However, when VHL is faulty, or missing from a cell, the cell produces high levels of VEGF and other growth factors that trigger angiogenesis [161] (see Figure 6.6). As a result, angiogenesis inhibitors target the underlying defect that drives clear cell RCC.

VEGF and VEGF Receptor Inhibitors as RCC Treatments

Angiogenesis inhibitors are important treatments for advanced clear cell RCC, and nine of them are licensed as RCC treatments (see Table 6.16). Response rates to angiogenesis inhibitors in trials are generally around 30%. However, when resistance develops and a second angiogenesis inhibitor is tried, the chance of the patient benefiting from it drops to around 20% [162, 163]. Sadly, treatment with angiogenesis inhibitors cannot cure people with advanced RCC – the cancer does inevitably start growing again. However, trials generally show that each angiogenesis inhibitor can hold metastatic clear cell RCC in check for around 8–10 months [162, 163].

Over the years, there have been a dizzying number of trials testing out the various

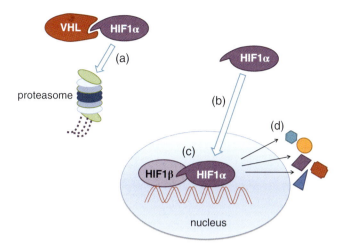

Figure 6.6 Mutations in VHL cause angiogenesis and trigger other changes [161]. **(a)** In healthy cells, and in normal oxygen conditions, VHL interacts with a second protein called HIF-1alpha (HIF-1α). This interaction leads to the destruction of HIF-1α by the proteasome. **(b)** In clear cell renal cell carcinoma cells, VHL is generally faulty or completely missing. Hence, HIF-1α isn't destroyed. Levels of HIF-1α therefore increase, and it moves into the nucleus, where it joins with a partner protein called HIF-1β. **(c)** Together, HIF-1α and HIF-1β form a transcription factor called HIF-1, which attaches to the control regions (promoters) of a variety of genes, causing their transcription. **(d)** In response, the cell produces more than 60 proteins, including VEGF (which drives angiogenesis), EPO (which tells the bone marrow to produce more red blood cells), GLUT1 (which transports glucose into the cell), ADM (which protects the cell from apoptosis), and TGF-α (which activates EGF receptors).
Abbreviations: VHL – von Hippel-Lindau; HIF – hypoxia inducible factor; VEGF – vascular endothelial growth factor; EPO – erythropoietin; GLUT1 – glucose transporter-1; ADM – adrenomedullin; TGF – transforming growth factor

angiogenesis inhibitors and comparing them to one another [166] (see Table 6.17 for examples of clinical trials results).

A few conclusions from these trials are [163]:

- Pazopanib and sunitinib give very similar results in trials, but pazopanib is preferred by patients because it gives less severe side effects.

- Cabozantinib may have an advantage over other angiogenesis inhibitors because of its ability to block MET and AXL, both of which are overproduced by RCCs that are resistant to angiogenesis inhibitors such as sunitinib. Trials with cabozantinib as a second-line treatment seem to bear this out, and it's also looking promising as a first-line treatment [171].

- Most combinations of VEGF inhibitors (such as combinations of bevacizumab with sunitinib, sorafenib, or everolimus) cause too many side effects to be tolerable for patients. The exception is the combination of lenvatinib with everolimus; this combination does cause more severe side effects than either drug alone, but it's still considered an acceptable combination.

mTOR Inhibitors as RCC Treatments

As well as drugs that directly target VEGF (bevacizumab) or VEGF receptors (sunitinib, sorafenib, pazopanib, axitinib, lenvatinib, and cabozantinib), two mTOR inhibitors are licensed as RCC treatments: everolimus and temsirolimus (see Chapter 3, Section 3.8.4). mTOR is involved in the PI3K/AKT/mTOR pathway, and it's therefore involved in growth factor signaling and the control of cell proliferation and survival. However, there is also a

Table 6.17 Examples of results from clinical trials that aimed to determine the best second-line treatment for people with metastatic renal cell carcinoma (RCC).

Treatments compared to one another	Objective response rate	Progression-free survival	Overall survival
Axitinib versus sorafenib [167]	19% versus 9%	6.7 months versus. 4.7 months	20.1 months versus 19.2 months*
Lenvatinib + everolimus versus everolimus [168]**	43% versus 6%	14.6 months versus 5.5 months	25.5 months versus 17.5 months
Cabozantinib versus everolimus [169]	21% versus 5%	7.5 months versus 3.9 months	21.4 months versus 16.5 months
Nivolumab versus everolimus [170]	25% versus 5%	4.6 months versus 4.4 months*	25.0 months versus 19.6 months

*These results were not deemed to be statistically significant (i.e., the difference between the two figures is too likely to be a chance finding to be considered important).
**This was a phase 2 trial, whereas all the other trials were phase 3.

strong connection between the PI3K/AKT/ mTOR pathway and angiogenesis. When the PI3K/AKT/mTOR pathway is active, it causes VEGF production by the cell via activating HIF-1,[33] and via an HIF-1-independent mechanism. The pathway also controls the production of other angiogenesis-promoting growth factors [172].

Because the PI3K/AKT/mTOR pathway is involved in cell proliferation, survival, and angiogenesis, you might expect mTOR inhibitors to be more effective than VEGF receptor inhibitors as RCC treatments. However, although they're useful treatments, mTOR inhibitors don't seem to be as effective as VEGF receptor inhibitors [163]. This might be because everolimus and temsirolimus can't completely block mTOR activity, or it might be because of another as yet unknown reason.

6.7.2 Immunotherapy for Kidney Cancer

Immunotherapies have been used as treatments for kidney cancer since the 1990s. However, until recently the treatments used were general boosters of the immune system such as interferon-alpha (IFN-α) or interleu-

kin-2 (IL-2; Aldesleukin; Proleukin) [173]. These treatments tend to benefit around 15% of people with RCC, and their effects can be long-lasting, but they often cause severe side effects [173].

Since 2005, when the first VEGF receptor inhibitor was licensed as a treatment for RCC, doctors have been using IFN-α and IL-2 less and less. However, their interest in immunotherapy as a treatment option for RCC remained. This continued interest was driven in part by past successes with IL-2 and IFN-α, and because (like malignant melanomas) RCCs occasionally spontaneously disappear without treatment [173]. Also, RCCs often contain lots of infiltrating white blood cells such as T cells, natural killer cells, dendritic cells, and macrophages. Hence, when scientists created checkpoint inhibitors, RCC was one of the first cancers in which they tested them out.

Monoclonal Antibody Checkpoint Inhibitors for RCC

The first (and as of December 2017 still the only) checkpoint inhibitor to be licensed as a treatment for RCC was nivolumab. The phase

---

[33] This is something that the loss of VHL activity also does – see Figure 6.6.

3 trial (called CheckMate 025) that led to its approval showed that nivolumab led to an improvement in OS, but not in PFS when compared with everolimus [174] (see Table 6.17). As I've said previously, checkpoint inhibitors can give strange PFS results because their benefits can be delayed and take several months to become apparent. The usefulness of nivolumab does become clearer when you look at the response rates and the OS results, with nivolumab providing a 5 month improvement over everolimus (25.0 versus 19.6 months).

PD-L1 Levels as a Biomarker for Checkpoint Inhibitors in RCC

As part of the CheckMate 025 trial, patients' tumors were analyzed for the presence of PD-L1. High PD-L1 levels often correlate with response to a checkpoint inhibitor, and many trials use cutoffs of PD-L1 levels when selecting patients to enter the trial. However, in some trials in RCC patients, there hasn't been any connection between PD-L1 level and the patient's response to a PD-1 or PD-L1 targeted antibody. For example, in the CheckMate 025 trial, 92% of tumor samples contained some amount of PD-L1. The PFS and OS times of patients in the trial were actually longer for the patients with less PD-L1 on their cancer cells than for the patients with more PD-L1 [174]. So the trial would seem to suggest that measuring PD-L1 levels might not be useful for predicting which RCC patients should receive a checkpoint inhibitor. However, it's still early days, and this situation might change.

Checkpoint Inhibitor Combinations for RCC

Because nivolumab has proved to be a useful RCC treatment, other checkpoint inhibitors are in phase 3 trials (summarized in Table 6.18). The first things you notice when you look at a list of ongoing trials are that:

1. Checkpoint inhibitors are now largely being investigated as first-line treatments for RCC, or as adjuvant treatments following surgery.
2. Many of the trials involve a combination of a checkpoint inhibitor with an angiogenesis inhibitor.

There are three reasons why checkpoint inhibitors are being combined with angiogenesis inhibitors:

1. We know that angiogenesis inhibitors are useful treatments for RCC, so it would be unethical not to include them in the trials – you can't withhold a treatment that's known to work.
2. Angiogenesis inhibitors and checkpoint inhibitors cause completely different side effects, and hence it should be safe to combine them together as they shouldn't exacerbate one another's toxicities.
3. It's hoped that the two treatments will synergize because the angiogenesis inhibitor will help the body's T cells travel into the tumor, where they are activated by the checkpoint inhibitor [175].

Other combinations under investigation include a PD-1 or PD-L1 antibody in combination with a CTLA-4 antibody, and a PD-1 antibody combined with an IDO inhibitor (see Chapter 5, Section 5.3.8 for more about IDO inhibitors).

Other Immunotherapy Strategies for RCC

As well as checkpoint inhibitors, other immunotherapy strategies have been tested in RCC, such as peptide vaccines and dendritic cell therapies (see Chapter 5, Section 5.6). For example, a peptide vaccine called IMA901 reached phase 3 trials. IMA901 contains a mixture of 10 fragments derived from proteins thought to be present in RCC cells, including MET and cyclin D1. The hope was that the protein fragments would be picked up by patients' dendritic cells, which would then activate T cells. However, there was no survival advantage when IMA901 was combined with sunitinib in the phase 3 trial [176].

Table 6.18 Summary of phase 3 trials of checkpoint inhibitors for people with renal cell carcinoma (RCC) as of December 2017.

Trial name	Details	Estimated study completion date
Pembrolizumab/Keytruda		
CLEAR	Lenvatinib + everolimus versus lenvatinib + pembrolizumab versus sunitinib as a first-line treatment for metastatic RCC (NCT02811861)	January 2020
KEYNOTE-426	Pembrolizumab + axitinib versus sunitinib as a first-line treatment for metastatic RCC (NCT02853331)	January 2020
KEYNOTE-564	Pembrolizumab as an adjuvant treatment for RCC (NCT03142334)	November 2022
KEYNOTE-679	Pembrolizumab + epacadostat vs. sunitinib or pazopanib for locally advanced or metastatic RCC (NCT03260894)	June 2023
Nivolumab/Opdivo		
PROSPER	Surgery with or without nivolumab for the treatment of localized RCC (NCT03055013)	July 2022
CheckMate 214	Nivolumab + ipilimumab versus sunitinib as a first-line treatment for RCC (NCT02231749)	September 2019
CheckMate 914	Nivolumab + ipilimumab vs. placebo for localized RCC following surgery (NCT03138512)	July 2023
CheckMate 025	Nivolumab vs. everolimus in pre-treated advanced or metastatic RCC (NCT01668784)	September 2018
CheckMate 9ER	Nivolumab + cabozantinib with or without ipilimumab vs. sunitinib for previously-untreated advanced or metastatic RCC (NCT03141177)	August 2022
Atezolizumab/Tecentriq		
IMmotion151	Atezolizumab + bevacizumab versus sunitinib as a first-line treatment for people with inoperable, locally advanced or metastatic RCC (NCT02420821)	July 2020
IMmotion010	Atezolizumab versus placebo as an adjuvant treatment after surgery (NCT03024996)	April 2024
Avelumab/Bavencio		
JAVELIN Renal 101	Avelumab + axitinib versus sunitinib as a first-line treatment for advanced or metastatic RCC (NCT02684006)	April 2021
Durvalumab/Imfinzi		
RAMPART	Durvalumab vs. durvalumab + tremelimumab vs. active monitoring for people with localized RCC, following surgery (NCT03288532)	December 2037

A dendritic cell therapy has also reached phase 3 trials. Called AGS-003 (also called rocapuldencel-T), the treatment involves isolating some immature dendritic cells from the patient's blood. These cells are then matured and genetically altered so that they produce proteins made by the patient's cancer cells, plus part of a protein called CD40 Ligand, which activates white blood cells. Hence, the treatment involves the manufacture of a tailor-made treatment for each patient [177]. Results published in September 2017 suggest some survival benefit for the vaccine over standard therapy [178].

6.7.3 Conclusions

Since 2005, nine angiogenesis inhibitors have been licensed as treatments for people with metastatic kidney cancer. These treatments have improved survival times, but the cancer inevitably becomes resistant. Hence, the added effectiveness of the everolimus + lenvatinib combination is exciting. The approval of nivolumab also leads us into a new era for RCC, in which the patient's immune system is leveraged in a more targeted way than with IFN-α and IL-2. The approval of nivolumab will no doubt be followed by the approval of other checkpoint inhibitors as more clinical trials conclude.

However, some questions remain to be answered, such as:

1. What's the best time to introduce a checkpoint inhibitor into a patient's treatment?
2. Will checkpoint inhibitors work better alone or when combined with an angiogenesis inhibitor?
3. Will some of the people who experience complete remissions with a checkpoint inhibitor be cured? Or will their cancer ultimately return?
4. What biomarker can we use to predict who will be helped by a checkpoint inhibitor?

6.8 TARGETED TREATMENTS FOR HEAD AND NECK CANCER

7,900 men and 3,500 women are diagnosed with head and neck cancer each year in the United Kingdom [179]. The vast majority of head and neck cancers are derived from the flat (squamous) cells that line the moist, mucosal surfaces inside the head and neck. They are therefore referred to as head and neck squamous cell carcinomas (HNSCC) [180].

91% of HNSCCs are potentially preventable [181]. They can be split into two groups: those caused by smoking and drinking alcohol, and those caused by infection with the human papilloma virus (HPV) and that are associated with oral sex. The number of cases of HNSCC has risen by almost 40% in the past 10 years [179]. But this hides the fact that the number of cases caused by smoking is decreasing, whereas the number linked to HPV infection is increasing [182]. HPV-positive and HPV-negative tumors contain different DNA mutations, behave differently, and carry different prognoses [183]. For example, people with HPV-positive HNSCC have an 80% chance of surviving five years, compared to a 50% chance for people with HPV-negative cancers [182].

Three targeted treatments are currently licensed for HNSCC: the first was cetuximab, an anti-EGFR antibody (for more on EGFR antibodies, see Chapter 3, Section 3.3.1). The other two, nivolumab and pembrolizumab, are checkpoint inhibitors (see Chapter 5, Section 5.3).

6.8.1 Targeting EGFR

90% of head and neck cancers have excess EGFR on their surface. High EGFR levels go hand in hand with resistance to radiotherapy and shortened survival times [184]. A wide range of trials have therefore been conducted in which anti-EGFR antibodies such as cetuximab, panitumumab, zalatumumab, and nimotuzumab have been used. These antibodies have been tested on their own, or combined with radiotherapy, chemotherapy, or both radiotherapy and chemotherapy (often abbreviated to chemoradiation) [185].

Trials with EGFR-Targeted Treatments

Trials with EGFR antibodies have shown that they can improve survival times when combined with radiotherapy for people with locally advanced HNSCC when compared to radiotherapy alone. But they don't improve survival times when the comparison is radiotherapy plus EGFR antibody versus chemoradiation; or when the comparison is chemoradiation plus EGFR antibody versus chemoradiation alone [185].

EGFR-targeted antibodies can also improve survival times when given to people with metastatic or recurrent HNSCC when combined with chemotherapy. For example, the EXTREME trial showed that the addition of cetuximab to chemotherapy improved the median survival time from 7.4 to 10.1 months [186].

Kinase inhibitors that target EGFR have also been investigated in HNSCC trials, but they've generally had little impact on survival [187]. The only EGFR kinase inhibitor currently in a phase 3 trials for HNSCC is afatinib.

Biomarkers of Response or Resistance to EGFR Antibodies

When treating *bowel cancer* with an EGFR-targeted antibody, the patient's tumor is first tested for the presence of *KRAS* mutations; *KRAS* mutations are present in 30%–50% of bowel cancers, and they cause resistance to EGFR antibodies. In contrast, *RAS* mutations (predominantly affecting *HRAS*) are present in only about 5% of newly diagnosed HNSCCs. But, *RAS* gene mutations (in *KRAS*, *NRAS* and *HRAS*) do appear to be present in a much higher proportion of HNSCCs in people whose cancers are resistant to EGFR antibodies [188]. This suggests that *RAS*-mutant cells are a cause of EGFR antibody resistance.

A large proportion of HNSCCs show signs of infection with HPV, and hence the presence or absence of HPV has been investigated as a possible marker of response or resistance to EGFR antibodies. However, the results of these investigations have been mixed. Some studies have suggested that only people with HPV-negative tumors benefit from EGFR antibodies, whereas other studies have found that benefit from EGFR antibodies is independent of whether or not the cells carry signs of HPV

infection [182]. So at the moment there's nothing useful to say.

Because the picture is rather mixed, we don't currently have any biomarkers that can predict either response or resistance to EGFR-targeted treatments when given to people with HNSCC.

6.8.2 Immunotherapy for Head and Neck Cancer

Scientists used to think of HNSCC as being a non-immunogenic cancer – that is, a cancer that is hidden from the immune system. The environment within HNSCCs is also highly immune suppressing, with lots of regulatory T cells and myeloid-derived suppressor cells (MDSCs), and very few B and T cells [189]. Also, in those HNSCCs that have arisen due to HPV infection, various virus proteins interfere with normal immune responses [189].

However, checkpoint inhibitors have given promising results in other cancers that used to be thought of as non-immunogenic, such as NSCLC. So, scientists are also investigating these treatments in HNSCC. In addition, because HPV is foreign to the body, scientists are investigating various ways of alerting the patient's immune system to its presence, and encouraging it to destroy virus-infected cancer cells

Monoclonal Antibody Checkpoint Inhibitors for HNSCC

A number of checkpoint inhibitors that target CTLA-4, PD-1, and PD-L1 have been tested in trials involving people with HNSCC, and a range of phase 3 trials are in progress (see Table 6.19). So far, most of the results that have come out are from relatively small trials. However, the results from a phase 3 trial with nivolumab (CheckMate 141) were published in November 2016 [190, 191] (see Table 6.20 for the results). In this trial, OS was 7.5 months in people with chemotherapy-resistant or metastatic HNSCC who received nivolumab

Table 6.19 Summary of phase 3 trials of checkpoint inhibitors for people with squamous cell carcinoma of the head and neck (HNSCC).

Trial name	Details	Estimated study completion date
Pembrolizumab/Keytruda		
KEYNOTE-048	Pembrolizumab alone vs. pembrolizumab + chemotherapy versus cetuximab + chemotherapy, as a first-line treatment for recurrent or metastatic HNSCC (NCT02358031)	January 2019
KEYNOTE-040	Pembrolizumab vs. standard of care for recurrent or metastatic HNSCC (NCT02252042)	June 2018
KEYNOTE-669	Pembrolizumab vs. pembrolizumab + epacadostat* vs. cetuximab + chemotherapy as a first-line treatment for recurrent or metastatic HNSCC (NCT03358472)	April 2021
KEYNOTE-412	Chemoradiation with or without pembrolizumab for locally advanced HNSCC (NCT03040999)	June 2023
Nivolumab /Opdivo		
CheckMate 141	Nivolumab vs. standard of care for people with recurrent or metastatic HNSCC (NCT02105636)	Sept 2018 – but stopped early in Jan 2016
CheckMate 651	Nivolumab + ipilimumab** vs. standard of care for people with recurrent or metastatic HNSCC (NCT02741570)	March 2020
	Nivolumab + BMS-986205* vs. cetuximab + chemotherapy as a first-line treatment for recurrent or metastatic HNSCC (NCT03386838)	July 2024
	Nivolumab vs. nivolumab + cisplatin, combined with radiotherapy, for locally advanced HNSCC (NCT03349710)	October 2022
CheckMate 9NA	Nivolumab + epacadostat* + chemotherapy vs. cetuximab + chemotherapy as a first-line treatment for recurrent or metastatic HNSCC (NCT03342352)	January 2023
Avelumab/Bavencio		
REACH	Avelumab + radiotherapy + cetuximab vs. standard of care for locally advanced HNSCC (NCT02999087)	January 2021
JAVELIN HEAD AND NECK 100	Avelumab + chemoradiation vs. chemoradiation for people with locally advanced HNSCC (NCT02952586)	May 2022
Durvalumab/Imfinzi		
KESTREL	Durvalumab with or without tremelimumab** vs. standard of care as a first-line treatment for recurrent or metastatic HNSCC (NCT02551159)	Oct 2018
EAGLE	Durvalumab with or without tremelimumab** vs. standard of care for people with recurrent or metastatic HNSCC (NCT02369874)	February 2018
	Radiothearpy combined with durvalumab or cetuximab for stage 3/4b HNSCC (NCT03258554)	December 2022

*epacadostat and BMS-986205 are both IDO inhibitors.
**Ipilimumab and tremelimumab are both antibodies that block the CTLA-4 checkpoint protein.

Table 6.20 Results from the Checkmate-141 involving 361 people with metastatic or recurrent HNSCC whose cancer had progressed within six months of receiving platinum-based chemotherapy.

	Nivolumab	Doctor's choice of methotrexate, docetaxel or cetuximab
Median OS	7.5 months	5.1 months
Median PFS	2.0 months	2.3 months
1 year survival	36%	16.6%
% progression-free at six months	19.7%	9.9%
Objective response rate	13.3%	5.8%
Incidence of grade 3 or 4 adverse events	13.1%	35.1%

Source: Ferris RL et al. (2016). Nivolumab for recurrent squamous-cell carcinoma of the head and neck. *N Engl J Med* **375**: 1856–1867.

compared to 5.1 months in people who received standard treatment with chemotherapy or cetuximab. Importantly, as in other cancers, many of the people who responded to nivolumab experienced long-lasting benefits, demonstrated by the one-year survival rate of 36% versus 16.6%.

Results from the CheckMate 141 trial also revealed that people whose cancers were HPV-positive, and those in whom more than 1% of their cancer cells had PD-L1 on their surface were most likely to benefit from nivolumab. However, the associations weren't clear-cut – some people with HPV-negative, PD-L1-negative tumors benefited from nivolumab as well [190].

A second PD-1 targeted antibody, pembrolizumab, is also licensed for HNSCC, but as of December 2017 only in the United States. This approval was based on the KEYNOTE-12 study, which gave a response rate of 18% in 132 people with chemotherapy-resistant or metastatic HNSCC [192]. A phase 3 trial of pembrolizumab, KEYNOTE-040, reported its initial results in September 2017 [193]. In that trial, the median overall survival was 8.4 versus 7.1 months in people who received pembrolizumab or standard of care (methotrexate, docetaxel, or cetuximab). However, in patients where at least 50% of their cancer

cells produced PD-L1, the median survival time was 11.6 months. And the response rate, which was only 14.6% among everyone who received pembrolizumab, was 26.6% in people who met the 50% threshold for PD-L1.

Other Immunotherapy Strategies for HNSCC

A wide variety of different immunotherapy strategies are being investigated in HNSCC, including a range of DNA and peptide vaccines [194]. These include several strategies that alert the body to the presence of HPV, including using modified bacteria and viruses. The hope is that the bacterium/virus will deliver virus proteins and trigger a strong response because the immune system perceives them as a disease-causing infection [189]. So far, these approaches have only been tested in phase 1 and phase 2 trials, but many are being tested in combination with checkpoint inhibitors to see if they can boost response rates.

6.8.3 Conclusions

After many years of little progress against HNSCC, there is currently optimism that survival times can be improved and a corresponding increase in the number of clinical trials. Early signs of promise with checkpoint inhibitors have led to at least 13 phase 3 trials investigating six PD-1, PD-L1, and CTLA-4 antibodies. Hopefully at least some of these trials will lead to meaningful benefits for an increasing proportion of people with HNSCC.

6.9 TARGETED TREATMENTS FOR BRAIN TUMORS

Around 11,000 people are diagnosed with a brain tumor or other tumor in the central nervous system (CNS) each year in the United Kingdom [195]. There are over 130 different types of brain and CNS tumors. However, the most common and most aggressive type of brain tumor is glioblastoma – an aggressive form of glioma. Gliomas are cancers derived from glial cells, the brain's support cells. Many different types of glial cells perform functions such as nourishing, protecting, stabilizing, and providing myelin to nerve cells (neurons) [196].

Reading about trials involving people with glioblastoma is often disheartening because so many different treatments have been trialled and failed. The only targeted treatment licensed for people with glioblastoma is bevacizumab, an angiogenesis inhibitor. Kinase inhibitors and monoclonal antibodies that target EGFR have also been investigated in numerous studies. More recently, checkpoint inhibitors and other immunotherapy approaches have entered trials.

6.9.1 Angiogenesis Inhibitors

A hallmark of glioblastomas is that they contain lots of blood vessels and high levels of VEGF [197]. Hence, it's logical that they would respond to treatment with an angiogenesis inhibitor. A huge range of different angiogenesis inhibitors have been investigated in trials including monoclonal antibodies and kinase inhibitors. To date, only bevacizumab has given good enough results to become a licensed treatment, although it's only licensed in the United States and not in Europe.

An example of the sort of impact that bevacizumab has on glioblastoma comes from the EORTC 26101 phase 3 trial. This trial investigated bevacizumab plus lomustine[34] versus lomustine alone in 437 people with glioblastoma who had previously been treated with standard chemotherapy and radiotherapy. The addition of bevacizumab improved PFS from 1.5 to 4.2 months, and OS from 8.6 to 9.1 months [198]. The survival benefit wasn't deemed significant.

6.9.2 Targeting EGFR

About 50% of glioblastomas contain mutations in the *EGFR* gene and/or high levels of EGFR protein [199]. The most common mutant version of EGFR found in glioblastomas is called variant III; in this version of the EGFR protein, the part that protrudes out of the cell and connects with EGF is missing. Variant III EGFR is profoundly overactive and no longer controlled by growth factors [200].

EGFR inhibitors such as gefitinib can penetrate the brain and limit the growth of brain metastases from NSCLC. This would suggest that kinase inhibitors will also penetrate the brain in people with glioblastoma. However, despite encouraging results from scientific studies using glioblastoma cells, clinical trials of EGFR inhibitors (e.g., gefitinib, erlotinib, and lapatinib) in people with glioblastoma have so far been rather disappointing [201].

Monoclonal antibodies (e.g., cetuximab and nimotuzumab) have also been investigated in trials. There have been a few signs of activity but again nothing very exciting [200, 201].

---

[34] Lomustine is a form of chemotherapy.

6.9.3 Immunotherapy for Glioblastoma

The glioblastoma microenvironment is highly immune suppressing [202]. Glioblastomas contain lots of signaling molecules (such as interleukin-10 and prostaglandin E2) that suppress white blood cells (even those in the person's bloodstream), and they lack immune-activating signaling molecules (such as interleukins 12 and 18). Also, glioblastoma cells remove proteins from their surface that might reveal them to the immune system. They also contain lots of regulatory T cells and tumor-associated macrophages, both of which suppress other types of white blood cells [203].

However, despite the immune-suppressing environment of glioblastoma, there are a couple of reasons why immunotherapies, and particularly checkpoint inhibitors, might be helpful treatments for them. First, most glioblastomas contain PD-L1, which is a sign that a PD-1 or PD-L1 antibody might be helpful. Second, ipilimumab and pembrolizumab (both checkpoint inhibitors) are known to have some impact on brain metastases from other tumors [201].

As well as checkpoint inhibitors, a variety of other immunotherapy approaches are being explored for glioblastoma. These include modified dendritic cells, CAR-modified T cells, and peptide vaccines [201]. It's difficult to say which, if any, of these approaches will ultimately become licensed treatments. Some immunotherapies, such as a peptide vaccine called rindopepimut, have already been withdrawn after disappointing clinical trial results; while for others, such as checkpoint inhibitors, although many trials are in progress [202], it's too early say what level of benefit they might be able to deliver. As I write this in December 2017, one dendritic cell treatment DCVax®-L is in a phase 3 trial [204]. There are also two phase 3 trials (Checkmate 498 and Checkmate 548) investigating nivolumab, a checkpoint inhibitor. In addition, there is growing optimism that CAR-modified T cell therapy might be both possible and effective, particularly if used in combination with other immunotherapy approaches [205].

6.9.4 Conclusions

Glioblastomas are one of the most difficult cancers to treat and one of the most lethal. Progress in developing new treatments has been incredibly slow, and pretty much every treatment that has been tested has failed to improve survival times. Currently, scientists are largely focusing their efforts on immunotherapy, but as yet no immunotherapy has delivered improved survival times in a phase 3 trial.

6.10 TARGETED TREATMENTS FOR BLADDER CANCER

Around 10,000 people are diagnosed with bladder cancer each year in the United Kingdom [206]. Over 90% of bladder cancers are urothelial carcinomas; the other 10% are squamous cell carcinomas (SCC) and adenocarcinomas.

For a long time, scientists thought that all urothelial carcinomas developed from the same kind of bladder cell. However, in the past few years, they have realized that this isn't the case. They've discovered that the slow-growing bladder cancers (called papillary cancers) that rarely invade into the muscle wall, and that account for about 80% of urothelial carcinomas, are very different from the muscle-invading bladder cancers that are responsible for most deaths [207]. They've also discovered that different types of bladder cancer develop from different bladder cells [208, 209] (see Figure 6.7).

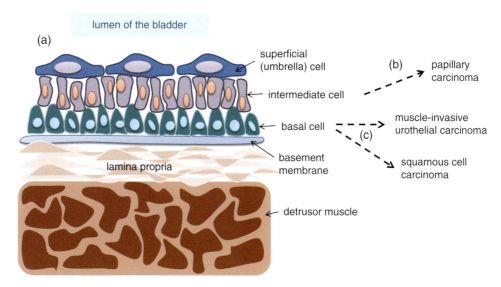

Figure 6.7 **Different types of bladder cancer develop from different cell types** [210]. **(a)** The lining of the bladder is made up of various layers of cells, which sit on top of a basement membrane. The basement membrane is surrounded by a layer called the lamina propria, which contains some muscle cells, nerve endings, blood vessels, elastic fibers, and connective tissue. Around this is a muscle layer called the detrusor muscle. **(b)** Intermediate cells give rise to the slow-growing, generally non-invasive bladder cancers called papillary carcinomas. **(c)** Basal cells give rise to fast-growing, invasive urothelial carcinomas and squamous cell carcinomas.

6.10.1 Immunotherapy for Bladder Cancer

Bladder cancers, particularly **fast-growing invasive bladder cancers, contain lots and lots of DNA mutations.** In fact, the only cancers that generally contain more mutations are lung cancers in smokers and melanoma skin cancers [211].[35] When cancers contain lots of mutations, this is often a sign that they will rapidly become resistant to treatment. But these days, it's also seen as a sign that the cancer might respond to immunotherapy. Therefore, there's huge interest in using immunotherapy against bladder cancer.

BCG Vaccine for Bladder Cancer

The number of mutations bladder cancers contain provides a reason why immunother-apy might work. On top of that, immunotherapy already has a track record in bladder cancer. Since the 1970s, a standard treatment for non-invasive bladder cancer has been to introduce the **BCG (Bacillus Calmette-Guerin) vaccine** directly into the person's bladder. The BCG vaccine, which contains living bacteria, was developed as a vaccine to protect people against tuberculosis. When injected into the bladder, BCG activates the patient's immune system and causes white blood cells to enter their tumor [212].

The **BCG vaccine is an effective treatment for non-invasive bladder cancer,** but it doesn't work for metastatic, invasive bladder cancers. Until recently, the only treatment options for these cancers were surgery and platinum-based chemotherapies such as

---

[35] There's also a relatively rare type of bowel cancer called MSI bowel cancer that has even more mutations. And there are some other rare cancers that exhibit MSI properties.

cisplatin. However, the results of clinical trials with checkpoint inhibitors have created a wave of excitement among scientists and doctors.

Monoclonal Antibody Checkpoint Inhibitors for Bladder Cancer

Checkpoint inhibitors are increasingly used as treatments for people with bladder cancer, particularly for people whose cancer has worsened despite chemotherapy. The first approval for a checkpoint inhibitor came in May 2016, when atezolizumab/Tecentriq, an anti-PD-L1 antibody, was licensed in the United States. In 2017, atezolizumab was also approved for use in Europe. These approvals were based on the results of the IMvigor 210

and IMvigor 211 trials (see Table 6.21). 2017 also saw the approval of nivolumab/Opdivo and pembrolizumab/Keytruda in the United States and Europe, and the approval of durvalumab/Imfinzi and avelumab/Bavencio in the United States. The nivolumab approval was based on a single-arm phase 2 study (CheckMate-275), which reported a response rate of 19.6% [213], and the approval of pembrolizumab followed the results of the phase 3 KEYNOTE-045 study. In KEYNOTE-045, pembrolizumab improved the survival time of bladder cancer patients compared to chemotherapy by around three months (10.3 months versus 7.4 months). The response rate in this trial was 21.1% with pembrolizumab versus 11.0% with chemotherapy [214]. The

Table 6.21   Results from the IMvigor 210 and IMvigor 211 clinical trials investigating atezolizumab/ Tecentriq for people with invasive bladder cancer, who had previously been treated with platinum-based chemotherapy.

IMvigor 2010 [217]

A phase 2 trial involving 310 patients with inoperable locally advanced or metastatic bladder cancer whose disease had worsened after receiving platinum-based chemotherapy

	Atezolizumab
Overall response rate	14.8%
Response rate in patients with ≥5% PD-L1 expression	26%
Response rate in patients with <5% PD-L1 expression	9.5%

IMvigor 211 [218]

A phase 3 trial of atezolizumab vs. chemotherapy (vinflunine, paclitaxel, or docetaxel) in 931 patients with locally advanced or metastatic bladder cancer whose disease had worsened after receiving platinum-based chemotherapy

	Atezolizumab	Chemotherapy
Overall survival in patients with ≥5% PD-L1 expression	11.1 months	10.6 months
Objective response rate in patients with ≥5% PD-L1 expression	23% (26 out of 113 patients)	22% (25 out of 116 patients)
Objective response rate in the entire study population	13.4%	13.4%
Median duration of response in patients with ≥5% PD-L1 expression	15.9 months	8.3 months
Median duration of response in the entire study population	21.7 months	7.4 months

approval of avelumab was based on another single-arm study called JAVELIN, in which avelumab gave a response rate of 13.3% in 242 patients [215]. Finally, the approval of dur-valumab was based on "Study 1108," which gave a response rate of 20.4% [216].

If the results of all these trials seem a bit confused, that's because they are. In some trials, there appeared to be a correlation between PD-L1 levels and patient benefit, but in others there wasn't. Also, in IMvigor211, people given chemotherapy did much better than those given similar chemotherapy in KEYNOTE-045. Also, pembrolizumab led to a survival benefit in KEYNOTE-045, whereas atezolizumab didn't in IMvigor211. However, commentators on these studies, and others, have repeatedly suggested that endpoints such as progression-free survival and overall survival can be misleading when response rates are low [219], and that perhaps duration of response gives a better indicator of the value of checkpoint inhibitors. The 21.7 month versus 7.4 month duration of response in IMvigor211 does seem to bear this out. In the KEYNOTE-045, the duration of response data wasn't mature at the point when the study was published.

In response to these promising trial results, many different phase 3 trials are investigating checkpoint inhibitors as treatments for blad-der cancer (Table 6.22). Some of these trials are for people with previously treated bladder cancer; some are for people who haven't yet been given any treatment.

As in other solid tumors, the focus of many future checkpoint inhibitor trials will be twofold: (1) to identify which patients are most likely to benefit by exploring biomark-ers such as PD-L1 levels and number of DNA mutations, and (2) to improve response rates by using checkpoint inhibitors in combination with one another and with other types of treatment.

6.10.2 Other Targeted Treatments for Bladder Cancer

The majority of bladder cancers contain muta-tions that make them potentially vulnerable to existing targeted treatments. Some of these mutations, such as *FGFR* gene mutations, are common in low-grade bladder cancers. *FGFR* mutations, *PIK3CA*[36] mutations, *HER2* muta-tions, and *EGFR* gene amplifications have also been found in muscle-invasive bladder cancer [220]. However, trials with treatments such as EGFR-targeted treatments (gefitinib, erlotinib, cetuximab, and panitumumab), HER2-targeted treatments (trastuzumab and lapat-inib), and FGFR inhibitors (dovitinib) have so far given patchy and mostly disappointing results [221]. This is partly because the high degree of intratumoral heterogeneity in blad-der cancers causes rapid drug resistance [211]. But, there's lots of work going on to find out if particular mutations, such as *FGFR3* muta-tions, make some bladder cancers vulnerable to FGFR inhibitors or other treatment combi-nations. And there are many trials in progress.

Targeting Angiogenesis

As with other solid tumors, bladder cancers depend on a blood supply for their growth and survival. Many different angiogenesis inhibitors have been tested in trials including antibodies (bevacizumab and ramucirumab) and kinase inhibitors (sorafenib, sunitinib, pazopanib, vandetanib, and cabozantinib). However, most of these trials have again given disappointing results [222].

---

[36] *PIK3CA* is the gene for the active part of PI3K; mutations in PIK3CA therefore cause the PI3K/AKT/mTOR pathway to be overactive.

Table 6.22 Phase 3 trials of checkpoint inhibitors in bladder cancer, as of December 2017.

Trial name	Details	Estimated study completion date
Atezolizumab/Tecentriq		
IMvigor 211	Atezolizumab versus chemotherapy in 932 patients with metastatic BC previously treated with chemotherapy (NCT02302807)	November 2017
IMvigor 010	Adjuvant atezolizumab versus observation in 700 patients with high-risk BC (NCT02450331)	May 2022
IMvigor 130	Atezolizumab alone or in combination with chemotherapy for 1,200 patients with untreated advanced or metastatic BC – NCT02807636	July 2020
Pembrolizumab/Keytruda		
KEYNOTE-045	Pembrolizumab versus chemotherapy for 542 patients with metastatic BC previously treated with chemotherapy (NCT02256436)	May 2017
AMBASSADOR	Pembrolizumab vs. observation in 739 people with muscle invasive and locally advanced BC (NCT03244384)	February 2019
KEYNOTE-698	Pembrolizumab with or without epacadostat in 648 patients with metastatic BC previously treated with chemotherapy (NCT03374488)	May 2021
KEYNOTE-361	Chemotherapy with or without pembrolizumab vs. pembrolizumab alone in 990 people with advanced or metastatic BC (NCT02853305)	May 2020
KEYNOTE-672	Pembrolizumab with or without epacadostat in 650 patients with cisplatin-ineligible advanced or metastatic BC (NCT03374488)	April 2021
Nivolumab/Opdivo		
CheckMate 274	Nivolumab versus placebo in 640 patients who have had surgery for invasive BC (NCT02632409)	May 2020
Avelumab/Bavencio		
JAVELIN bladder 100	Maintenance treatment with avelumab versus best support care in 668 patients whose BC did not worsen during or following chemotherapy (NCT02603432)	July 2020
Durvalumab/Imfinzi		
DANUBE	Durvalumab with or without tremelimumab vs. chemotherapy as a first-line treatment in 1200 patients with inoperable BC (NCT02516241)	September 2019

Abbreviations: BC – bladder cancer

6.10.3 Conclusions

Things are currently looking up for people with bladder cancer. It's still early days, but there are exciting signs that checkpoint inhibitors will be effective treatments for some patients. The many phase 3 trials that are currently taking place will hopefully clarify the level of benefit and who should receive them. Studies into the gene mutations that bladder cancer cells contain are also opening up new lines of investigation.

6.11 TARGETED TREATMENTS FOR PANCREATIC CANCER

Pancreatic cancer is **one of the most deadly of all cancers.** It is diagnosed in around 9,600 people each year in the United Kingdom, and causes 8,800 deaths [223]. Only 20% of people survive for a year after their diagnosis, and only 3% of people survive for five years [224].

The vast majority (90%–95%) of pancreatic cancers are aggressive pancreatic ductal adenocarcinomas (PDACs), which develop from acinar cells (or occasionally from ductal cells or centro-acinar cells) [225] (see Figure 6.8). A much rarer group of pancreatic cancers are the slower-growing pancreatic neuroendocrine tumors (pNETs), which develop from cells in the islets of Langerhans that produce insulin or glucagon. Other rare types of pancreatic cancer are the pancreatic acinar cell carcinomas and intraductal papillary mucinous neoplasms.

PDACs often contain mutations in four key genes that drive their growth and survival. These four genes are KRAS, TP53, SMAD4, and CDKN2A [227] (see Figure 6.9a, b, and c). However, when it comes to treating pancreatic cancer, one of the greatest obstacles is the cancer's microenvironment (Figure 6.9d).

Pancreatic cancer cells live alongside millions of white blood cells and structural cells such as fibroblasts and stellate cells [228]. The white blood cells produce growth factors and other signaling proteins that protect cancer cells from treatment. In addition, the fibroblasts and stellate cells produce vast quantities of fibrous proteins that they secrete to create a dense network called desmoplasia. On top of this, there are very few blood vessels in pancreatic cancers, and those that do exist are squashed and flattened. Hence, even potentially very effective drugs have no little or no impact on pancreatic cancer because they simply don't reach the heart of the tumor. And, because of the lack of blood vessels, cancer cells that want to escape do so by traveling inside nerve bundles, where cancer drugs cannot reach them [229].

6.11.1 Targeting EGFR

Pancreatic cancer cells often have EGF receptors (EGFR) on their surface [230]. The only targeted cancer treatment ever to show any effectiveness against pancreatic cancer is erlotinib (Tarceva), an EGFR inhibitor (see

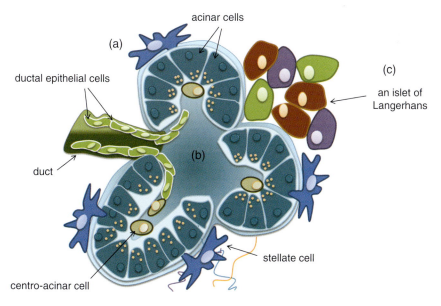

Figure 6.8 Normal pancreas biology [226]. **(a)** In the pancreas there are millions of tiny clusters of cells called acini, in which clusters of acinar cells surround a central space **(b)**. Acinar cells secrete digestive enzymes into the central space, which then feeds into a duct, which eventually combines with other ducts and releases digestive enzymes into the intestine. **(c)** Interspersed with the acini are groups of cells called islets of Langerhans that produce hormones. In each islet are four types of cells that produce four hormones: insulin, glucagon, pancreatic polypeptide, and somatostatin. **(d)** Stellate cells produce useful structural proteins that support the pancreas's other cells.

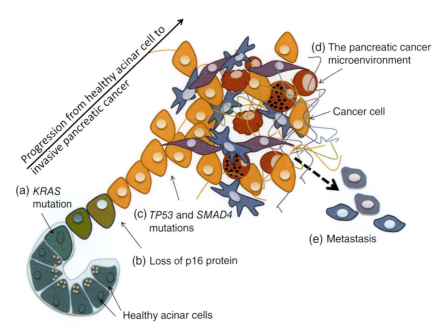

Figure 6.9 **Progression from healthy acinar cell to invasive pancreatic cancer. (a)** The most common mutation in early, pre-cancerous pancreatic cells is a *KRAS* mutation, which causes a healthy acinar cell to become more ductal cell-like in appearance. **(b)** *KRAS* mutations are followed by loss of p16 protein. **(c)** Invasive pancreatic cancer cells also commonly contain mutations in *TP53* and *SMAD4*. **(d)** Cancer cells, immune cells and stromal cells communicate and cooperate to create a complex, fibrous microenvironment. **(e)** During the development of pancreatic cancer, some cells detach from the tumor and move into nerves, lymph, and blood vessels, leading to metastasis.

Chapter 3, Section 3.3). I've spoken about this drug previously in relation to lung cancers with *EGFR* gene mutations, against which it works well, often keeping the cancer in check for a year or so. But the picture is very different in pancreatic cancer, in which it only improved survival from 5.91 to 6.24 months when added to chemotherapy – a difference of about 10 days [231]. Clinical trials with other targeted agents have generally shown no benefit at all [232].

6.11.2 Other Approaches in Development

Perhaps one of the most promising lines of attack against pancreatic cancer is to create drugs that are designed to penetrate the tumor better than existing drugs. One example is nab-paclitaxel (Abraxane), a form of paclitaxel chemotherapy in which the drug is used to coat albumin [233].[37] Nab-paclitaxel is much more water soluble than the original chemotherapy, and has an easier job of getting in and out of blood vessels [234]. In a clinical trial, patients given Nab-paclitaxel plus gemcitabine had a median survival of 8.5 months compared to 6.7 months in patients given gemicabine alone [235]. A similar treatment is irinotecan hydrochloride liposome (Onivyde), in which the chemotherapy irinotecan is contained in tiny fat particles called liposomes. Other drugs have been created that have novel delivery mechanisms or that are activated by the low oxygen levels found inside pancreatic cancers [236].

---

[37] Albumin is the most abundant protein floating free in our blood.

One treatment approach that might be applicable for a small proportion of people with pancreatic cancer is the PARP inhibitors. PARP inhibitors are licensed treatments for women with ovarian cancer who have a mutated *BRCA1* or *BRCA2* gene. And people (not just women) with inherited *BRCA* gene mutations are also at a higher risk of developing pancreatic cancer. In fact, *BRCA2* mutations are found in about 17% of pancreatic cancers in people who have a family history of the disease [237]. In 2015, researchers conducted a clinical trial that included 23 people with pancreatic cancer known to have *BRCA* gene mutations. In five (22%) of these people, treatment with a PARP inhibitor (olaparib) caused their tumor to shrink [238]. Olaparib is now the subject of a phase 3 trial (called POLO), which is recruiting 145 people with pancreatic cancer who have inherited *BRCA* mutations. Other PARP inhibitors (e.g., veliparib and rucaparib) are also in pancreatic cancer trials.

6.11.3 Immunotherapy for Pancreatic Cancer

Pancreatic cancers generally contain millions of white blood cells. However, many of these white blood cells are immune suppressing, such as MDSCs [239]. These MDSCs prevent any T cells, which are also present in pancreatic cancer, from mounting an anti-cancer immune response. In addition, dendritic cells present in pancreatic cancers are prevented from doing their normal, helpful job of picking up cancer cell debris and taking it to T cells in lymph nodes.

So far, numerous trials with immunotherapies such as peptide vaccines and checkpoint inhibitors have given very mixed results. And those that have given promising results in early trials have failed to do the same when trialled in larger groups of patients. As a result, at the moment it's unclear whether any of these approaches have a future as

treatments for pancreatic cancer [240]. However, a quick search of ClinicalTrials.gov reveals 38 phase 2 trials with PD-1 and PD-L1 antibodies. So over the next couple of years we might get a better idea as to whether any of these antibodies might be useful alone, or in combination with other treatments.

One glimmer of hope in pancreatic cancer is that a small proportion of them, possibly around 1%–2%, are MSI-high [241]. That is, they contain thousands of DNA mutations because they contain defects in a DNA repair process called mismatch repair. As I mentioned in Section 6.5.5, cancers with defects in mismatch repair are often sensitive to treatment with a checkpoint inhibitor. In a study investigating the usefulness of pembrolizumab (a PD-1-targeted checkpoint inhibitor) in 83 people with various MSI-high solid tumors, five out of eight people with pancreatic cancer responded to treatment, and in a further person their disease stabilized [242]. The number of people with pancreatic cancer involved in this study was obviously very small. But the result does suggest that, as in other cancers, people with pancreatic cancers that contain extremely high numbers of DNA mutations might benefit from treatment with a checkpoint inhibitor.

6.11.4 Conclusions

As with glioblastoma, clinical trials testing out new treatments for people with pancreatic cancer have generally failed to improve survival times. Two important reasons why this cancer is so difficult to treat, and why most treatments fail, are:

1. Late diagnosis due to a lack of obvious symptoms
2. The impenetrable cancer microenvironment

Hence, even the tiny survival improvement that erlotinib gave in trials was enough to see it become a licensed treatment.

At the moment, the majority of clinical trials involving people with pancreatic cancer are focused on novel delivery mechanisms of chemotherapy, PARP inhibitors for the small proportion of cases linked to inherited faulty *BRCA* genes, and combinations of immunotherapies with one another or with chemotherapy or radiotherapy.

6.12 FINAL THOUGHTS

Having summarized progress in the use of targeted cancer treatments for the ten most common cancers in the United Kingdom, you can see that we've made more progress against some cancers than others. And it also becomes apparent that some treatment approaches have brought about bigger benefits for patients than others. The difference in the degree of benefit seems to sometimes be to do with the limitations of the treatment approach (e.g., angiogenesis inhibitors) and sometimes to do with the treatment's target (e.g., whether the target protein is mutated or simply overproduced). I've summarized some of my thoughts on various treatment approaches below.

6.12.1 Angiogenesis Inhibitors

For most people with solid tumors the benefits of adding an angiogenesis inhibitor to chemotherapy tend to be fairly modest. For example, in bowel, lung, breast, and glioblastomas, the survival benefit tends to be in the region of a couple of months or so. The exceptions to this are kidney cancer and, perhaps, *EGFR*-mutated lung cancer.

In kidney cancer, the benefits of angiogenesis inhibitors, even when used on their own, are very clear and relatively long-lasting.

Many different angiogenesis inhibitors have proved effective in phase 3 trials, and seven of them are licensed treatments. In *EGFR*-mutated lung cancer, the improvement in PFS when you add an angiogenesis inhibitor to an EGFR-inhibitor appears to be very important.[38] However, so far we only have the results of one phase 2 trial, so this benefit is not yet certain.

6.12.2 Treatments That Target EGF Receptors (EGFR and HER2)

Treatments that target EGFR and HER2 have brought about important benefits to women with HER2-positive breast cancer and to people (often non-smokers) with *EGFR*-mutated NSCLC. In these cases, the gene for the receptor is either amplified (in *HER2*-mutated breast cancer) or mutated and overactive (in *EGFR*-mutated NSCLC). Thus, there is a clear difference between the person's cancer cells and the cells in the rest of their body.

Where the effectiveness of EGFR-targeted treatments have been more modest is in cancers where EGFR is present in high levels, but the receptor is wild type (i.e., unmutated). In these cancers, such as bowel cancer and head and neck cancer, EGFR-targeted antibodies do benefit some people, but often in fewer numbers and to a lesser extent than in *EGFR*-mutated NSCLC. However, various discoveries, such as that EGFR antibodies work better for people with left-sided than right-sided bowel cancers, have opened up new opportunities for using these treatments more precisely and to greater effect in future.

---

[38] It's not possible to talk about improvements in OS because the combination was tested as the patients' first line of treatment. Hence, when their cancer progressed, they will have been offered further treatments such as chemotherapy, a third-generation EGFR inhibitor, or a checkpoint inhibitor. So, when they died, it wouldn't be possible to discern what impact their initial treatment had on their survival time.

6.12.3 Targeting the MAPK Pathway

The MAPK pathway comprises Ras, Raf, MEK, and ERK proteins. So far, only B-Raf and MEK inhibitors have proved their worth as cancer treatments, and they are important treatments for people with **BRAF-mutated malignant melanoma**. Through detailed analysis of how the MAPK pathway operates in *BRAF*-mutated lung cancers and bowel cancers, they are looking promising for these cancers too.

Despite the fact that 30% of cancers contain mutations in *RAS* genes, scientists still haven't been able to create any powerful, specific Ras inhibitors.

6.12.4 Targeting the PI3K/AKT/mTOR Pathway

Despite decades of research and vast evidence showing the importance of this pathway in cancer, it still feels like we're still **at the beginning of the journey toward creating PI3K/AKT/mTOR pathway inhibitors.**

So far, the only licensed drugs that block this pathway are the two indirect mTOR inhibitors, temsirolimus and everolimus, and two PI3K inhibitors given to people with chronic lymphocytic leukemia and non-Hodgkin lymphoma (see Chapter 7, Section 7.4.4). However, the creation of a range of PI3K inhibitors that can block individual versions of PI3K, and the creation of many powerful AKT and mTOR inhibitors, will surely lead to more successes in clinical trials.

6.12.5 CDK Inhibitors

CDK inhibitors have been around for many years, but it's only recently that we've seen drugs developed that can selectively block just a couple of them at a time (e.g., CDK 4 and 6). These **selective CDK inhibitors are still at the beginning of their journey.** So far these treatments have been licensed only for

breast cancer. But there's plenty of optimism that CDK4/6 inhibitors will be effective against many other cancers as well.

6.12.6 PARP Inhibitors

In this chapter, I've only mentioned PARP inhibitors briefly, and mostly in relation to triple-negative breast cancer, prostate cancer, and pancreatic cancer. But where they've already proved their worth is in the treatment of ovarian cancer (Chapter 4, Section 4.3). Put simply, **they seem to be effective against cancers that have great problems repairing DNA damage.** And because many cancers share this feature, PARP inhibitors are being explored in many different cancer types.

6.12.7 Monoclonal Antibody Checkpoint Inhibitors

When I first began writing this book in January 2015, the potential of these treatments was only just beginning to become clear. Now, three years later, they're licensed treatments for many different solid tumors (e.g., malignant melanoma, lung cancer, head and neck cancer, bladder cancer, and kidney cancer) and Hodgkin lymphoma. No doubt by the time you read this there will be more approvals to add to the list. At the moment, trial after trial gives tantalizing results: a combination of a modest response rate (somewhere between 10% and 30%) with an incredibly long duration of response in some of the people who benefit. This duration of response is much longer than you would generally expect to see with other antibodies or kinase inhibitors.

My hope is that in the next few years, scientists and doctors will manage to pin down biomarkers that can be used to predict who will respond to these treatments, and discover how to increase the proportion of people who benefit. Hopefully, researchers will find was to increase response rates to checkpoint inhibitors by increasing (1) **the visibility of cancers** to the immune system, (2) **the number of T cells** in patients' tumors, and (3) **the activity of these T cells.** Looking at the results of recent clinical trials, the biomarkers will probably be different from cancer to cancer, as will the strategies to boost the proportion of people who benefit.

6.12.8 Other Immunotherapy Strategies

So far, peptide and DNA vaccines, modified dendritic cells, and modified T cells **haven't made much of an impact on the treatment of people with solid tumors.** The immune-suppressing environment within solid tumors is a major obstacle, as is the cost of some of these treatments. However, various trials are under way in which various immunotherapies are being combined, such as peptide vaccines combined with checkpoint inhibitors, and these might give better results.

REFERENCES

1 Cancer Research UK (2016). Breast Cancer Incidence Statistics. [online] Available at: http://www.cancerresearchuk.org/health-professional/cancer-statistics/statistics-by-cancer-type/breast-cancer [Accessed January 3, 2018].

2 Giordano SH (2005). A review of the diagnosis and management of male breast cancer. *The Oncologist* **10**(7): 471–479.

3 Cancer Research UK (2016). Triple Negative Breast Cancer. [online] Available at: http://www.cancerresearchuk.org/about-cancer/breast-cancer/stages-types-grades/types/triple-negative-breast-cancer [Accessed January 3, 2018].

4 Marino M et al. (2006). Estrogen signaling multiple pathways to impact gene transcription. *Curr Genomics* **7**(8): 497–508.

5 McDonnell DP and Wardell SE (2010). The molecular mechanisms underlying the pharmacological actions of ER modulators: Implications for new drug discovery in breast cancer. *Curr Op Pharmacol* **10**(6): 620–628.

6 Reinert T and Barrios CH (2015). Optimal management of hormone receptor positive metastatic breast cancer in 2016. *Ther Adv Med Oncol* **7**(6): 304–320.

7 Smith IE and Dowsett M (2003). Aromatase inhibitors in breast cancer. *N Engl J Med* **348**: 2431–2442.

8 Lambertini M et al. (2017). Ovarian function suppression in premenopausal women with early-stage breast cancer. *Curr Treat Options Oncol* **18**(1): 4.

9 Turner NC et al. (2017). Advances in the treatment of advanced oestrogen-receptor-positive breast cancer. *Lancet* **389**(10087): 2403–2414.

10 Osborne CK and Schiff R (2011). Mechanisms of endocrine resistance in breast cancer. *Annu Rev Med* **62**: 233–247.

11 U.S. Department of Health and Human Services Food and Drug Administration (2007). Guidance for Industry Clinical Trial Endpoints for the Approval of Cancer Drugs and Biologics. [online] Available at: https://www.fda.gov/downloads/drugsGuidanceComplianceRegulatoyInformation/Guidance/UCM071590.pdf [Accessed January 3, 2018].

12 Eisenhauer EA et al. (2009). New response evaluation criteria in solid tumours: Revised RECIST guideline (version 1.1). *Eur J Cancer* **45**(2): 228–247.

13 Wolchok JD (2009). Guidelines for the Evaluation of immune therapy activity in solid tumors: Immune-related response criteria. *Clin Cancer Res* **15**(23): 7412–7420.

14 Merlano M et al. (2016). Immune-related response criteria: Light and shadows. *ESMO Open* **1**: e000082.

15 There's lots of information about clinical trials on the Roche website: Roche. What is a clinical trial and how does a trial work? [online]. Available at: https://www.roche.com/research_and_development/who_we_are_how_we_work/clinical_trials/what_is_a_clinical_trial.htm [Accessed January 3, 2018].

16 Finn RS et al. (2016). Palbociclib and letrozole in advanced breast cancer. *N Engl J Med* **375**: 1925–1936.

17 Christofanilli M et al. (2016). Fulvestrant plus palbociclib versus fulvestrant plus placebo for treatment of hormone-receptor-positive, HER2-

negative metastatic breast cancer that progressed on previous endocrine therapy (PALOMA-3): Final analysis of the multicentre, double-blind, phase 3 randomised controlled trial. *Lancet Oncol* **17**(4): 425–439.

18 Hortobagyi GN et al. (2016). Ribociclib as first-line therapy for HR-positive, advanced breast cancer. *N Engl J Med* **375**: 1738–1748.

19 Sledge GW Jr. et al. (2017). MONARCH 2: Abemaciclib in combination with Fulvestrant in women with HR+/HER2– Advanced breast cancer who had progressed while receiving endocrine therapy. *J Clin Oncol* **35**(25): 2875–2884.

20 For an overview of the progress made in treating HER2-positive breast cancer and the role of trastuzumab, see: Loibl S, Gianni L (2017). HER2-positive breast cancer. *Lancet* **389**: 2415–2419.

21 Swain SM et al. (2015). Pertuzumab, trastuzumab, and docetaxel in HER2-positive metastatic breast cancer. *N Eng J Med* **372**: 724–734.

22 Verma S et al. (2012). Trastuzumab emtansine for HER2-positive advanced breast cancer. *N Engl J Med* **367**(19): 1783–1791.

23 Generics and Biosimilars Initiative (2017). Biosimilars of Trastuazumab. [online] Available at: http://www.gabionline.net/Biosimilars/General/Biosimilars-of-trastuzumab [Accessed January 3, 2018].

24 European Medicines Agency. Ontruzant. Summary of opinion (initial authorisation). http://www.ema.europa.eu/docs/en_GB/document_library/Summary_of_opinion_-_Initial_authorisation/human/004323/WC500234791.pdf [Accessed December 27, 2017].

25 For a discussion of margetuximab, see: Bucco D (2017). Pegram Sheds Light on Margetuximab in HER2+ Breast Cancer. OncLive. [online] Available at: http://www.onclive.com/web-exclusives/pegram-sheds-light-on-margetuximab-in-her2-breast-cancer [Accessed January 3, 2018].

26 Gelmon KA (2015). Lapatinib or Trastuzumab Plus Taxane therapy for human epidermal growth factor receptor 2–positive advanced breast cancer: Final results of NCIC CTG MA.31. *J Clin Oncol* **33**(14): 1574–1583.

27 European Medicines Agency. Tyverb (lapatinib). [online] Available at: http://www.ema.europa.eu/ema/index.jsp?curl=pages/medicines/human/medicines/000795/human_med_001120.jsp&mid=WC0b01ac058001d124 [Accessed January 3, 2018].

28 Martin M et al. (2017). Neratinib after trastuzumab-based adjuvant therapy in HER2-positive breast cancer (ExteNET): 5-year analysis of a randomised, double-blind, placebo-controlled, phase 3 trial. *Lancet Oncol* **18**(12): 1688–1700.

29 Awada A et al. (2016). Neratinib plus paclitaxel vs trastuzumab plus paclitaxel in previously untreated metastatic ERBB2-positive breast cancer: The NEfERT-T randomized clinical trial. *JAMA Oncol* **2**(12): 1557–1564.

30 Aalders KC et al. (2017). Anti-angiogenic treatment in breast cancer: Facts, successes, failures and future perspectives. *Cancer Treat Rev* **53**: 98–110.

31 Department of Health and Human Services Food and Drug Administration (2011). Proposal to Withdraw Approval for the Breast Cancer Indication for AVASTIN (Bevacizumab). Decision of the Commissioner. [online] Available at: https://www.fda.gov/downloads/NewsEvents/Newsroom/UCM280546.pdf [Accessed January 3, 2018].

32 Kotoula V et al. (2017). The fate of BRCA1-related germline mutations in triple-negative breast cancer. *Am J Cancer Res* **7**(1): 98–114.

33 Bianchini G et al. (2016). Triple-negative breast cancer: Challenges and opportunities of a heterogeneous disease. *Nat Rev Clin Oncol* **13**: 674–690.

34 Robson M et al. (2017). Olaparib for metastatic breast cancer in patients with a germline BRCA mutation. *N Engl J Med* **377**: 523–533.

35 Litton J et al. (2017). EMBRACA: A phase 3 trial comparing talazoparib, an oral PARP inhibitor, to physician's choice of therapy in patients with advanced breast cancer and a germline BRCA mutation. San Antonio Breast Cancer Symposium: Abstract GS6-07. Presented December 8, 2017.

36 Gyawali B (2017). The OlympiAD trial: Who won gold? *ecancer* **11**:ed75 10.3332/ecancer.2017.ed75

37 Tutt A et al. (2014). The TNT trial. San Antonio Breast Cancer Symposium. Abstract S3-01. Presented December 11, 2014.

38 Cancer Research UK (2016). Breast Cancer Mortality Trends over Time (Females). [online] Available at: http://www.cancerresearchuk.org/health-professional/cancer-statistics/statistics-by-cancer-type/breast-cancer/mortality#heading-Two [Accessed January 3, 2018].

39 Cancer Research UK (2016). Prostate Cancer Incidence Statistics. [online] Available at: http://www.cancerresearchuk.org/health-professional/cancer-statistics/statistics-by-cancer-type/prostate-cancer [Accessed January 3, 2018].

40 Shore ND (2015). Radium-223 dichloride for metastatic castration-resistant prostate cancer: The urologist's perspective. *Urology* **85**(4): 717–724.

41 Wilson EM (2010). Androgen receptor molecular biology and potential targets in prostate cancer. *Ther Adv Urol* **2**(3): 105–117.

42 Chen Y (2009). Antiandrogens and androgen depleting therapies in prostate cancer: Novel agents for an established target. *Lancet Oncol* **10**(10): 981–991.

43 Crawford ED and Hou AH (2009). The role of LHRH antagonists in the treatment of prostate cancer. *Oncology* **23**(7): 626–630.

44 Chen Y (2009). Antiandrogens and androgen depleting therapies in prostate cancer: Novel agents for an established target. *Lancet Oncol* **10**(10): 981–991.

45 Boudadi K and Antonarakis ES (2016). Resistance to novel antiandrogen therapies in metastatic castration-resistant prostate cancer. *Clin Med Insights Oncol* **10**(Suppl 1): 1–9.

46 Lord CJ and Ashworth A (2016). BRCAness revisited. *Nat Rev Cancer* **16**: 110–120.

47 Palmbos PL and Hussain MH (2016). Targeting PARP in prostate cancer: Novelty, pitfalls, and promise. *Oncology* **30**(5): 377–385.

48 Rodrigues DN et al. (2017). The molecular underpinnings of prostate cancer: Impacts on management and pathology practice. *J Pathol* **241**(2): 173–182.

49 King, S. (2014). ViewPoints: Dendreon's House Comes Crashing Down, with Provenge Providing Flimsy Foundations. [online] Firstwordpharma.com. Available at: https://www.firstwordpharma.com/node/1245029?tsid=17 [Accessed January 3, 2018].

50 Modena A et al. (2016). Immune checkpoint inhibitors and prostate cancer: A new frontier? *Oncol Rev* **10**(1): 293.

51 Kwon ED (2014). Ipilimumab versus placebo after radiotherapy in patients with metastatic castration-resistant prostate cancer that had progressed after docetaxel chemotherapy (CA184-043): A multicentre, randomised, double-blind, phase 3 trial. *Lancet Oncol* **15**(7): 700–712.

52 Cancer Research UK (2016). Lung Cancer Incidence Statistics. [online] Available at: http://www.cancerresearchuk.org/health-professional/cancer-statistics/statistics-by-cancer-type/lung-cancer/incidence#heading-Zero [Accessed January 3, 2018].

53 Cancer Research UK (2016). Lung Cancer Risk Factors. [online] Available at: http://www.cancerresearchuk.org/health-professional/cancer-statistics/statistics-by-cancer-type/lung-cancer#heading-Three [Accessed January 3, 2018].

54 Markman M (2016). Genetics of Non-Small Cell Lung Cancer. [online] Available at: http://emedicine.medscape.com/article/1689988-overview#a1 [Accessed January 3, 2018].

55 Swanton C and Govindan R (2016). Clinical implications of genomic discoveries in lung cancer. *N Engl J Med* **374**: 1864–1873.

56 The Cancer Genome Atlas Network (2012). Comprehensive genomic characterization of squamous cell lung cancers. *Nature* **489**(7417): 519–525.

57 The Cancer Genome Atlas Network (2014). Comprehensive molecular profiling of lung adenocarcinoma. *Nature* **511**(7511): 543–550.

58 Strickler A (2017). Rovalpituzumab Tesirine Active and Safe in Small Cell Lung Cancer. [online] Available at: http://www.onclive.com/web-exclusives/rovalpituzumab-tesirine-active-and-safe-in-small-cell-lung-cancer [Accessed January 3, 2018].

59 Information from: European Medicines Agency: http://www.ema.europa.eu and National

Cancer Institute: https://www.cancer.gov/about-cancer/treatment/drugs/lung

60 Chong CR and Janne PA (2013). The quest to overcome resistance to EGFR-targeted therapies in cancer. *Nat Med* **19**(11): 1389–1400.

61 Lynch TJ et al. (2004). Activating mutations in the epidermal growth factor receptor underlying responsiveness of non–small-cell lung cancer to gefitinib. *N Engl J Med* **350**(21): 2129–2139.

62 Burotto M et al. (2015). Gefitinib and Erlotinib in metastatic non-small cell lung cancer: A meta-analysis of toxicity and efficacy of randomized clinical trials. *Oncologist* **20**(4): 400–410.

63 Liang W et al. (2014). Network meta-analysis of erlotinib, gefitinib, afatinib and icotinib in patients with advanced non–small-cell lung cancer harboring EGFR mutations. *PLoS One* **9**(2): e85245.

64 Lim SH et al. (2014). Comparison of clinical outcomes following gefitinib and erlotinib treatment in non–small-cell lung cancer patients harboring an epidermal growth factor receptor mutation in either Exon 19 or 21. *J Thoracic Oncol* **9**(4): 506–511.

65 Park K et al. Afatinib versus gefitinib as first-line treatment of patients with EGFR mutation positive non–small-cell lung cancer (LUX-Lung 7): A phase 2B, open-label, randomised controlled trial. *Lancet Oncol* **17**(5): 577–589.

66 Urata Y et al. (2016). Randomized phase III study comparing gefitinib with erlotinib in patients with previously treated advanced lung adenocarcinoma: WJOG 5108L. *J Clin Oncol* **34**(27): 3248–3257.

67 Tan DSW et al. (2016). The International association for the study of lung cancer consensus statement on optimizing management of egfr mutation–positive non-small cell lung cancer: Status in 2016. *J Thoracic Oncol* **11**(7): 646–963.

68 Ke E-E and Wu Yi-Long (2016). EGFR as a pharmacological target in EGFR-mutant non–small-cell lung cancer: Where do we stand now? *Trends Pharmacol Sci* **37**(11): 887–903.

69 Hata AN et al. (2016). Tumor cells can follow distinct evolutionary paths to become resistant to epidermal growth factor receptor inhibition. *Nat Med* **22**: 262–269.

70 Mok TM et al. (2016). Osimertinib or platinum–pemetrexed in EGFR T790M–positive lung cancer. *N Engl J Med* **376**: 629–640.

71 Soria J-C et al. (2018). Osimertinib in untreated *EGFR*-mutated advanced non–small-cell lung cancer. *N Engl J Med* **378**: 113–125.

72 Thatcher N et al. (2015). Necitumumab plus gemcitabine and cisplatin versus gemcitabine and cisplatin alone as first-line therapy in patients with stage IV squamous non–small-cell lung cancer (SQUIRE): An open-label, randomised, controlled phase 3 trial. *Lancet Oncol* **16**(7): 765–774.

73 Paz-Ares (2016). Correlation of EGFR-expression with safety and efficacy outcomes in SQUIRE: A randomized, multicenter, open-label, phase III study of gemcitabine–cisplatin plus necitumumab versus gemcitabine–cisplatin alone in the first-line treatment of patients with stage IV squamous non–small-cell lung cancer. *Ann Oncol* **27**(8): 1573–1579.

74 Goldstein DA et al. (2015). Necitumumab in metastatic squamous cell lung cancer: Establishing a value-based cost. *JAMA Oncol* **1**(9): 1293–1300.

75 Hagen T (2015). Necitumumab Assigned "Low Value" in Lung Cancer by Emory and Georgia Tech. [online] OncLive. Available at: http://www.onclive.com/publications/oncology-business-news/2015/september-2015/necitumumab-assigned-low-value-in-lung-cancer-by-emory-and-georgia-tech [Accessed January 4, 2018].

76 Hirsch FR et al. (2016). New and emerging targeted treatments in advanced non–small-cell lung cancer. *Lancet* **388**: 1012–1024.

77 Wu J et al. (2016). Second- and third-generation ALK inhibitors for non-small cell lung cancer. *J Hematol Oncol* **9**: 19.

78 Peters S et al. (2017). Alectinib versus crizotinib in untreated ALK-positive non–small-cell lung cancer. *N Engl J Med* **377**(9):829–838.

79 Lovly C et al. (2015). BRAF in Non-Small Cell Lung Cancer (NSCLC). [online] *My Cancer Genome*. Available at: https://www.mycancergenome.org/content/disease/lung-cancer/braf/ [Accessed January 4, 2018].

80 Planchard D et al. (2016). Dabrafenib plus trametinib in patients with previously treated

BRAF[V600E]-mutant metastatic non-small cell lung cancer: An open-label, multicentre phase 2 trial. *Lancet Oncol* **17**(7): 984–993.

81   ESMO (2017). EMA Recommends Extensions of Indications for Dabrafenib and Trametinib: Combination is indicated for the treatment of adult patients with advanced NSCLC with a BRAF V600 mutation. [Online] European Society for Medical Oncology. Available at: http://www.esmo.org/Oncology-News/EMA-Recommends-Extensions-of-Indications-for-Dabrafenib-and-Trametinib [Accessed January 4, 2018].

82   Middleton G et al. (2015). The National Lung Matrix Trial: Translating the biology of stratification in advanced non–small-cell lung cancer. *Ann Oncol* **26**(12): 2464–2469.

83   Reviewed in: Villaruz LC and Socinski MA (2015). The role of anti-angiogenesis in non–small-cell lung cancer: An update. *Curr Oncol Rep* **17**(6): 26.

84   Raphael J et al. (2017). Antiangiogenic therapy in advanced non–small-cell lung cancer: A meta-analysis of phase III randomized trials. *Clin Lung Can* **18**(4): 345–353.

85   Aggarwal C et al. (2012). Antiangiogenic agents in the management of non-small cell lung cancer: Where do we stand now and where are we headed? *Cancer Biol Ther* **13**(5): 247–263.

86   Seto T et al. (2014). Erlotinib alone or with bevacizumab as first-line therapy in patients with advanced non-squamous non–small-cell lung cancer harbouring EGFR mutations (JO25567): An open-label, randomised, multicentre, phase 2 study. *Lancet Oncol* **15**(11): 1236–1244.

87   Garon EB et al. (2014). Ramucirumab plus docetaxel versus placebo plus docetaxel for second-line treatment of stage IV non–small-cell lung cancer after disease progression on platinum-based therapy (REVEL): A multicentre, double-blind, randomised phase 3 trial. *Lancet* **384**(9944): 665–673.

88   Bronte G et al. (2016). Nintedanib in NSCLC: Evidence to date and place in therapy. *Ther Adv Med Oncol* **8**(3): 188–197.

89   Sundar R et al. (2015). Nivolumab in NSCLC: Latest evidence and clinical potential. *Ther Adv Med Oncol* **7**(2): 85–96.

90   Schvartsman G et al. (2016). Checkpoint inhibitors in lung cancer: Latest developments and clinical potential. *Ther Adv Med Oncol* **8**(6): 460–473.

91   Nishino M et al. (2017). Monitoring immune-checkpoint blockade: Response evaluation and biomarker development. *Nat Rev Clin Oncol* **14**: 655–668.

92   Leventakos K and Mansfield AS (2014). Reflections on immune checkpoint inhibition in non-small cell lung cancer. *Transl Lung Cancer Res* **3**(6): 411–413.

93   Borghaei H et al. (2015). Nivolumab versus docetaxel in advanced nonsquamous non–small-cell lung cancer. *N Engl J Med* **373**: 1627–1639.

94   Reck M et al. (2016). Pembrolizumab versus chemotherapy for PD-L1–positive non–small-cell lung cancer. *N Engl J Med* **375**(19): 1823–1833.

95   Carbone DP et al. (2017). First-line Nivolumab in Stage IV or recurrent non–small-cell lung cancer. *N Engl J Med* **376**: 2415–2426.

96   Kelly K (2016). Immune Checkpoint Inhibitors March to First-Line Treatment in Advanced NSCLC. [online] Asco Post. Available at: http://www.ascopost.com/issues/september-25-2016/immune-checkpoint-inhibitors-march-to-first-line-treatment-in-advanced-nsclc/ [Accessed January 4, 2018].

97   Langer CJ et al. (2016). Carboplatin and pemetrexed with or without pembrolizumab for advanced, non-squamous non–small-cell lung cancer: A randomised, phase 2 cohort of the open-label KEYNOTE-021 study. *Lancet Oncol* **17**(11): 1497–1508.

98   Antonia SJ et al. (2017). Durvalumab after chemoradiotherapy in stage III non–small-cell lung cancer. *N Engl J Med* **377**: 1919–1929.

99   ASCO Post (2017). AACR 2017: 5-Year Survival Rate for Nivolumab-Treated Advanced Lung Cancer Higher Than Historical Rate in Early-Phase Trial. [online] Available at: http://www.ascopost.com/News/55480 [Accessed January 4, 2018].

100 Paglialunga L et al. (2016). Immune checkpoint blockade in small cell lung cancer: Is there a light at the end of the tunnel? *ESMO Open* **1**: e000022.

101 Antonia SJ et al. Nivolumab alone and nivolumab plus ipilimumab in recurrent small-cell lung can-

cer (CheckMate 032): A multicentre, open-label, phase 1/2 trial. *Lancet* **17**(7): 883–895.

102 Ott P et al. (2016). OA05.01. Pembrolizumab in patients with extensive-stage small cell lung cancer: Updated survival results from key-note-028. *J Thoracic Oncol* **12**(1) Suppl, Page S259.

103 Cancer Research UK (2016). Bowel Cancer Incidence Statistics. [online] Available at: http://www.cancerresearchuk.org/health-professional/cancer-statistics/statistics-by-cancer-type/bowel-cancer/incidence#heading-Zero [Accessed January 4, 2018].

104 Spano J-P et al. (2005). Impact of EGFR expression on colorectal cancer patient prognosis and survival. *Ann Oncol* **16**(1): 102–108.

105 Information from: European Medicines Agency: http://www.ema.europa.eu and National Cancer Institute: https://www.cancer.gov/about-cancer/treatment/drugs/lung

106 Muller MF et al. (2016). Molecular pathological classification of colorectal cancer. *Virchows Arch* **469**: 125–134.

107 For a beautiful diagram showing the anatomical distribution of bowel cancers in men and women, see: Cancer Research UK (2015). Bowel Cancer Incidence by Anatomical Site. [online] Available at: http://www.cancerresearchuk.org/health-professional/cancer-statistics/statistics-by-cancer-type/bowel-cancer/incidence#heading-Four [Accessed January 4, 2018].

108 Kim S-E et al. (2015). Sex- and gender-specific disparities in colorectal cancer risk. *World J Gastroenterol* **21**(17): 5167–5175.

109 Dienstmann R et al. (2015). Overcoming resistance to anti-EGFR therapy in colorectal cancer. *Am Soc Clin Oncol Educ Book*. e149–56. doi: 10.14694/EdBook_AM.2015.35.e149.

110 Neumann J et al. (2009). Frequency and type of KRAS mutations in routine diagnostic analysis of metastatic colorectal cancer. *Pathol Res Pract* **205**(12): 858–862.

111 Dienstmann R et al. (2017). Consensus molecular subtypes and the evolution of precision medicine in colorectal cancer. *Nat Rev Cancer* **17**(2): 79–92.

112 De Roock W et al. (2010). Effects of KRAS, BRAF, NRAS, and PIK3CA mutations on the efficacy of cetuximab plus chemotherapy in chemotherapy-refractory metastatic colorectal cancer: A retrospective consortium analysis. *Lancet Oncol* **11**: 753–762.

113 Richman SD et al. (2017). How close are we to standardised extended *RAS* gene mutation testing? The UK NEQAS evaluation. *J Clin Pathol* **70**: 58–62.

114 Holch JW et al. (2017) The relevance of primary tumour location in patients with metastatic colorectal cancer: A meta-analysis of first-line clinical trials. *Eur J Cancer* **70**: 87–98.

115 Sartore-Bianchi A et al. (2016). Dual-targeted therapy with trastuzumab and lapatinib in treatment-refractory, KRAS codon 12/13 wild-type, HER2-positive metastatic colorectal cancer (HERACLES): A proof-of-concept, multicentre, open-label, phase 2 trial. *Lancet* **17**(6): 738–746.

116 Sforza V et al. (2016). Mechanisms of resistance to anti-epidermal growth factor receptor inhibitors in metastatic colorectal cancer. *World J Gastroenterol* **22**(28): 6345–6361.

117 Gong J et al. (2016). RAS and BRAF in metastatic colorectal cancer management. *J Gastrointest Oncol* **7**(5): 687–704.

118 Sanz-Garcia E et al. (2017). BRAF mutant colorectal cancer: Prognosis, treatment, and new perspectives. *Ann Oncol* **28**(11): 2648–2657.

119 Hurwitz H et al. (2004). Bevacizumab plus irinotecan, fluorouracil, and leucovorin for metastatic colorectal cancer. *N Engl J Med* **350**(23): 2335–2342.

120 Richelmann R and Grothey A (2017). Antiangiogenic therapy for refractory colorectal cancer: Current options and future strategies. *Ther Adv Med Oncol* **9**(2): 106–126.

121 Saltz LB et al. (2008). Bevacizumab in combination with oxaliplatin-based chemotherapy as first-line therapy in metastatic colorectal cancer: A randomized phase III study. *J Clin Oncol* **26**(12): 2013–2019.

122 Van Cutsem E et al. (2012). Addition of aflibercept to fluorouracil, leucovorin, and irinotecan improves survival in a phase III randomized trial in patients with metastatic colorectal cancer previously treated with an oxaliplatin-based regimen. *J Clin Oncol* **30**: 3499–3506.

123 Tabernero J et al. (2015). Ramucirumab *versus* placebo in combination with second-line FOLFIRI in patients with metastatic colorectal

carcinoma that progressed during or after first-line therapy with bevacizumab, oxaliplatin, and a fluoropyrimidine (RAISE): A randomised, double-blind, multicentre, phase III study. *Lancet Oncol* **16**: 499–508.

124 Grothey A et al. (2013). Regorafenib monotherapy for previously treated metastatic colorectal cancer (CORRECT): An international, multicentre, randomised, placebo-controlled, phase 3 trial. *Lancet* **381**(9863): 303–312.

125 For a discussion about this, see: Venook AP (2015). Bevacizumab vs EGFR antibodies in metastatic colorectal cancer. *Clin Adv Hematol Oncol* **13**(2): 90–92.

126 Le DT et al. (2015). PD-1 blockade in tumors with mismatch-repair deficiency. *N Engl J Med* **372**: 2509–2520.

127 Boland CR and Goel A (2010). Microsatellite instability in colorectal cancer. *Gastroenterology* **138**(6): 2073–2087.

128 Passardi A et al. (2017) Immune checkpoints as a target for colorectal cancer treatment. *Int J Mol Sci* **18**(6): 1324.

129 Overman MJ et al. (2017). Nivolumab in patients with metastatic DNA mismatch repair-deficient or microsatellite instability-high colorectal cancer (CheckMate 142): An open-label, multicentre, phase 2 study. *Lancet Oncol* **18**(9): 1182–1191.

130 U.S. Food and Drug Administration (2017). FDA approves first cancer treatment for any solid tumor with a specific genetic feature. [online] Available at: www.fda.gov/newsevents/newsroom/pressannouncements/ucm560167.htm [Accessed December 29, 2017].

131 Goldstein J et al. (2014). Multicenter retrospective analysis of metastatic colorectal cancer (CRC) with high-level microsatellite instability (MSI-H). *Ann Oncol* **25**(5): 1032–1038.

132 Bendell JC (2016). Clinical activity and safety of cobimetinib (cobi) and atezolizumab in colorectal cancer (CRC). *J Clin Oncol* **34**; suppl; abstract 3502.

133 Adams R et al. (2016). FOCUS4-D: Results from a Randomised, Placebo Controlled Trial of AZD8931 (An Inhibitor of Signalling by HER1, 2, and 3) in Patients with Advanced or Metastatic Colorectal Cancer in Tumours That Are Wildtype for BRAF, PIK3CA, KRAS & NRAS. www.

focus4trial [online] Available at: www.focus4trial.org/NCRI_2016_Poster_FOCUS4-D_v1.0.pdf [Accessed December 29, 2017].

134 Cancer Research UK. (2016). Skin Cancer Statistics. [online] Available at: http://www.cancerresearchuk.org/health-professional/cancer-statistics/statistics-by-cancer-type/skin-cancer [Accessed December 29, 2017].

135 Cancer Research UK. (2016). Skin Cancer Survival Statistics. [online] Available at: http://www.cancerresearchuk.org/health-professional/cancer-statistics/statistics-by-cancer-type/skin-cancer/survival#heading-Three [Accessed December 29, 2017].

136 COSMIC; Catalogue of Somatic Mutations in Cancer. http://cancer.sanger.ac.uk/cosmic/

137 Holderfield M et al. (2015). Targeting RAF kinases for cancer therapy: BRAF mutated melanoma and beyond. *Nat Rev Cancer* **14**(7): 455–467.

138 Shain AH et al. (2015). The genetic evolution of melanoma from precursor lesions. *N Engl J Med* **373**: 1926–1936.

139 Shain AH and Bastian BC (2016). From melanocytes to melanomas. *Nat Rev Cancer* **16**: 345–358.

140 Information from: European Medicines Agency: http://www.ema.europa.eu and National Cancer Institute: https://www.cancer.gov/about-cancer/treatment/drugs/lung

141 Holderfield M et al. (2014). Mechanism and consequences of RAF kinase activation by small-molecule inhibitors. *Br J Cancer* **111**: 640–645.

142 Medina TM & Lewis KD (2016). The evolution of combined molecular targeted therapies to advance the therapeutic efficacy in melanoma: A highlight of vemurafenib and cobimetinib. *Onco Targets Ther* **9**: 3739–3752.

143 Reviewed in Eroglu Z and Ribas A (2016). Combination therapy with BRAF and MEK inhibitors for melanoma: Latest evidence and place in therapy. *Ther Adv Med Oncol* **8**(1): 48–56.

144 Kemper K et al. (2015). Intra- and inter-tumor heterogeneity in a vemurafenib-resistant melanoma patient and derived xenografts. *EMBO Mol Med* **7**(9): 1104–1118.

145 Kim S-E et al. (2015). Sex- and gender-specific disparities in colorectal cancer risk. *World J Gastroenterol* **21**(17): 5167–5175.

146 Samatar AA and Poulikakos (2014). Targeting RAS–ERK signalling in cancer: Promises and challenges. *Nat Rev Drug Discov* **13**(12): 928–942.

147 Haanen JBAG (2013). Immunotherapy of melanoma. *EJC Suppl* **11**(2): 97–105.

148 Flaherty KT (2015). Gauging the long-term benefits of ipilimumab in melanoma. *J Clin Oncol* **33**(17): 1865–1866.

149 Johnson DB et al. (2015). Nivolumab in melanoma: Latest evidence and clinical potential. *Ther Adv Med Oncol* **7**(2): 97–106.

150 Daud AI et al. (2016). Programmed death-ligand 1 expression and response to the anti-programmed death 1 antibody pembrolizumab in melanoma. *J Clin Oncol* **34**(34): 4102–4109.

151 Larkin J et al. (2015). Combined nivolumab and ipilimumab or monotherapy in untreated melanoma. *N Engl J Med* **373**: 23–34.

152 OncLive website (2017). Nivolumab/ Ipilimumab Combo Shows Modest OS Benefit in Advanced Melanoma in Updated Phase III Findings. [online] Available at: www.onclive.com/conference-coverage/aacr-2017/nivolumabipilimumab-combo-shows-modest-os-benefit-in-advanced-melanoma-in-updated-phase-iii-findings?p=1 [Accessed December 29, 2017].

153 Franklin C et al. (2016). Immunotherapy in melanoma: Recent advances and future directions. *Eur J Surg Oncol* 2016 Sep 2. pii: S0748-7983(16)30866-6.

154 Schadendorf D et al. (2015) Pooled analysis of long-term survival data from phase II and phase III trials of ipilimumab in unresectable or metastatic melanoma. *J Clin Oncol* **33**(17): 1889–1894.

155 NHS Choices (September 2013). More Data on Survival with New Skin Cancer Drug. [online] Available at: http://www.nhs.uk/news/2013/09September/Pages/More-data-on-survival-with-new-skin-cancer-drug.aspx [Accessed January 4, 2018].

156 Andtbacka RH et al. (2015). Talimogene laherparepvec improves durable response rate in patients with advanced melanoma. *J Clin Oncol* **33**(25): 2780–2788.

157 Cancer Research UK (2016). Kidney Cancer Incidence Statistics. [online] Available at: http://www.cancerresearchuk.org/health-professional/cancer-statistics/statistics-by-cancer-type/kidney-cancer#heading-Zero [Accessed January 4, 2018].

158 Cancer Research UK (2016). Kidney Cancer Risk Factors. [online] Available at: http://www.cancerresearchuk.org/health-professional/cancer-statistics/statistics-by-cancer-type/kidney-cancer/risk-factors [Accessed January 4, 2018].

159 Cancer Research UK (2016). Kidney Cancer: Types and Grades. [online] Available at: http://www.cancerresearchuk.org/about-cancer/kidney-cancer/stages-types-grades/types-grades [Accessed January 4, 2018].

160 Jayson GC et al. (2016). Antiangiogenic therapy in oncology: Current status and future directions. *Lancet* **388**: 518–529.

161 Semenza GL (2003). Targeting HIF-1 for cancer therapy. *Nat Rev Cancer* **3**: 721–732.

162 Stukalin I et al. (2016). Contemporary treatment of metastatic renal cell carcinoma. *Onc Rev* **10**: 295.

163 Zarrabi K et al. (2017). New treatment options for metastatic renal cell carcinoma with prior antiangiogenesis therapy. *J Hematol Oncol* **10**: 38.

164 NCI Drug Dictionary: https://www.cancer.gov/publications/dictionaries/cancer-drug

165 Stukalin I et al. (2016). Contemporary treatment of metastatic renal cell carcinoma. *Onc Rev* **10**: 295.

166 Minguet J et al. (2015). Targeted therapies for treatment of renal cell carcinoma: Recent advances and future perspectives. *Cancer Chemother Pharmacol* **76**: 219–233.

167 Rini BI et al. (2011) Comparative effectiveness of axitinib versus sorafenib in advanced renal cell carcinoma (AXIS): A randomised phase 3 trial. *Lancet* **378**: 1931–1939.

168 Motzer RJ et al. (2015). Lenvatinib, everolimus, and the combination in patients with metastatic renal cell carcinoma: A randomised, phase 2, open-label, multicentre trial. *Lancet Oncol* **16**(5): 1473–1482.

169 Choueiri TK et al. (2015). Cabozantinib versus everolimus in advanced renal-cell carcinoma. *N Engl J Med* **373**:1814–1823.

170 Motzer RJ et al. (2015). Nivolumab versus everolimus in advanced renal-cell carcinoma. *N Engl J Med* **373**: 1803–1813.

171 Davenport L (2016). Cabozantinib Could Be First-Line Choice in Advanced RCC. Medscape. [online] Available at: http://www.medscape.com/viewarticle/870077 [Accessed January 4, 2018].

172 Karar J and Maity A (2011). PI3K/AKT/mTOR pathway in angiogenesis. *Front Mol Neurosci* **4**: 51.

173 Raman R and Vaena D (2015). Immunotherapy in metastatic renal cell carcinoma: A comprehensive review. *Biomed Res Int* **2015**: 367354.

174 Motzer RJ et al. (2015). Nivolumab versus everolimus in advanced renal-cell carcinoma. *N Engl J Med* **373**: 1803–1813.

175 Wallin JJ et al. (2016). Atezolizumab in combination with bevacizumab enhances antigen-specific T-cell migration in metastatic renal cell carcinoma. *Nat Commun* **7**: 12624.

176 Reviewed in: Greef B and Eisen T (2016). Medical treatment of renal cancer: New horizons. *Br J Cancer* **115**(5): 505–516.

177 Agarwal N (2016). Vaccine Therapy in Metastatic Renal Cell Carcinoma: Past, Present, and Future. The Asco Post [Online] Available at: www.ascopost.com/issues/november-25-2016/vaccine-therapy-in-metastatic-renal-cell-carcinoma-past-present-and-future/ [Accessed January 4, 2018].

178 OncLive website (2017). Longer Follow-Up Shows Survival Increase With Rocapuldencel-T in mRCC. [Online] Available at: http://www.onclive.com/web-exclusives/longer-followup-shows-survival-increase-with-rocapuldencelt-in-mrcc [Accessed March 3, 2018].

179 Cancer Research UK. (2016). Oral Cancer Incidence. [online] Available at: http://www.cancerresearchuk.org/health-professional/cancer-statistics/statistics-by-cancer-type/oral-cancer#heading-Zero [Accessed January 4, 2018].

180 For more information on head and neck cancers and a diagram showing where they can arise, see: National Cancer Institute (2013). Head and Neck Cancers. [online] https://www.cancer.gov/types/head-and-neck/head-neck-fact-sheet [Accessed January 4, 2018].

181 Cancer Research UK. (2016). Oral Cancer Risk Factors. [online] Available at: http://www.cancerresearchuk.org/health-professional/cancer-statistics/statistics-by-cancer-type/oral-cancer/risk-factors#heading-Eleven [Accessed January 4, 2018].

182 Dok R and Nuyts S (2016). HPV positive head and neck cancers: Molecular pathogenesis and evolving treatment strategies. *Cancers* **8**: 41.

183 Kang H et al. (2015). Emerging biomarkers in head and neck cancer in the era of genomics. *Nat Rev Clin Oncol* **12**: 11–26.

184 Sacco AG and Worden FP (2016). Molecularly targeted therapy for the treatment of head and neck cancer: A review of the ErbB family inhibitors. *Onco Targets Ther* **9**: 1927–1943.

185 For a summary of trials, see: Machiels J-P and Schmitz S (2015). Epidermal growth factor receptor inhibition in squamous cell carcinoma of the head and neck. *Hematol Oncol Clin North Am* **29**(6): 1011–1032.

186 Vemorken JB et al. (2008). Platinum-based chemotherapy plus cetuximab in head and neck cancer. *N Engl J Med* **359**: 1116–1127.

187 Echarri MJ et al. (2016). Targeted therapy in locally advanced and recurrent/metastatic head and neck squamous cell carcinoma (LA-R/M HNSCC). *Cancers* **8**: 27.

188 Braig F et al. (2016). Liquid biopsy monitoring uncovers acquired RAS-mediated resistance to cetuximab in a substantial proportion of patients with head and neck squamous cell carcinoma. *Oncotarget* **7**(28): 42988–42995.

189 Ferris RL (2015). Immunology and immunotherapy of head and neck cancer. *J Clin Oncol* **33**(29): 3293–3304.

190 Ferris RL et al. (2016). Nivolumab for Recurrent squamous-cell carcinoma of the head and neck. *N Engl J Med* **375**: 1856–1867.

191 For a discussion of the results, see: Goodman A (2016). Nivolumab: New Standard of Care for Progressive Head and Neck Cancer After Platinum Therapy. ASCO Post. [online] Available at: http://www.ascopost.com/issues/may-10-2016/nivolumab-new-standard-of-care-for-progressive-head-and-neck-cancer-after-platinum-therapy/ [Accessed January 4, 2018].

192 Algazi AP and Grandis JR (2017). Head and neck cancer in 2016: A watershed year for improvements in treatment? *Nat Rev Clin Oncol* **14**: 76–78.

193 ESMO (2017). ESMO 2017 Press Release: KEYNOTE-040 Evaluates Pembrolizumab in Head and Neck Cancer. [online] Available at: http://www.esmo.org/Press-Office/Press-Releases/KEYNOTE-040-Evaluates-Pembrolizumab-in-Head-and-Neck-Cancer [accessed December 29, 2017].

194 Bann DV et al. (2015). Novel immunotherapeutic approaches for head and neck squamous cell carcinoma. *Cancers* **8**: 87.

195 Cancer Research UK. (2015). Brain, Other CNS and Intracranial Tumours Incidence Statistics [online] Available at: http://www.cancerresearchuk.org/health-professional/cancer-statistics/statistics-by-cancer-type/brain-other-cns-and-intracranial-tumours/incidence#heading-Four [Accessed January 4, 2018].

196 Purves D et al. (2001). Neuroglial cells. In: Neuroscience. 2nd edition. Sunderland (MA). Sinauer Associates. Available at: https://www.ncbi.nlm.nih.gov/books/NBK10869/ [Accessed January 4, 2018].

197 Tanaka S et al. (2013). Diagnostic and therapeutic avenues for glioblastoma: No longer a dead end? *Nat Rev Clin Oncol* **10**: 14–26.

198 Wick W et al. (2016). EORTC 26101 phase III trial exploring the combination of bevacizumab and lomustine in patients with first progression of a glioblastoma. *J Clin Oncol* **34**: 2016 (suppl; abstr 2001).

199 Cancer Genome Atlas Research Network(2008). Comprehensive genomic characterization defines human glioblastoma genes and core pathways. *Nature* **455**: 1061–1068.

200 Padfield E et al. (2015). Current therapeutic advances targeting EGFR and EGFRvIII in glioblastoma. *Front Oncol* **5**: 5.

201 Polivka J et al. (2017). Advances in experimental targeted therapy and immunotherapy for patients with glioblastoma multiforme. *Anticancer Res* **37**: 21–34.

202 For an overview, see: Lim M et al. (2016). Current state of immune-based therapies for glioblastoma. *Am Soc Clin Oncol Educ Book* **35**: e132–139.

203 Dunn-Pirio AM and Vlahovic G (2017). Immunotherapy approaches in the treatment of malignant brain tumors. *Cancer* **123**: 734–750.

204 Northwest Biotherapeutics. DCVax® Technology. [online] Available at: https://www.nwbio.com/dcvax-technology/ [Accessed January 4, 2018].

205 Targeted Oncology (2017). Engineering Chimeric Antigen Receptor T Cells to Treat Glioblastoma. [online] Available at: http://www.targetedonc.com/publications/targeted-therapies-cancer/2017/2017-august/engineering-chimeric-antigen-receptor-t-cells-to-treat-glioblastoma [Accessed January 3, 2018]

206 Cancer Research UK. (2016). Bladder Cancer Incidence. [online] Available at: http://www.cancerresearchuk.org/health-professional/cancer-statistics/statistics-by-cancer-type/bladder-cancer#heading-Zero [Accessed January 4, 2018].

207 Wu X-R (2005). Urothelial tumorigenesis: A tale of divergent pathways. *Nat Rev Cancer* **5**: 713–725.

208 Van Batavia J et al. (2014). Bladder cancers arise from distinct urothelial sub-populations. *Nature Cell Biol* **16**: 982–991.

209 Dancik GM et al. (2014). A cell of origin gene signature indicates human bladder cancer has distinct cellular progenitors. *Stem Cells* **32**(4): 974–982.

210 Van Batavia J et al. (2014). Bladder cancers arise from distinct urothelial sub-populations. *Nature Cell Biol* **16**: 982–991.

211 Li R et al. (2016). New discoveries in the molecular landscape of bladder cancer. *F1000Research* **5**: 2875.

212 Redelman-Sidi G et al. (2014) The mechanism of action of BCG therapy for bladder cancer – a current perspective. *Nature Rev Urol* **11**: 153–162.

213 Sharma P et al. (2017). Nivolumab in metastatic urothelial carcinoma after platinum therapy (CheckMate 275): A multicentre, single-arm, phase 2 trial. *Lancet Oncol* **18**(3): 312–322.

214 Bellmunt J et al. (2017). Pembrolizumab as second-line therapy for advanced urothelial carcinoma. *N Engl J Med* **376**: 1015–1026.

215 Bavencio (avelumab) injection prescribing information, EMD Serono, Inc, May 2017. [online] Available at https://www.accessdata.fda.gov/drugsatfda_docs/label/2017/761078s000lbl.pdf [Accessed January 3, 2018].

216 Powles T et al. (2017). Updated efficacy and tolerability of durvalumab in locally advanced or metastatic urothelial carcinoma. *J Clin Oncol* **35**(Suppl 6S; abstract 286).

217 Rosenberg JE at al. (2016). Atezolizumab in patients with locally advanced and metastatic urothelial carcinoma who have progressed following treatment with platinum-based chemotherapy: A single-arm, multicentre, phase 2 trial. *Lancet* **387**(10031): 1909–1920.

218 Powles T et al. (2017). Atezolizumab versus chemotherapy in patients with platinum-treated locally advanced or metastatic urothelial carcinoma (IMvigor211): A multicentre, open-label, phase 3 randomised controlled trial. *Lancet* 2017 Dec 18. pii: S0140-6736(17)33297-X [Epub ahead of print].

219 Massari F and Di Nunno V (2017). Atezolizumab for platinum-treated metastatic urothelial carcinoma. *Lancet* 2017 Dec 18. pii: S0140-6736(17)33298-1 [Epub ahead of print].

220 The Cancer Genome Atlas Network (2014). Comprehensive molecular characterization of urothelial bladder carcinoma. *Nature* **507**: 315–322.

221 Cheetham PJ and Petrylak DP (2016). New agents for the treatment of advanced bladder cancer. *Oncology* **30**(6): 571–579.

222 Narayanan S and Srinivas S (2017). Incorporating VEGF-targeted therapy in advanced urothelial cancer. *Ther Adv Med Oncol* **9**(1): 33–45.

223 Research UK. (2016). Pancreatic cancer statistics. [online] Available at: http://www.cancerresearchuk.org/health-professional/cancer-statistics/statistics-by-cancer-type/pancreatic-cancer [Accessed January 4, 2018].

224 Research UK. (2014). Pancreatic Cancer Survival Statistics. [online] Available at: http://www.cancerresearchuk.org/health-professional/cancer-statistics/statistics-by-cancer-type/pancreatic-cancer/survival#heading-Zero [Accessed January 4, 2018].

225 Kopp JL et al. (2012). Identification of Sox9-dependent acinar-to-ductal reprogramming as the principal mechanism for initiation of pancreatic ductal adenocarcinoma. *Cancer Cell* **22**(6): 737–750.

226 Bardeesy N and DePinho RA (2002). Pancreatic cancer biology and genetics. *Nat Rev Cancer* **2**: 897–909.

227 Jones S et al. (2008). Core signaling pathways in human pancreatic cancers revealed by global genomic analyses. *Science* **321**(5897): 1801–1806.

228 von Ahrens D et al. (2017). The role of stromal cancer-associated fibroblasts in pancreatic cancer. *J Hematol Oncol* **10**: 76.

229 Feig et al. (2012). The pancreas cancer microenvironment. *Clin Cancer Res* **18**: 4266–4276.

230 Karandish F and Malik S (2016). Biomarkers and targeted therapy in pancreatic cancer. *Biomark Cancer* **8**(Suppl 1): 27–35.

231 Moore MJ et al. (2007). Erlotinib plus gemcitabine compared with gemcitabine alone in patients with advanced pancreatic cancer: A phase III trial of the National Cancer Institute of Canada Clinical Trials Group. *J Clin Oncol* **25**: 1960–1966.

232 For some examples of negative trials, see Paez D et al. (2012). Pancreatic cancer: Medical management (novel chemotherapeutics). *Gastroenterol Clin N Am* **41**: 189–209.

233 Paal K et al. (2001). High affinity binding of paclitaxel to human serum albumin. *FEBS J* **268**(7): 2187–2191.

234 Miele E et al. (2009). Albumin-bound formulation of paclitaxel (Abraxane®ABI-007) in the treatment of breast cancer. *Int J Nanomedicine* **4**: 99–105.

235 Von Hoff DD et al. (2013). Increased survival in pancreatic cancer with nab-paclitaxel plus gemcitabine. *N Engl J Med* **369**(18): 1691–1703.

236 Adiseshaiah PP et al. (2016). Nanomedicine strategies to overcome the pathophysiological barriers of pancreatic cancer. *Nat Rev Clin Oncol* **13**: 750–765.

237 Murphy KM et al. (2002). Evaluation of candidate genes MAP2K4, MADH4, ACVR1B, and BRCA2 in familial pancreatic cancer: Deleterious BRCA2 mutations in 17%. *Cancer Res* **62**: 3789–3793.

238 Kaufman B et al. (2015). Olaparib monotherapy in patients with advanced cancer and a germline BRCA1/2 mutation. *J Clin Oncol.* **33**(3): 244–250.

239 Chang JH et al. Role of immune cells in pancreatic cancer from bench to clinical application. *Medicine (Baltimore)* **95**(49): e5541.

240 For a discussion on the future of immunotherapy for pancreatic cancer see: OncLive (2016). Immunotherapy in Pancreatic Cancer. [online] Available at: http://www.onclive.com/insights-archive/pancreatic-cancer-outcomes/immunotherapy-in-pancreatic-cancer [Accessed January 3, 2018].

241 Lupinacci RM et al. (2018). Prevalence of microsatellite instability in intraductal papillary mucinous neoplasms of the pancreas. *Gastroenterology* **154**(4): 1061–1065.

242 Le DT et al. (2017). Mismatch-repair deficiency predicts response of solid tumors to PD-1 blockade. *Science* **357**(6349): 409–413.

CHAPTER 7

Targeted Treatments for Hematological Cancers

IN BRIEF

The treatment of hematological cancers is changing rapidly due to the creation of new monoclonal antibody treatments, new kinase inhibitors, and other innovative treatment approaches.

As with targeted treatments for solid tumors, in order to understand the treatments being developed for hematological cancers, it's important to know a bit about the proteins found on the surface of the cancer cells, how the cells communicate, and what gene defects drive their behavior.

Some of the treatments described in this chapter have been in use for over twenty years, such as Bcr-Abl inhibitors for chronic myeloid leukemia, and CD20 targeted antibodies for B-cell non-Hodgkin lymphoma and chronic lymphocytic leukemia. Some of the treatments for these cancers are more targeted than others. For example, treatments like BTK (Bruton's tyrosine kinase) inhibitors impact a single pathway and have a clearly defined mechanism; whereas others, such as proteasome inhibitors and thalidomide derivates, have many mechanisms of action. With some of the treatments, we still don't entirely know why they work (e.g., thalidomide), why not everyone benefits from them (e.g., PI3Kδ inhibitors), or whether they will prove sufficiently beneficial to become licensed treatments (e.g., KIT inhibitors).

As in other chapters, I have focused on treatments that are already licensed for use in Europe and the United States, or that are likely to be licensed in the coming months.

7.1 INTRODUCTION

In this chapter, I will be dealing with drugs that are currently exclusively (or almost exclusively) used to treat hematological cancers (primarily leukemias, lymphomas, and multiple myeloma[1]). I will focus on treatments that are either already licensed in Europe and/or the United States, or that are close to becoming so.

---

[1] There are other blood cancers. There are also blood disorders that behave a bit like cancer and that sometimes become cancer. I don't have room for everything, so I'm just going to focus on treatments for leukemias, lymphomas, and multiple myeloma.

A Beginner's Guide to Targeted Cancer Treatments, First Edition. Elaine Vickers.
© 2018 John Wiley & Sons Ltd. Published 2018 by John Wiley & Sons Ltd.

In order to explain targeted treatments for cancers that develop from white blood cells, I do need to go into a bit of detail about the immune system. But I will be selective and, as ever, there will be a lot of things that I will leave out because they're not relevant to the targeted treatment approaches I'm going to describe. However, in order to explain the treatments that do now exist, I need to mention various immunology concepts such as **B cell activation, cell communication**, and a variety of **CD antigens.**

As with Chapter 5, you might find it helpful to learn a bit about the immune system before reading this chapter. Or you might wish to have a textbook to hand while you read. If so, I highly recommend *How the Immune System Works* by Lauren Sompayrac [1]. If you'd like more detail, an undergraduate textbook such as *Janeway's Immunobiology* [2] would be ideal.

As in chapter 6, I include in this chapter brief results from a selection of clinical trials. However, I'm giving you this information purely to give you a flavor of the degree of benefit that each treatment is able to bring. And I don't attempt to cover all the treatment options and combinations that are used to treat the many different hematological cancers. Instead, I go through each type of treatment in turn, and provide brief details as to which cancers the treatments are most relevant for.

7.2 A BIT ABOUT HEMATOLOGICAL CANCERS

Hematological cancers are all caused by **faulty mature or immature white blood cells or hematopoietic stem cells**[2] (see Figure 7.1 [3–6]). The type of cancer the faulty white

blood cell causes, and how it behaves and responds to treatment, depends on factors like:

- How **mature or immature** the cell was when it went wrong
- What **combination of mutations** or other faults the cell contains
- **Where it was** when it went wrong (e.g., the bone marrow or a lymph node)
- Whether it was **in the process of responding** to an infection when it went wrong
- Whether it had responded to an infection **in the past**
- Whether the infection the cell had responded to **is still around** (e.g., most MALT lymphomas are linked to an ongoing *H. pylori* infection [7])

For example, a very immature white blood cell that has just begun to specialize to become a myeloid cell[3] might give rise to acute myeloid leukemia; whereas if a fully mature B lymphocyte (B cell) living in a lymph node goes wrong, it's likely to cause a non-Hodgkin lymphoma.

As you might imagine, there are lots of different types of hematological cancer. For a quick summary of some of the most important types, see Table 7.1.

As well as being derived from white blood cells and hematopoietic stem cells, hematological cancers have other important characteristics. I've listed a few of these below as they will hopefully help you make sense of the treatments that have been developed.

7.2.1 Most of Them Are Derived from B Cells

As you can see from Table 7.2, the majority of leukemias, lymphomas, and other blood cancers diagnosed in the United Kingdom

---

[2] Hematopoietic stem cells live in our bone marrow, where they make all our red blood cells (erythrocytes) and white blood cells (leukocytes).

[3] Myeloid cells include macrophages, neutrophils, basophils, mast cells, eosinophils, erythroblasts, and megakaryocytes (basically, almost anything that isn't a B cell or a T cell).

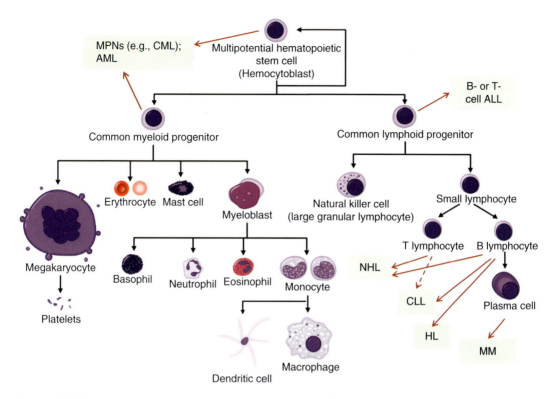

Figure 7.1 Diagram of hematopoiesis showing the cell of origin of common hematological cancers. Stem cells create progenitor cells that gradually specialize and become mature myeloid or lymphoid white blood cells. If a stem cell or immature myeloid progenitor cell goes wrong, this may cause a myeloproliferative neoplasm (MPN) such as chronic myeloid leukemia (CML), or it could cause acute myeloid leukemia (AML). If an immature lymphocyte goes wrong, this may lead to a B cell or T cell acute lymphoblastic leukemia (B cell or T cell ALL). Mature T cells rarely lead to cancer; in the rare cases when this happens, they may cause one of various types of T cell non-Hodgkin lymphoma (T cell NHL). Mature B cells are the cell of origin of the vast majority of chronic lymphocytic leukemias (CLL); they also cause B cell non-Hodgkin lymphomas (NHL) and Hodgkin lymphoma (HL). When B cells are releasing antibodies to fight an infection, they are known as plasma cells. Multiple myeloma (MM) is a cancer of plasma cells. Original figure taken from Wikipedia: https://en.wikipedia.org/wiki/Haematopoiesis#/media/ File:Hematopoiesis_simple.svg

are of **B cell origin**. Only a minority are T cell cancers or cancers derived from myeloid cells.

B cells seem to be more prone to going wrong than other white blood cells for a couple of reasons. First, because of the processes they go through in order to mature and become a fully functional B cell. And second, because of the activation steps they go through when they've recognized an infection and want to fight it off by producing antibodies. **As they mature in the bone marrow, B cells deliberately cut up and rejoin various segments of antibody genes** to create a complete antibody gene (a process called VDJ recombination). And then **when they react to an infection, they cut up, rejoin, and mutate their antibody genes** to change what type of antibody they make and to improve the interaction between their

Table 7.1 Summary of some of the most common hematological cancers diagnosed in the United Kingdom.

Disease	Features [8, 9]
Acute myeloid leukemia (AML)	
Who gets it	• It accounts for about 15% of childhood leukemias, but it's most common in people over 65 years of age.
Behavior	• Aggressive.*
Location	• Cancer cells are made in the bone marrow and enter the blood.
Cell features	• Cancer cells commonly contain mutations in two growth factor receptors (FLT3 and KIT) [10]. • Cancer cells commonly have CD33 and CD123 on their surface [11].
Five-year survival	• Five-year survival rates are much better in children under 14 years (around 65%) than in adults over 65 years (around 5%).
Acute lymphoblastic leukemia (ALL)	
Who gets it	• It's the most common leukemia in children. • The most common age at diagnosis is between 0 and 4 years old.
Behavior	• Aggressive.*
Location	• Cancer cells are made in the bone marrow and enter the blood.
Cell features	• Cancer cells often contain >50 chromosomes. • 75% develop from faulty B cells and have CD19, CD20, and CD22 on their surface [12].
Five-year survival	• Five-year survival rates are much better in children under 14 years (around 90%) than in adults over 65 years (around 15%).
Chronic myeloid leukemia (CML)	
Who gets it	• Risk increases very gradually with age; around 48% of cases are diagnosed in people of age 65 and over.
Behavior	• Indolent.*
Location	• Cancer cells are made in the bone marrow and enter the blood.
Cell features	• Cancer cells usually contain a fusion protein called Bcr-Abl due to a translocation between chromosomes 9 and 22 (see Section 7.5) .
Five-year survival	• Due to the creation of Bcr-Abl inhibitors, the life expectancy of people with CML is now approaching that of the general population [13].
Chronic lymphocytic leukemia (CLL)	
Who gets it	• Risk of CLL increases rapidly from around the age of 45–49; around 60% of cases are diagnosed in people over 70 years.
Behavior	• Indolent.*
Location	• Cancer cells are made in the bone marrow and enter the blood, but they can also build up in the lymph nodes and spleen. • This disease is the same thing as "small lymphocytic lymphoma" – doctors use this name if some of the cancer cells are found in lymph nodes.
Cell features	• Surface proteins include CD20 and CD19. • Up to 80% contain characteristic chromosomal abnormalities such as 13q14 deletion, trisomy 12, 11q23 deletion, or 17p13 deletion. • 11q23 and 17p13 deletions are associated with aggressive disease and shorter survival times [14]; 17p13 is the location on chromosome 17 where the *TP53* gene is found. • CLL can be split into two groups depending on whether the cancer cell have unmutated or mutated antibody genes; those with unmutated genes are generally more aggressive [15].
Five-year survival	• Five-year survival rates are around 70% for men and 75% for women.

Table 7.1   (Continued)

Non-Hodgkin lymphoma (NHL)

- There are over 60 different types of NHL.
- These cancers develop in the lymph nodes or other lymph tissues; they can therefore occur pretty much anywhere in the body.
- Surface proteins include CD20 and CD19.

- **Follicular lymphoma**
  - Indolent.*
  - Generally occurs in adults over 50 years.
  - Five-year survival is around 87%.
  - Cancer cells almost always contain a particular translocation: t(14;18)(q32;q21).

- **Mantle cell lymphoma**
  - Has features of both indolent* and aggressive* lymphomas.
  - Mostly affects men over 50 years.
  - Five-year survival is around 40%.

- **Diffuse large B cell lymphoma**
  - Aggressive.*
  - There are two main sub-types: germinal center B cell-like (GCB) and activated B cell-like (ABC).
  - The most common age to be diagnosed is around 60.
  - Five-year survival is around 60%.

- **Marginal zone lymphomas**
  - This is a group of slow-growing NHLs.
  - Five-year survival is around 78%.
  - One type of marginal zone lymphoma, called MALT lymphomas, are commonly associated with chronic infection with a bacterium or virus such as helicobacter pylori or hepatitis C virus (MALT lymphoma = mucosa-associated lymphoid tissue lymphoma); these lymphomas commonly start in the stomach.

- **Burkitt's lymphoma**
  - Aggressive.*
  - Mostly occur in children and young adults.
  - They sometimes occur in people with a compromised immune system, such as transplant patients and people with HIV/AIDS.
  - Five-year survival is around 56%.

- **T cell lymphomas**
  - Aggressive.*
  - A group of different lymphomas that develop from T cells (all the others mentioned develop from B cells).
  - Five-year survival is around 48%.

Hodgkin lymphoma

Who gets it	• It is most commonly diagnosed in 20- to 24-year-olds or in those over 70.
Behavior	• Aggressive.*
Location	• The cancer cells develop in the lymph nodes; it can start in any of the lymph nodes in the body.
Cell features	• Cancer cells of the most common type of Hodgkin lymphoma, classical Hodgkin lymphoma, are called Reed Sternberg (RS) cells. • RS cells only comprise about 1% of the cells in Hodgkin lymphoma; the other cells are lymphocytes such as regulatory T cells [16]. • RS cells have proteins such CD30, CD15, CD40, CD80, and CD25 on their surface [17].
Five-year survival	• Five-year survival is about 90% but decreases with age.

(Continued)

Table 7.1 (Continued)

Disease	Features [8, 9]
Multiple Myeloma	
Who gets it	• Risk increases rapidly from around the age of 55–59.
Behavior	• Usually preceded by a condition called Monoclonal Gammopathy of Undetermined Significance (MGUS) which doesn't normally cause symptoms. • 1% of MGUS become multiple myeloma each year [18].
Location	• Develop from plasma cells in the bone marrow (bone marrow is found inside many of the larger bones in our body).
Cell features	• Cancer cells commonly have proteins such as CS1/SLAMF7, CD38, CD40, and HM1.24 on their surface [18]. • Multiple myeloma cells produce vast quantities of a single antibody; this antibody isn't helpful and can't fight infections.
Five-year survival	• Five-year survival is about 50%.
Myeloproliferative neoplasms (MPNs)	

	• These are a group of disorders that develop from faulty immature myeloid white blood cells in the bone marrow (they technically include chronic myeloid leukemia – CML).
	 • The most common types (other than CML) are:
	   • Polycythemia vera (PV)
	   • Essential thrombocythemia (ET)
	   • Myelofibrosis (MF)
	 • Doctors debate over whether these conditions are cancers or not.

Behavior	• They are usually very slow growing.
Who gets them	• Most people who develop MPNs are over 60 years.
Cell features	• The faulty cells often contain mutations in the JAK2 gene.
Five-year survival	• Five-year survival varies from 93% (for PV and ET) to 41% for MF.

*Aggressive cancers are fast growing and would cause death quickly if left untreated. Indolent cancers (also described as low-grade or chronic) tend to develop very slowly. A person may have a chronic leukemia or indolent lymphoma for months or years without having many symptoms. And it may be many months or years before their disease gets worse and needs aggressive treatment.

antibody and its target. These processes are called **class switching** and **somatic hyper-mutation**[4] (the life of a B cell is summarized in Figure 7.2). Not surprisingly, if the B cell doesn't perform these processes 100% accurately, it may accidently cut and mutate its DNA in ways that ultimately cause it to become a cancer cell [6].

By the way, when we talk about a person's CLL having mutated or unmutated antibody genes, we're describing whether or not the B cell had already responded to an infection at the point it became a cancer cell. CLLs with **mutated** antibody genes are those derived from cells that have responded to an infection, and that have gone through the processes of

---

[4] If you want to learn more about these processes, I would suggest looking it up in an immunology textbook, as I don't want to go into it here. The important things to notice are that (1) in order to become fully mature and respond to an infection, a B cell has to perform processes in which it swaps around and mutates its own DNA, and (2) when these processes go wrong, a B cell has taken one step along a path to becoming a cancer cell.

Table 7.2 The cell of origin of various hematological cancers.

Type of cancer	Cell of origin	Expected number of cases each year in the United Kingdom [19]
Acute myeloid leukemia (AML)	Hematopoietic stem cells and immature myeloid cells [20]	2420
B cell Acute lymphoblastic leukemia (B cell ALL)	Common lymphoid progenitor cells and immature B cells [21]	550
T cell Acute lymphoblastic leukemia (T cell ALL)	Common lymphoid progenitor cells and immature T cells [21]	160
Chronic myeloid leukemia (CML)	Hematopoietic stem cells and immature myeloid cells [3]	600
Chronic lymphocytic leukemia (CLL)	Mature B cell [22]	4,130
B cell non-Hodgkin lymphoma (B cell NHL)	Mature B cell [23]	9,820
T cell non-Hodgkin lymphoma (T cell NHL)	Mature T cell or natural killer cell [24]	640
Hodgkin lymphoma	Mature B cell [6]	1730
Multiple myeloma	Mature B cell (specifically plasma cells) [6]	4,070
Proportion of cancers in this table that are of:	**B cell origin**	84%
	T cell origin	3%
	Myeloid cell origin	13%

class switching and somatic hypermutation. These CLLs are less aggressive than CLLs with **unmutated** antibody genes, which are derived from B cells that haven't responded to an infection [15].

Another important feature of B cell cancers is that, like healthy B cells, they have **thousands of identical antibodies/B cell receptors (BCRs) on their surface** (see Box 7.1) (a notable exception to this is the cancer cells of Hodgkin lymphoma [6]). Importantly, in many B cell lymphomas and leukemias (particularly in CLL and NHLs), the BCR, and the signaling pathways it controls, are overactive. This realization has led to **treatments that block BCR signaling**, such as Bruton's tyrosine kinase (BTK) inhibitors and PI3Kδ inhibitors such as ibrutinib (Imbruvica) and idelalisib (Zydelig). I'll come back to this in Section 7.4.

7.2.2 Certain Chromosome Translocations Are Common to Each Type and Sub-type

Chromosome translocations are a common feature of hematological cancers.[5] Many types, and sub-types, of hematological cancers have **characteristic translocations** that exist alongside other mutations and abnormalities (Table 7.3 lists a few of the most common translocations). And it seems that for some hematological cancers, a translocation between two chromosomes was the first mutation that occurred in an otherwise normal cell that put it on the path to becoming a cancer cell [25].

Knowing what translocations have taken place in a patient's cancer can provide important information as to the likely future course of their cancer, how aggressive it's going to be, and whether it will respond to certain

---

[5] They're common in solid tumors too.

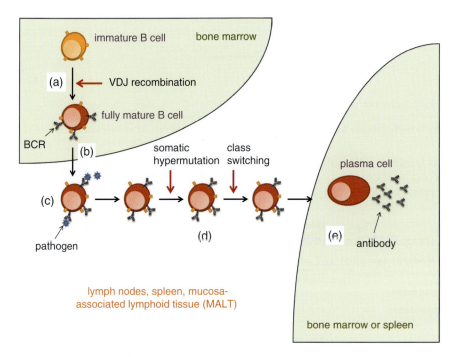

Figure 7.2 The maturation and activation of B cells is a multi-step process. (a) As a B cell matures, it creates a unique B cell receptor (BCR) by a process called VDJ recombination. A fully mature B cell has thousands of copies of its unique BCR on its surface. **(b)** Mature B cells leave the bone marrow (where they are created) and travel to lymph nodes and other immune tissues. **(c)** Mature B cells are constantly coming into contact with bacteria, viruses, and other pathogens. **(d)** If a B cell comes into contact with an infection its BCR can recognize, it might it go through a multi-step activation process involving somatic hypermutation and class switching. **(e)** Finally, the B cell becomes a full-fledged plasma cell capable of releasing its BCR (now called an antibody) into the bloodstream. Plasma cells are mostly found in the bone marrow and spleen.
Abbreviations: BCR – B cell receptor

Box 7.1   B cell receptors (BCRs), antibodies, and immunoglobulins

BCRs, immunoglobulins, and antibodies are virtually the same thing – they are the specialized proteins made by B cells that get released into the blood when the B cell fights an infection. The only difference between the B cell receptor (BCR) and an antibody is that the BCR is tethered to the surface of a B cell by two other proteins called Igα and Igβ (also called CD79a and b) (see Figure 7.3). We tend to use the name "antibody" to refer to BCRs that have been released into the blood and that are now fighting infections. But we generally refer to the genes that code for antibodies as the "immunoglobulin (Ig) genes." Mature B cells have thousands of copies of their BCR on their surface. When they respond to an infection, they become antibody-producing plasma cells that manufacture tens of thousands of copies of their BCR and release them as antibodies into the blood.

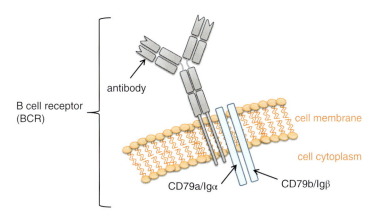

Figure 7.3 **The B cell receptor (BCR).** The BCR is made up of an antibody (also known as an immuno-globulin – Ig) tethered to the surface of the B cell by two proteins known as CD79a and CD79b (also known as Igα and Igβ) that span the cell membrane.
Abbreviations: BCR – B cell receptor; Ig – immunoglobulin

treatments. The discovery of translocations has also led to the discovery of important genes and proteins that have since led scientists to create new treatments. Sometimes, such as in chronic myeloid leukemia (CML), mantle cell lymphoma, and follicular lymphoma, there's just one specific translocation found in the cancer cells of virtually every person. In other cancers, you find a range of different translocations.

Some translocations, like the t(9;22)(q34;q11) translocation (see Box 7.2) found in CML cells, or the t(15;17)(q22;q21) translocation found in acute promyelocytic leukemia (APL[6]) cells, cause the cancer cells to make a **fusion protein**. The abnormal protein forces the cell to multiply and/or prevents it from maturing properly.

Other translocations, like those found in non-Hodgkin lymphomas (NHLs) and multiple myeloma, force the cell to **overproduce a cancer-causing protein**. These translocations often involve chromosome 14 at position q32.[7]

This is the location of powerful promoters and enhancers[8] that control genes (known as immunoglobulin H – IgH – genes) necessary for making BCRs (see Figure 7.4 for an explanation of gene promoters and enhancers). Not surprisingly, in mature B cells IgH genes are very active because they're constantly making copies of their BCRs. Hence, if you splice together a promoter or enhancer for an IgH gene with the protein-coding region of an oncogene (a gene that contains the instructions to make a protein that promotes cell growth, proliferation, and survival), you will cause overproduction of the cancer-causing protein (Figure 7.5). Oncogenes affected by this sort of translocation include the genes for making Myc (a multi-purpose protein that controls many cell functions), Bcl-2 (a survival protein), and various cyclins (they control the cell cycle).

However, do remember that translocations aren't the only mutations found in hematological cancer cells. For example, in the cancer

---

[6] APL is a very rare form of acute myeloid leukemia.
[7] "q" tells you that the chromosome break is in the long arm of the chromosome rather than in the short (p) arm.
[8] If you want to know how promoters and enhancers control how much protein is made from genes, see: http://www.nature.com/scitable/topicpage/gene-expression-14121669.

Table 7.3 Some common translocations found in hematological cancer cells.

Disease	Translocation	Consequence
Acute myeloid leukemia (AML)	t(8;21)(q22;q22)	Creates the RUNX1-RUNX1T1 (also called AML1-ETO) fusion protein that disrupts core-binding protein (CBF)
	inv(16)(p13;q22)*	
	t(16;16)(p13;q22)	Creates a CBFbeta-MYH11 fusion protein that disrupts CBF
	t(4;11)(q21;q23)	Creates an MLL fusion protein (common in infants and children)
	t(9;11)(p21;q23)	Creates an MLL fusion protein (common in infants and children)
Acute promyelocytic leukemia**	t(15;17)(q22;q21)	PML-RARα fusion protein
Acute lymphoblastic leukemia (ALL)	t(12;21)(p13;q22)	ETV6-RUNX1 fusion protein (common in children)
	t(4;11)(q21;q23)	Creates an MLL fusion protein (common in infants)
	t(9;22)(q34;q11)	Bcr-Abl fusion protein (common in adults with ALL)
Chronic myeloid leukemia (CML)	t(9;22)(q34;q11)	Bcr-Abl fusion protein
Chronic lymphocytic leukemia (CLL)	various	Around a third of cases contain translocations but no individual translocation is particularly common [26]
Non-Hodgkin lymphoma (NHL):		
Follicular lymphoma	t(14;18)(q32;q21)	Overproduction of Bcl-2
Mantle cell lymphoma	t(11;14)(q13;q32)	Overproduction of cyclin D1
Diffuse large B cell lymphoma	t(14;18)(q32;q21)	Overproduction of Bcl-2
	t(3;v)(q27;v)	Overproduction of BCL6 (v = various)
	t(8;14)(q24;32)	Overproduction of Myc
MALT lymphoma	t(1;14)(p22;q32)	Overproduction of BCL10
	t(11;18)(q21;q21)	Overproduction of MALT1
	t(14;18)(q32;q21)	Overproduction of Bcl-2
	t(3;14)(p14;q32)	Overproduction of FOXP1
Burkitt's lymphoma	t(8;14)(q24;q32)	Overproduction of Myc
	t(2;8)(p12;q24)	Overproduction of Myc
	t(8;22) (q24;q11)	Overproduction of Myc
Hodgkin lymphoma		Translocations are rare
Multiple myeloma	t(11;14)(q13;q32)	Overproduction of cyclin D1
	t(4;14)(p16;q32)	Overproduction of FGFR3 and MMSET

*This is technically an inversion rather than a translocation; a section of chromosome 16 is snipped out, flipped over, and reinserted back into the chromosome.
**Acute promyelocytic leukemia is a rare sub-type of AML.
Abbreviations: CBF – core-binding protein; MALT – mucosa-associated lymphoid tissue

Source: De Kouchkovsky I, Abdul-Hay M (2016). Acute myeloid leukemia: A comprehensive review and 2016 update. *Blood Cancer J* **6**, e441; doi:10.1038/bcj.2016.50
Rowley JD (2008). Chromosomal translocations: Revisited yet again. *Blood* **112**: 2183.
Moorman AV (2016). New And Emerging Prognostic And Predictive Genetic Biomarkers In B-Cell Precursor Acute Lymphoblastic Leukemia. *Haematologica* **101**: 407–416; doi:10.3324/haematol.2015.141101.
Baliakas P et al. (2014). Chromosomal translocations and karyotype complexity in chronic lymphocytic leukemia: A systematic reappraisal of classic cytogenetic data. *Am J Hematol* **89**(3): 249–255.
Kuppers R (2005). Mechanisms of B-cell lymphoma pathogenesis. *Nat Rev Cancer* **5**: 251–262.
Troppan K et al. (2015). Molecular pathogenesis of MALT lymphoma. *Gastroenterology Research & Practice* **2015**:102656. doi: 10.1155/2015/102656.
Jares P, Colomer D, Campo E (2007). Genetic and molecular pathogenesis of mantle cell lymphoma: Perspectives for new targeted therapeutics. *Nat Rev Cancer* **7**: 750–762.
Molyneux EM et al. (2012). Burkitt's lymphoma. *Lancet* **379**: 1234–1244.
Kuppers R (2008). The biology of Hodgkin's lymphoma. *Nat Rev Cancer* **9**: 15–27.
Bergsagel PL, Kuehl WM (2001). Chromosome translocations in multiple myeloma. *Oncogene* **20**(40): 5611–5622.

Box 7.2   The conventions of writing down translocations

When someone writes **t(9;22)(q34;q11)**, they are giving you detailed information about the translocation that has taken place. First, **t** stands for translocation. Second, the translocation involves chromosomes 9 and 22. The term **q34** tells you that it was the long arm (rather than **p** – the short arm) of chromosome 9 that broke, specifically at position 34. And **q11** tells you that it was the long arm of chromosome 22 that broke, at position 11. All chromosomes have a long arm and a short arm, which are separated by a narrow region of the chromosome called the centromere [27].

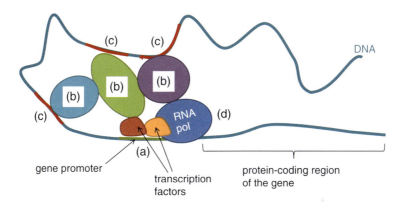

Figure 7.4 Genes are controlled by promoters and enhancers. (a) Immediately in front of the instructions for making a **protein**, each gene contains a promoter, where proteins called transcription factors (shown as red and orange blobs) attach to the gene's DNA. **(b)** In order for a gene to be active, and used to make a protein, other proteins need to interact with the transcription factors on the gene's promoter. These other proteins include additional transcription factors and co-activators (shown as turquoise, green, and purple circles). **(c)** The additional proteins attach to distant locations on the chromosome called **enhancers**. **(d)** When all the necessary transcription factors and co-activators are attached to the gene's promoter and enhancers, RNA pol is recruited to the gene, and it transcribes the gene into mRNA, which is then used by a ribosome to make protein.
Abbreviations: RNA pol – RNA polymerase

cells of chronic lymphocytic leukemia (CLL), the region of chromosome 17 that contains the *TP53* gene[9] is commonly deleted or mutated. Lack of functional p53 protein in CLL cells causes the disease to be aggressive and resistant to chemotherapy [28].

7.2.3 They Have CD Antigens on Their Surface

All the proteins (and other large, complex molecules) found on the surface of our white blood cells have been allocated a number known as a "CD antigen" number.[10] (CD

---

[9] The *TP53* gene contains the instructions to make the p53 protein, which is probably our cells' most important tumor suppressor protein.
[10] For a table of some of the most common ones, as well as a full list, see: https://www.bdbiosciences.com/documents/cd_marker_handbook.pdf.

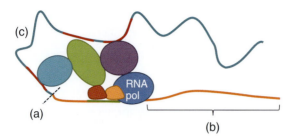

Figure 7.5 Translocations in hematological cancer cells often result in an oncogene being positioned next to control regions from an immunoglobulin gene. (a) The splice site where the two broken chromosomes have fused together. The translocation has fused together **(b)** the protein-coding region of an oncogene such as *MYC* or *BCL2* (which would normally be inactive in B cells) with **(c)** the control region from an immunoglobulin gene that contains several enhancer elements.
Abbreviations: RNA pol – RNA polymerase

stands for "cluster of differentiation," but it doesn't mean anything very much.) CD numbers correspond to the order in which the proteins were discovered (CD1 came first, then CD2 was discovered, then CD3 …). Scientists agreed on the idea of numbering the proteins found on white bloods cells in 1982 when they decided on the identity of CD antigens 1 to 15. They've now discovered and numbered over 370 CD antigens; regular workshops are held to discuss and number the CD antigens found since the previous meeting.

So the number assigned to a CD antigen doesn't tell you anything about that antigen (other than give you a rough idea of when it was discovered). But the range of CD antigens on the surface of a white blood cell can tell you things like:

- What type of white blood cell it is (e.g., only B cells have CD20 on their surface)
- Whether it's a mature, fully functioning white blood cell, or an immature one, or somewhere in between
- What its job is

- Whether, if it's a B or T cell, it has recognized and responded to an antigen[11]

Each type of white blood cell (WBC) has a wide variety of different CD antigens on its surface. Many of these proteins help our WBCs communicate with one another. Other CD antigens transport things in and out of the cell, help the cell move through the bloodstream and into tissues, or help it destroy invaders.

It's worth noting a couple more things about CD antigens at this point:

- They're found on the surface of WBCs and they are therefore accessible to monoclonal antibody (mAb) treatments.
- Many of them are not necessary for the survival of the WBC that they are found on; therefore, blocking them with an antibody won't necessarily kill the cell.
- Each type of WBC has a very particular set of CD antigens on its surface. If a cell goes wrong and becomes a cancer cell, the cancer cell often has (more or less) the same CD antigens on its surface as its healthy counterparts.

---

[11] In case you've forgotten, an antigen is anything (usually a protein, complex carbohydrate, or complex fat molecule) that an antibody can potentially attach to and that can trigger an immune response. Antigens include proteins, carbohydrates, and fats found on the surface of bacteria, viruses, transplanted organs, and parasitical worms. Some proteins on the surface of cancer cells can also behave as antigens. Although "antigen" and "CD antigen" sound like they're very similar to one another, it's probably easiest to think of them as two entirely different things: "antigens" being things that antibodies attach to and that can trigger an immune response, and "CD antigens" being proteins and other large molecules found on the surface of white blood cells.

7.2.4 Targeted Treatments Licensed for Hematological Cancers

Table 7.4 summarizes the licensed targeted treatments for hematological cancers that I explain in this chapter. They include anti-body-based treatments and kinase inhibitors (such as BTK, PI3K, and Bcr-Abl inhibitors) that are used to treat various cancers. I've also included proteasome inhibitors and thalidomide and its derivatives, which are important treatments for multiple myeloma. There are also three HDAC inhibitors (belinostat/Beleodaq, panobinostat/Farydak, and vorinostat/Zolinza). However, I only

Table 7.4 Targeted treatments licensed for people with hematological cancers, as of December 2017.

Drug (marketing name)	Description	Approvals in the United States and Europe [30]
Antibody-based treatments for NHL and CLL		
Alemtuzumab (Campath; MabCampath; Lemtrada[12])	Anti-CD52 monoclonal antibody	FDA-approved for B cell CLL (removed from European and US markets in 2012)
90Y- Ibritumomab tiuxetan (Zevalin)	Anti-CD20 radiolabeled monoclonal antibody	Approved in United States and Europe for B cell NHL
Obinutuzumab (Gazyvaro; Gazyva)	Anti-CD20 monoclonal antibody	Approved in United States and Europe for CLL and follicular lymphoma
Ofatumumab (Arzerra)	Anti-CD20 monoclonal antibody	Approved in United States and Europe for CLL
Rituximab (MabThera; Rituxan)	Anti-CD20 monoclonal antibody	Approved in United States and Europe for CLL and B cell NHL
Rituximab biosimilar[13]: Blitzima	Anti-CD20 monoclonal antibody	Licensed in Europe in July 2017 for CLL and B cell NHL
Rituximab biosimilar: Ritemvia	Anti-CD20 monoclonal antibody	Licensed in Europe in July 2017 for B cell NHL
Rituximab biosimilar: Rituzena (previously Tuxella)	Anti-CD20 monoclonal antibody	Licensed in Europe in July 2017 for CLL and B cell NHL
Rituximab biosimilar: Rixathon	Anti-CD20 monoclonal antibody	Licensed in Europe in June 2017 for CLL and B cell NHL
Rituximab biosimilar: Riximyo	Anti-CD20 monoclonal antibody	Licensed in Europe in June 2017 for CLL
Rituximab biosimilar: Truxima	Anti-CD20 monoclonal antibody	Licensed in Europe in February 2017 for CLL and B cell NHL
[131]I-Tositumomab (Bexxar)	Anti-CD20 radiolabeled monoclonal antibody	FDA-approved for follicular NHL but no longer marketed
Antibody-based treatments for multiple myeloma		
Daratumumab (Darzalex; HuMax-CD38)	Anti-CD38 monoclonal antibody	Approved in United States and Europe for multiple myeloma
Elotuzumab (Empliciti)	Anti-CD319 monoclonal antibody (CD319 is usually known as CS1/ SLAMF7)	Approved in United States and Europe for multiple myeloma

(Continued)

[12] It's called Lemtrada when it's given to people with multiple sclerosis, but it's still alemtuzumab.
[13] The patents on rituximab expired in 2013 in Europe and in 2016 in the United States; this has led many companies to create rituximab biosimilars – copycat versions of the rituximab antibody.

Table 7.4 (Continued)

Drug (marketing name)	Description	Approvals in the United States and Europe [30]
Antibody-based treatments for other hematological cancers		
Blinatumomab (Blincyto)	Bi-specific antibody that attaches to CD19 and CD3	Approved in United States and Europe for adults with ALL
Inotuzumab ozogamicin (Besponsa)	Anti-CD22 drug-linked monoclonal antibody	Approved in United States and Europe for adults with CD22-positive ALL
Brentuximab vedotin (Adcetris)	Anti-CD30 drug-linked monoclonal antibody	Approved in US and Europe for anaplastic large cell lymphoma and Hodgkin lymphoma
Denileukin diftitox (Ontak)	Part of the diphtheria toxin linked to human interleukin-2*	FDA-approved for cutaneous T cell lymphoma
Gemtuzumab ozogamicin (Mylotarg)	Anti-CD33 drug-linked monoclonal antibody	FDA-approved for CD33-positive AML
Siltuximab (Sylvant)	Anti-interleukin 6 monoclonal antibody	Approved in United States and Europe for Multicentric Castleman disease[14]
Pembrolizumab (Keytruda)	Anti-PD-1 monoclonal antibody	Approved in US and Europe for Hodgkin lymphoma
Nivolumab (Opdivo)	Anti-PD-1 monoclonal antibody	Approved in US and Europe for Hodgkin lymphoma
B cell receptor signaling inhibitors		
Ibrutinib (Imbruvica)	Blocks BTK, a kinase involved in B cell receptor signaling	Approved in United States and Europe for CLL, mantle cell lymphoma, and Waldenström macroglobulinemia
Acalabrutinib (Calquence)	Blocks BTK, a kinase involved in B cell receptor signaling	Approved in the United States for mantle cell lymphoma
Idelalisib (Zydelig)	Blocks PI3Kδ, a kinase involved in B cell receptor signaling	Approved in United States and Europe for CLL and follicular lymphoma
Copanlisib (Aliqopa)	Blocks various forms of PI3K, including PI3Kδ	Approved in the United States for follicular lymphoma.
Bcr-Abl inhibitors		
Bosutinib (Bosulif)	Targets Bcr-Abl, a fusion protein found in CML (and some ALL) cancer cells	Approved in United States and Europe for CML
Dasatinib (Sprycel)	Targets Bcr-Abl, a fusion protein found in CML (and some ALL) cancer cells	Approved in United States and Europe for CML, and Bcr-Abl positive ALL
Imatinib (Glivec; Gleevec)	Targets Bcr-Abl, a fusion protein found in CML (and some ALL) cancer cells	Approved in United States and Europe for CML, and Bcr-Abl positive ALL (and for some other cancers)
Nilotinib (Tasigna)	Targets Bcr-Abl, a fusion protein found in CML (and some ALL) cancer cells	Approved in United States and Europe for CML
Ponatinib (Iclusig)	Targets Bcr-Abl, a fusion protein found in CML (and some ALL) cancer cells	Approved in United States and Europe for CML and Bcr-Abl positive ALL *Note*: It is only approved for people whose cancer cells contain the T315I mutation in Bcr-Abl

[14] Multicentric Castleman disease is a rare disease that, although not technically a cancer, behaves much like one and often turns into a lymphoma.

Table 7.4   (Continued)

Drug (marketing name)	Description	Approvals in the United States and Europe [30]
Proteasome inhibitors		
Bortezomib (Velcade)**	Blocks the proteasome	Approved in the United States and Europe for multiple myeloma and mantle cell lymphoma
Carfilzomib (Kyprolis)	Blocks the proteasome	Approved in the United States and Europe for multiple myeloma
Ixazomib (Ninlaro)	Blocks the proteasome	Approved in the United States and Europe for multiple myeloma
HDAC inhibitors		
Belinostat (Beleodaq)	Blocks histone deacetylases (HDACs)	Approved in the United States for peripheral T cell lymphomas
Panobinostat (Farydak)	Blocks histone deacetylases (HDACs)	Approved in the United States and Europe for multiple myeloma
Vorinostat (Zolinza)	Blocks histone deacetylases (HDACs)	Approved in the United States for cutaneous T cell lymphomas
Thalidomide and derivatives		
Lenalidomide (Revlimid)	Various mechanisms	Approved in the United States and Europe for multiple myeloma, mantle cell lymphoma, and myelodysplastic syndromes
Pomalidomide (Imnovid)	Various mechanisms	Approved in the United States and Europe for multiple myeloma
Thalidomide (Thalomid; Thalidomide Celgene)	Various mechanisms	Approved in the United States and Europe for multiple myeloma
JAK-STAT pathway inhibitors		
Ruxolitinib (Jakavi; Jakafi)	Blocks JAK1 and JAK2	Approved in the United States and Europe for myelofibrosis and polycythaemia vera
Bcl-2 inhibitors		
Venetoclax (Venclexta; Venclyxto)	Blocks Bcl-2	Approved in the United States and Europe for CLL
IDH2 (isocitrate dehydrogenase-2) inhibitors		
Enasidenib (Idhifa)	Blocks IDH2, a mitochondrial enzyme	Approved in the United States for IDH2-mutated AML
FLT3 inhibitors		
Midostaurin (Rydapt)	Blocks FLT3 and other kinases	Approved in the United States and Europe for FLT3-mutated AML and mast cell leukemia
CAR-modified T cell therapy		
Tisagenlecleucel (Kymriah)	The patient's T cells are modified to target CD19	Approved in the United States for children and young adults with ALL
Axicabtagene ciloleucel (Yescarta)	The patient's T cells are modified to target CD19	Approved in the United States people with various types of B cell NHL

*This technically isn't an antibody-based treatment, but it targets a CD antigen (IL-2 is the ligand for the IL-2 receptor – the receptor is also known as CD25).
**There are also three generic versions of bortezomib: Bortezomib Accord, Bortezomib Hospira and Bortezomib Sun.
Abbreviations: ALL – acute lymphoblastic leukemia; AML – acute myeloid leukemia; CML – chronic myeloid leukemia; CLL – chronic lymphocytic leukemia; NHL – non-Hodgkin lymphoma; BTK – Bruton's tyrosine kinase; PI3Kδ – phosphatidylinositol-3-kinase-delta; JAK – Janus kinase; STAT – signal transducer and activator of transcription

explain one of them in this chapter: panobinostat for multiple myeloma in Section 7.6.3. I don't explain the others, partly because of the rarity of the cancers they are licensed for, and partly because their mechanism of action is both incredibly complicated and unclear [29]. Some of the latest treatments to be licensed are two CAR-modified T cell therapies. I described the science behind these treatments, and provided some clinical trial results, in Chapter 5, Section 5.4.2.

7.3 ANTIBODY-BASED TREATMENTS THAT TARGET CD ANTIGENS

Monoclonal antibody-based treatments are the most widely used targeted treatments for hematological cancers. The first antibody treatment created, and still the most extensively used, is rituximab (Mabthera). It attaches to CD20 on the surface of B cells and is used for the treatment of B cell leukemias and lymphomas. Since the creation of rituximab, scientists have created many more monoclonal antibody (mAb) treatments that attach to other CD antigens. They have also attached drugs and radioactive particles to antibodies, and created new antibody-based proteins, in order to increase the treatment's ability to destroy cancer cells. In addition, in 2017, six rituximab "biosimilars" were licensed in Europe as CLL and B cell NHL treatments. If you're hazy as to what a biosimilar is, I described them in Chapter 2, Section 2.2.5.

7.3.1 Types of mAb Treatments for Hematological Cancers

As I mentioned back in Chapter 2, antibody-based treatments come in a variety of types (see Figure 7.6 for an illustration showing the different types listed below):

- "Naked" antibodies (e.g., rituximab, alemtuzumab, ofatumumab): These are plain antibodies with nothing attached to them (Figure 7.6a). They can be mouse, chimeric,

humanized, or fully human. Scientists have discovered that fully human and humanized antibodies are often less likely to get destroyed by the patient's immune system than mouse or chimeric antibodies, and be safer for the patient [31].

- Conjugated antibodies (e.g., gemtuzumab ozogamicin, brentuximab vedotin, ibritumomab tiuxetan, and inotuzumab ozogamicin): These antibodies (Figure 7.6b) are being used to deliver either chemotherapy (known as drug-linked antibodies or antibody-drug conjugates), or a radioactive particle (known as radiolabeled antibodies or radioimmunotherapies). In each case, chemists have fused the drug or radioactive particle to the antibody (see Figure 7.7 for an illustration of how gemtuzumab ozogamicin, a drug-linked antibody, is designed to work). The antibody then delivers the drug/particle to the target cells.

- Bi-specific antibodies (e.g., blinatumomab) The antigen-binding regions of two different antibodies are fused back to back so that the resulting antibody tethers together two different types of WBC (Figure 7.6c). (There's more on this approach in Section 7.5.)

- Immunotoxins (e.g., moxetumomab pasudotox) The antigen-binding region of an antibody is fused to part of a bacterial toxin (Figure 7.6d). As with conjugated antibodies, after the drug/toxin attaches to a target cell, it becomes internalized within the cell and then breaks apart to release the toxin.

Many mAbs are licensed as treatments for various hematological cancers (see Table 7.4 for a summary), and many more are in late phase clinical trials. The various mAb treatments listed in Table 7.4 work in a variety of different ways, but they have some properties in common:

- They attach to healthy WBCs as well as to cancer-causing WBCs; therefore, they cause immune suppression and make the patient susceptible to infections.

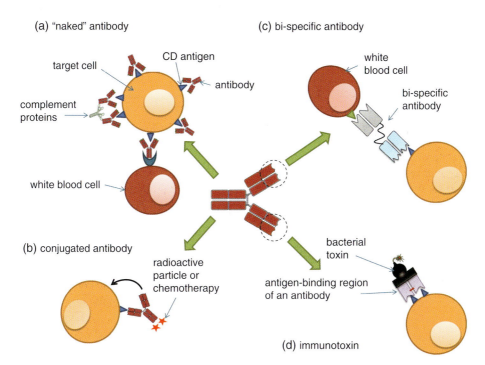

Figure 7.6 Different types of monoclonal antibody therapies. (a) "Naked" antibodies are intact antibodies that have not been modified by adding or removing anything. They work by directly killing the target cell, by attracting complement proteins in the bloodstream, or by attracting white blood cells that destroy the target cell. **(b)** Conjugated antibodies are antibodies that have had another entity, such as a chemotherapy or radioactive particle, attached to them. **(c)** Bi-specific antibodies are made from the antigen-binding regions of two different antibodies that have been linked to one another. **(d)** Immunoxins are constructed from the antigen-binding region of an antibody, which is fused to part of a bacterial toxin.

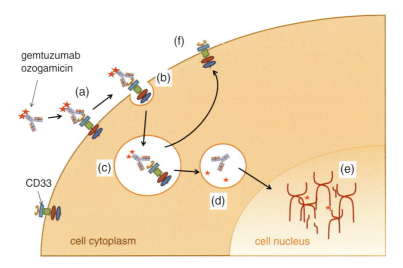

Figure 7.7 Drug-linked antibodies: mechanism of action. (a) The drug-linked antibody (in this case, gemtuzumab ozogamicin) attaches to CD33, a cell surface receptor present in 90% of acute myeloid leukemias. **(b)** The cell membrane folds inward. **(c)** The entire mAb-CD33 complex is internalized into a vesicle. **(d)** The chemotherapy breaks away from the antibody. **(e)** The chemotherapy (calicheamicin) causes double-strand breaks in the cell's DNA, killing the cell. **(f)** If the cell doesn't immediately die, CD33 is recycled back to the cell surface, ready for more drug-linked antibody to attach to it.

- The "naked" antibodies (i.e., those that **aren't** fused to chemotherapy, a radioactive particle, or a toxin) often have limited ability to kill cells outright. So, in order to kill cancer cells, **they need to recruit and activate healthy WBCs and/or complement proteins**.

- All mAbs are large proteins that are destroyed by stomach acids; therefore, **they have to be given subcutaneously or intravenously**.

- All mAbs have the potential to **trigger an immune reaction**; this can cause symptoms such as chills, fever, an itchy rash, feeling sick, breathlessness, wheezing, headaches, and changes in blood pressure [32].

7.3.2 CD Antigens Targeted by Monoclonal Antibodies

When creating new mAb treatments for hematological cancers, scientists have learned from experience that some CD antigens make better targets than others, because:

- Some of them are **not consistently found** on the surface of cancer-causing WBCs – so if you treat a patient with a mAb targeted against that CD antigen, not all the cancer cells will be killed (cells that lack the antigen will survive).

- **Some CD antigens are shed** from the surface of cancer-causing WBCs into the bloodstream, limiting the effectiveness of antibodies targeted against those CD antigens.

- Some of them are on the surface of cancer-causing WBCs, but as soon as an antibody attaches to them, the whole complex (CD antigen + antibody) is **transported inside the cell**. An antigen where this happens might make a good target for a conjugated antibody or an immunotoxin, where you

need the antibody to get inside the cell to deliver its payload and exert its effects. But it's not going to be much good as a target of a naked antibody, where you need the antibody to hang around on the surface long enough to attract healthy WBCs and activate complement proteins.[15]

Scientists are exploring a huge variety of CD antigens as targets for future cancer treatments. I've listed below ten CD antigens that have already proved to be useful targets.

CD19 [33, 34]

- **Examples of treatments that target it:** Blinatumomab, SAR3419, MEDI-551, CAR-modified T cells.

- **What is it?** It is found together with BCRs on the surface of B cells; it seems to fine-tune the activity of BCRs.

- **What cancer cells is it found on?** It is found on the surface of cancer cells in lots of different B cell leukemias and lymphomas, including acute lymphoblastic leukemia (ALL).

- **The good:** CD19 is found on a wider range of B cells leukemias and lymphomas than CD20. Therefore, treatments that target CD19 look promising for people whose cancer has stopped responding to treatments that target CD20.

- **The bad:** Not all leukemia cells have CD19 on their surface and, like CD30, CD19 gets transported inside the cell when an antibody attaches to it. These might be the reasons why the first anti-CD19 antibodies tested didn't work very well.

- **Current opportunities:** The lack of effectiveness of many anti-CD19 antibodies has led to new approaches such as the creation of blinatumomab, a bi-specific antibody (see Section 7.3.6). Scientists are also

---

[15] Complement proteins are a group of 20 or so proteins that float about in our bloodstream. They're activated by antibodies. When activated, they group together and kill cells by punching holes in their outer membrane. They also help activate various types of white blood cells.

developing CAR-modified T cells; this involves removing some of the patient's T cells from their blood, inserting into the T cells a gene for a T cell receptor-like protein that attaches to CD19, and then putting the modified T cells back into the patient's body (there's more on this in Chapter 5, Section 5.4.2).

CD20 [35]

- **Examples of treatments that target it:** Rituximab, ofatumumab, ocrelizumab, obinutuzumab, veltuzumab, and rituximab biosimilars.
- **What is it?** CD20 is found on our body's more mature B cells. It is a protein that crisscrosses the cell membrane four times. It is involved in the transport of calcium into B cells and it plays an important role in the development of B cells in the bone marrow.
- **What cancer cells is it found on?** It's found on cancer cells that started out life as normal B cells, including the majority of B cell leukemias and NHLs.
- **The good:**
  - Because of the distribution of CD20, mAbs that target it can be used as treatments for various types of NHL and CLL; they might also be helpful against ALL.
  - Even when an antibody attaches to CD20, it remains on the surface of the cell (it doesn't get shed or internalized), so the antibody has plenty of time to attract in nearby healthy WBCs which can attack the cancer-causing WBCs.
  - Rituximab, the first anti-CD20 mAb, has brought about meaningful, long-lasting improvements in survival times and quality of life for many people with NHL or CLL.
- **The bad:**
  - CD20 is found on the surface of lots of healthy B cells; many of these cells are

destroyed by anti-CD20 treatments, so the patient's immune system becomes suppressed.
- Also, when someone is being treated with a mAb that targets CD20, eventually you'll see cancer cells appearing that don't have CD20 on their surface and that are therefore unaffected by the treatment.
- **Current opportunities:** Many scientists are trying to create antibodies that are better than rituximab. Also, because rituximab's patent has expired, various companies have created biosimilars that could be cheaper than the original.

CD22 [36]

- **Examples of treatments that target it:** Epratuzumab, inotuzumab ozogamicin, BL22, moxetumomab pasudotox, CAR-modified T cells.
- **What is it?** It is found together with BCRs on the surface of B cells; it affects B cell activity and survival, and it's also involved in cell adhesion.
- **What cancer cells is it found on?** Because it's found on the surface of B cells at different stages of their development, it's also found on the surface of many different B cell leukemias and lymphomas.
- **The good/bad:** Like CD30, CD22 gets transported inside the cell when an antibody attaches to it, so conjugated anti-CD22 antibodies may be more effective than naked antibodies.
- **Current opportunities:** The antibody epratuzumab is being tried out as a naked antibody. It is also being tried as conjugated antibody and has been fused to radioactive particles, chemotherapy, and toxins. Moxetumomab pasudotox is looking exciting for hairy cell leukemia. Moxetumomab pasudotox contains the antigen-binding region of an antibody (known as the Fv), which is fused to part of a toxic protein

(a toxin) from the *Pseudomonas* bacterium [37]. Ant-CD22 antibodies might work well in combination with rituximab. CD22 is also being explored as a target for CAR-modified T cell therapy.

CD25 [38]

- **Examples of treatments that target it**: Denileukin diftitox, LMB-2, CHT25, and daclizumab (anti-Tac).
- **What is it?** It is one-half (known as the alpha-subunit) of the receptor for interleukin-2, and it's found on the surface of some activated B and T cells but not on resting cells (which make up the majority of our B and T cells).
- **What cancer cells is it found on?** Various B and T cell leukemias and lymphomas, including the cancer-causing cells in Hodgkin lymphoma (these are known as Reed Sternberg cells).
- **The good/bad**: It might be that naked anti-CD25 antibodies aren't able to kill enough cancer cells to be helpful, and therefore conjugated antibodies might be necessary.
- **Current opportunities**: Various conjugated antibodies are being explored as well as denileukin diftitox, which is made from interleukin-2 fused to the diphtheria toxin. Most clinical trials with CD25-targeted treatments are in people with peripheral T cell lymphoma [39], for which there are very few effective treatments.

CD30 [40, 41]

- **Examples of treatments that target it**: Brentuximab vedotin
- **What is it?** It's a cell surface receptor (part of the TNF-family of receptors, to be more precise).
- **What cancer cells is it found on?** It's found on cancer cells from Hodgkin lymphoma

and anaplastic large cell lymphoma, and on a subset of B cell NHL.

- **The good**: It's found in relatively low levels on the surface of healthy WBCs; therefore, drugs that target it cause relatively few side effects.
- **The bad**: Naked anti-CD30 treatments didn't seem to have a strong enough impact on cancer-causing WBCs to bring any benefit to patients – this is partly because CD30 is transported inside the cell when an antibody attaches to it.
- **Current opportunities**: Conjugated antibodies such as brentuximab vedotin have proved successful in trials because these work best when the antibody and its target both get transported inside the cell. Brentuximab vedotin is also in several trials for people with T cell lymphomas, mast cell leukemia, and various NHLs.

CD33 [42]

- **Examples of treatments that target it**: Gemtuzumab ozogamicin, lintuzumab, and CAR-modified T cells [43].
- **What is it?** A receptor protein found on immature myeloid WBCs.[16]
- **What cancer cells is it found on?** It's found on the surface of acute myeloid leukemia (AML) cells.
- **The good**: There is clear evidence that the anti-CD33 drug-linked antibody gemtuzumab ozogamicin can help people with AML, and there aren't many other effective treatment options available.
- **The bad**: Gemtuzumab ozogamicin causes lots of side effects, particularly liver toxicity. It was withdrawn from the market in 2010 because of this.
- **Current opportunities**: Even after its market withdrawal, doctors kept on using gemtuzumab ozogamicin in trials. As a result of

---

[16] These immature WBCs are found in the bone marrow; given the right signals, they move elsewhere in the body and mature to become macrophages, dendritic cells, neutrophils, basophils, and eosinophils.

these trials, it received a new license as a treatment of AML in the United States in 2017. It has also been submitted to the EMA for a license in Europe.

CD38 [44, 45]

- **Examples of treatments that target it**: Daratumumab, isatuximab (SAR650984), MOR03087, and MOR202.
- **What is it?** A protein found on the surface of some WBCs, including activated B and T cells and plasma cells. It helps to control the amount of calcium[17] inside the cell; healthy adults have relatively little of it on their WBCs.
- **What cancer cells is it found on?** It's found on multiple myeloma cells.
- **The good**: Because there's relatively little CD38 on healthy WBCs, drugs that target CD38 should cause minimal side effects.
- **The bad**: It's still relatively early days, so we don't yet know how best to use anti-CD38 antibodies.
- **Current opportunities**: An anti-CD38 antibody (daratumumab) is now a licensed treatment for people with multiple myeloma (see Section 7.3.4). Work continues to find out how to use it to best effect.

CD52 [46, 47]

- **Examples of treatments that target it**: Alemtuzumab.
- **What is it?** No one knows exactly what it does, but it's found on the surface of many different WBCs, including B and T cells.
- **What cancer cells is it found on?** CLL, myeloproliferative disorders, and some NHLs.
- **The good**: CD52 is found on lots of different hematological cancers, so antibodies that target it could be helpful for many people.

- **The bad**: It's found on both B cells and T cells, which means that when you attack cells with CD52 on their surface, you cause severe immune suppression. This is the main drawback of anti-CD52 mAb treatments like alemtuzumab, because of which they're being used less and less.
- **Current opportunities**: Anti-CD52 mAbs such as alemtuzumab are still being explored as cancer treatments; however, the company behind alemtuzumab is now focusing on its use in multiple sclerosis.

CD194 (Usually Known as the Chemokine Receptor CCR4) [48]

- **Examples of treatments that target it**: Mogamulizumab.
- **What is it?** It's the receptor for a chemokine – a signaling molecule produced by some WBCs. When chemokines attach to receptors on the surface of WBCs, they cause the cell to move and home in on the source of the chemokine. CCR4 is a chemokine receptor found on T cells.
- **What cancer cells is it found on?** T cell leukemias and lymphomas.
- **The good**: There are far fewer treatment options for people with T cell leukemias and lymphomas than B cell leukemias and lymphomas. CCR4 looks to be an exciting new target for treatments that will help people with T cell cancers.
- **The bad**: It's still early days, so we don't yet know how best to use anti-CCR4 antibodies.
- **Current opportunities**: Anti-CCR4 mAbs are being explored as treatments for peripheral T cell lymphoma and T cell leukemias.

CD319 (Usually Known as CS1/SLAMF7) [49]

- **Examples of treatments that target it**: Elotuzumab.

---

[17] Calcium is vitally important for B cells (and for all our other cells for that matter). Many receptors on the surface of B cells influence the cell's behavior by altering the level of calcium inside it.

- **What is it?** A receptor protein found on the surface of plasma cells (these are antibody-releasing B cells) and on natural killer (NK) cells.
- **What cancer cells is it found on?** Multiple myeloma (the cancer cells of multiple myeloma are plasma cells that have gone wrong).
- **The good**: CS1/SLAMF7 isn't found on most healthy WBCs; therefore, drugs that target it don't suppress the patient's immune system. Elotuzumab, an anti-CS1/SLAMF7 antibody, triggers an immune response against multiple myeloma cells.
- **The bad**: It's still early days, so we don't yet know how best to use anti-CS1/SLAMF7 antibodies.
- **Current opportunities**: An anti-CS1/SLAMF7 antibody (elotuzumab) is now a licensed treatment for people with multiple myeloma (see Section 7.3.4). Work continues to find out how to use it to best effect.

7.3.3 CD20-Targeted mAbs for B Cell NHL and CLL

By far the most common target of mAb treatments for hematological cancers is CD20. The first CD20-targeted antibody licensed as a cancer treatment was rituximab. Because it has proved to be a very successful and important treatment for B cell NHL and CLL, many companies have made their own CD20-targeted antibodies.

Rituximab (Mabthera)

Rituximab was the first mAb ever licensed as a cancer treatment back in 1997. Since that time, it has become a standard treatment for CLL and B cell NHL (specifically, for follicular lymphoma and diffuse large B cell lymphoma) [50]. As you can tell by the "xi" in its name, rituximab is a chimeric antibody. As such, it contains lots of amino acids that are from an original mouse antibody.

There is a variety of evidence from experiments on cells, animals, and human patients that rituximab can kill B cells, including cancer-causing B cells, through a variety of mechanisms [51] (illustrated in Figure 7.8). Scientists think that two things that rituximab does best are to **attract and activate healthy WBCs such as macrophages and NK cells** (Figures 7.8a and b) and to **trigger complement proteins** (Figure 7.8c). It is less able to directly trigger cell death (Figure 7.8d) [52].

Sadly, not everyone treated with rituximab benefits from it. And some people benefit initially, but then their cancer becomes resistant. Hence, many scientists and doctors have attempted to create more powerful anti-CD20 antibodies, such as [53]:

- Radiolabeled anti-CD20 antibodies, for example, ibritumomab tiuxitan and tositumomab
- Second-generation humanized and fully human antibodies
- Third-generation "glyco-engineered" antibodies

These antibodies are summarized in Figure 7.9.

We also have a new group of antibodies known as the "rituximab biosimilars,". These are copycat versions of rituximab that should be equally as effective as the original.

Radiolabeled Anti-CD20 Antibodies (Radioimmunotherapies)

These treatments exploit antibodies as delivery devices (this is illustrated in Figure 7.10). The goal is to **deliver a cell-killing dose of radioactivity** direct to the cancer cells. Two radiolabeled antibodies have been licensed for use for over ten years: ^{90}Y-Ibritumomab tiuxitan (Zevalin) and ^{131}I-Tositumomab (Bexxar). ^{90}Y (yttrium-90) and ^{131}I (iodine-131) are both radioactive isotopes that emit β-particles (high-speed, high-energy electrons) that travel a distance of 1–5 mm from

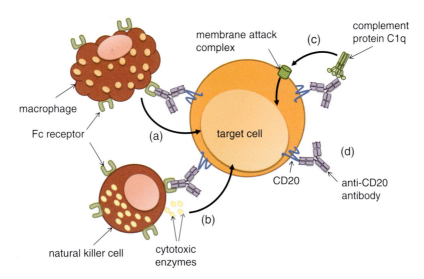

Figure 7.8 Naked anti-CD20 antibodies: mechanisms of action. Naked antibodies such as rituximab destroy target cells through four main mechanisms. **(a)** Attachment of antibody to CD20 attracts white blood cells such as macrophages and natural killer (NK) cells. These connect with the antibody via their Fc receptors. Macrophages destroy antibody-coated target cells via a process called phagocytosis. **(b)** NK cells (and macrophages) kill target cells by releasing cytotoxic (cell-killing) enzymes. Together, mechanisms (a) and (b) are called "antibody-dependent cell-mediated cytotoxicity" (ADCC). **(c)** Complement proteins in the bloodstream attach to the Fc portion of the antibody. This triggers formation of the membrane attack complex (MAC) made up of multiple different complement proteins. The MAC destroys the integrity of the cell membrane and causes cell death – known as complement-dependent cell cytotoxicity (CDC). **(d)** When antibodies attach to CD20, this can trigger signaling pathways within the cell that cause cell death.

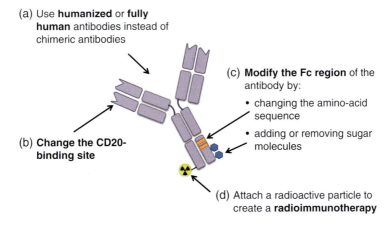

Figure 7.9 Improving the effectiveness of anti-CD20 antibodies. Scientists have harnessed various techniques to try and improve on rituximab and create more powerful, more specific, and longer-lasting anti-CD20 antibodies that are less likely to trigger an immune response. Mechanisms to improve these characteristics include **(a)** creating humanized or fully human antibodies, which should have reduced visibility to the patient's immune system; **(b)** changing the antigen-binding region of the antibody so that it attaches more tightly to CD20, or attaches to a different part of CD20; **(c)** modifying the Fc portion of the antibody to increase its ability to attract white blood cells and trigger antibody-dependent cellular cytotoxicity (ADCC); **(d)** attach a radioactive isotope to the antibody and use it to deliver doses of radioactivity to CD20 positive cells.

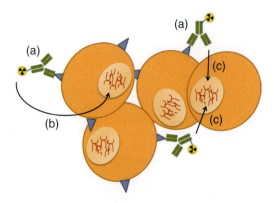

Figure 7.10 Mechanism of action of radioimmunotherapies. **(a)** A radioactively labeled antibody
such as ibritumomab, which carries radioactive
yttrium-90, binds to CD20 on the surface of B cells.
(b) The radioactivity causes double-strand breaks
in the cell's DNA, killing the cell. **(c)** Neighboring
cells, even those with very little CD20 on their
surface, are killed by a bystander effect.

the antibody. ^{131}I also emits γ radiation, which
travels much further, allowing the ^{131}I-labeled
antibody to be used for both treating and
imaging cancer.

However, despite both treatments proving
their worth in clinical trials, neither is widely
used [54]. Barriers to using these treatments
include safety issues (for patients and medical
staff) and the need for staff trained in the use
of radioactive substances [55]. In addition,
since the creation of Bexxar and Zevalin, many
other treatments (such as those listed below)
have been created for the same group of
patients – those with B cell NHL.

Second-Generation Antibodies: Humanized and Fully Human

Examples are ofatumumab, veltuzumab, and
ocrelizumab.

These are naked, humanized, or fully
human monoclonal antibodies that are very
similar to rituximab. However, scientists predicted that because these antibodies contain
fewer mouse amino acids than rituximab,
they would be less likely to cause allergy

reactions and would last in the body longer
[56]. They are also designed to attach more
strongly to CD20 than rituximab, making
them more potent. In addition, ofatumumab
binds to a different part of CD20 than rituximab, and it is designed to stick to complement
proteins better and therefore to trigger more
complement-dependent cytotoxicity [57].
Ofatumumab is licensed as a treatment for
people with newly diagnosed CLL and for
people with CLL whose disease has relapsed
following other treatments.

Third-Generation Antibodies: Bioengineered

Examples are obinutuzumab, ublituximab,
ocaratuzumab, PRO131921, AME-133v,
TRU015, and KM3065.

The Fc region (see Chapter 2, Section 2.2 for
more on this) of these antibodies has been
modified to increase their ability to attract
and activate WBCs such as NK cells. This can
be done by either altering the amino acid
sequence of the antibody or altering the sugar
molecules that are attached to it (this is known
as glyco-engineering) [58]. Obinutuzumab
has also been engineered to be better at triggering cancer cell death [59]. Obinutuzumab
is licensed in the United States and Europe as
a treatment for people with follicular lymphoma or CLL.

Second- and Third-Generation Antibodies – Are They Always Better?

It's important to remember that just because a
treatment has been designed to be better than
an original (in this case rituximab), it doesn't
always follow that it actually is better. Many
trials have taken place in which antibodies
such as ofatumumab and obinutuzumab have
been given to people with CLL and NHL, so
we have a wealth of information about these
treatments.

In some trials, such as the CLL11 trial (in
which obinotuzumab + chlorambucil was

compared to rituximab + chlorambucil or chlorambucil alone in 781 patients with CLL), the newer antibody did turn out to be superior in terms of response rates and survival times [60]. In addition, we know from the GADOLIN trial that obinutuzumab is helpful against follicular lymphomas that are resistant to rituximab [61]. However, in other trials, the newer antibody gave very similar results to rituximab. For example, in the GUASS trial in indolent lymphoma patients, obinutuzumab and rituximab gave very similar progression-free survival (PFS) results [62]. Also, in the ORCHAARD trial, ofatumumab plus chemotherapy was compared to rituximab plus chemotherapy as a treatment for people with diffuse large B cell lymphoma. Results from the trial showed no significant difference in overall survival (OS) or PFS for the two treatment combinations [63].

As a result, rituximab, and therefore also rituximab biosimilars, are still very important treatments for many people with CLL, follicular lymphoma and diffuse large B cell lymphoma.

Rituximab Biosimilars

Examples are Blitzima, Ritemvia, Rituzena, Rixathon, Riximyo and Truxima.

The patents on rituximab expired in 2013 in Europe and in 2016 in the United States. Rituximab sales are worth billions of pounds each year, and as a consequence many companies have created biosimilar versions of rituximab (see Chapter 2, Section 2.2.5 for more on biosimilars) in the hope of gaining a share of the rituximab market [64]. Several of these antibodies are licensed in countries such as Russia, India, and Argentina. In 2017, six rituximab biosimilars were licensed for use in Europe (called Truxima, Rixathon, Riximyo, Blitzima, Ritemvia, and Rituzena) [65, 66]. Truxima, Rixathon, Blitzima, and Rituzena are licensed to treat the same conditions as rituximab, which includes two types of B cell NHL

(follicular lymphoma and diffuse large B cell lymphoma) and CLL. Riximyo and Ritemvia is licensed for NHL but not CLL (look up rituximab on the EMA website for further details).

7.3.4 Antibody Treatments for Multiple Myeloma

CS-1/SLAMF7-Targeted Antibodies

CS1/SLAMF7 is a cell surface receptor found on both multiple myeloma cells and NK cells [67]. Antibodies directed against SLAMF7 have no direct cytotoxic effect on multiple myeloma cells [68], so their dominant mechanism of action is via attaching to SLAMF7, recruiting WBCs such as NK cells and macrophages and triggering ADCC (antibody-dependent cell cytotoxicity) in a similar way to other naked antibodies such as rituximab (see Figure 7.11). SLAMF7 antibodies may also attach to SLAMF7 on NK cells, directly triggering their activity [68]. Elotuzumab (Empliciti) became the first licensed SLAMF7 antibody in 2016. It doesn't have any activity against multiple myeloma when used on its own, but is effective when combined with other treatments such as dexamethasone and lenalidomide [69]. For example, in the ELOQUENT-2 phase 3 trial, which involved 646 patients with relapsed multiple myeloma, the proportion of patients alive after 2 years was 41% for people given dexamethasone, lenalidomide, and elotuzumab, but 27% for people given only dexamethasone plus lenalidomide. The overall response rate was 79% versus 66% [70].

CD38-Targeted Antibodies

CD38 is a cell surface enzyme (an ectoenzyme) that controls calcium levels inside the cell. It's found in low levels on various healthy WBCs and in high levels on multiple myeloma cells [71, 72]. Daratumumab (Darzalex), a CD38-targeted antibody, was licensed as a treatment for multiple myeloma in the United States in

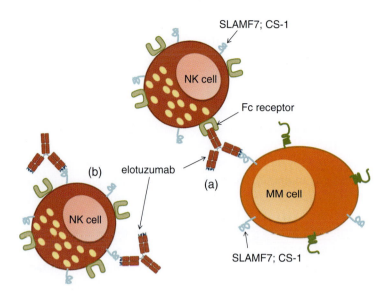

Figure 7.11 Mechanisms of action of elotuzumab. (a) Elotuzumab attaches to SLAMF7 (also called CS-1), which is found on the surface of multiple myeloma cells. Once bound, it activates white blood cells such as natural killer (NK) cells by interacting with their Fc receptors. The activated white blood cell releases toxic granules that kill the cancer cell. **(b)** Elotuzumab also attaches directly to SLAMF7 on the surface of NK cells and increases their activity.
Abbreviations: NK – natural killer

2015 and in Europe in 2016. It can target CD38 kill multiple myeloma cells in a similar way to rituximab: by **attracting and activating macrophages and NK cells, and by activating complement proteins.** CD38 antibodies can also **directly trigger the death of multiple myeloma cells** [72].

Clinical trials, particularly the CASTOR and POLLUX phase 3 trials, have shown that Daratumumab is effective when combined with other treatments. For example, in the CASTOR trial, 498 people with relapsed multiple myeloma were given dexamethasone and bortezomib, with or without daratumumab. After 12 months, 60.7% of people given daratumumab in their treatment combination were still progression-free (i.e., their disease hadn't got any worse), compared to just 26.9% in the group of people who didn't receive daratumumab. In addition, the response rate in the trial was 82.9% in the daratumumab group compared to 63.2% in the control group [73]. In the similar POLLUX

trial, daratumumab was added to lenalidomide and dexamethasone. Again, adding daratumumab to the combination improved the proportion of patients who were progression-free after a year from 60.1% to 83.2%. The addition of daratumumab also boosted the response rate from 76.4% to 92.9% [74].

Trial results also show that daratumub can be helpful when given on its own, even in people who have received many other lines of treatment (reviewed in [71]). A second CD38 antibody, isatuximab, is in multiple phase 3 trials.

7.3.5 Antibody Treatments for Hodgkin Lymphoma

CD30-Targeted Antibodies

CD30 is a member of a family of receptor proteins called the tumor necrosis factor receptor (TNFR) family. It's found on a few different subsets of WBCs such as activated B and T cells, and on the Reed Sternberg (RS) cells that drive Hodgkin lymphoma [75]. Brentuximab vedotin (Adcetris) is a **CD30-targeted antibody that is chemically linked to a chemotherapy called monomethyl auristatin E.** As with gemtuzumab ozogamicin (see Figure 7.7), when brentixumab vedotin attaches to CD30, it is drawn inside the cell and its chemotherapy is released [75].

Brentuximab vedotin was licensed as a treatment for people with Hodgkin lymphoma in the United States in 2011 and in Europe in 2012. These approvals were largely due to the results a phase 2 trial called SG035-003, which involved 102 people with relapsed Hodgkin lymphoma who had previously received an autologous stem cell transplant (ASCT). In this trial, the response rate was 75%, with 34% of patients going into complete remission [76]. There's also been a phase 3 trial, called AETHERA. This trial involved 329 people who were at high risk of relapse following an ASCT. Patients were given either brentuximab vedotin or a placebo. PFS improved from 24.1 months with placebo to 42.9 months with brentuximab vedotin [77].

PD-1-Targeted Antibodies

In RS cells, part of chromosome 9 is commonly amplified (i.e., repeated many times). This region of chromosome 9 contains the genes for PD-L1, PD-L2, and JAK2. As a result, RS cells usually overproduce all three proteins [78]. As we found out in Chapter 5 (in Section 5.3.4), PD-1 is found on the surface of activated T cells. When PD-1 connects with PD-L1 or PD-L2, the T cell's ability to fight infections or cancer cells is suppressed (Figure 7.12a). PD-1-targeted antibodies can interfere with this interaction and **activate T cells that are in the vicinity of RS cells** (Figure 7.12b).

During 2016 and 2017, the PD-1 antibodies nivolumab (Opdivo) and pembrolizumab (Keytruda) were both licensed as treatments

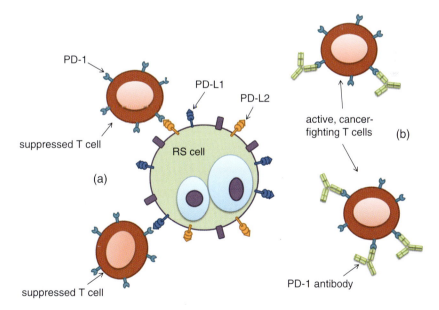

Figure 7.12 Mechanism of action of a PD-1 antibody against Hodgkin lymphoma (HL). **(a)** The cancer cells of HL – Reed Sternberg (RS) cells – commonly have PD-L1 and PD-L2 on their surface. These proteins interact with PD-1 on the surface of cytotoxic T cells, and this suppresses the T cells' activity. **(b)** By attaching to PD-1, a PD-1 antibody prevents the T cell from being suppressed. The T cell is therefore now able to attack and destroy RS cells.

Abbreviations: RS – Reed Sternberg; PD-1 – programmed cell death protein-1; PD-L1 – programmed death ligand-1; PD-L2 – programmed death ligand-2

for people with Hodgkin lymphoma in the United States and Europe. In the clinical trials that investigated PD-1 antibodies for people with Hodgkin lymphoma, the response rates have been extremely high (in the region of 70%–90%) [79–81]. This is higher than the response rates you see when they're given to people with solid tumors like melanoma skin cancer or non-small cell lung cancer. The high response rates probably reflect the fact that in Hodgkin lymphoma PD-L1 and PD-L2 levels are being driven by a mutation present in all the cancer cells. This is in contrast to solid tumors, in which PD-L1 (and occasionally PD-L2) is only generally found on a subset of cancer cells and expression levels vary in different parts of the tumor [82].

There's also some evidence that the combination of brentuximab vedotin plus nivolumab will be more effective than either treatment alone [83].

7.3.6 Antibody Treatments for ALL

Blinatumomab (Blincyto)

Blinatumomab was the first antibody-based treatment to be licensed for people with ALL. It is a bi-specific T cell engager – BiTE – which is a type of bi-specific antibody (see Chapter 5, Section 5.5). Blinatumomab is made from the scFv[18] of an antibody that attaches to CD3, linked to the scFV of an antibody that attaches to CD19 (see Figure 5.13). CD3 is a group of proteins associated with the T cell receptor and it is therefore always present on the surface of T cells. CD19, as I've mentioned before, is found on the surface of cancer cells that cause ALL and other B cell leukemias and lymphomas.

When blinatumomab attaches to CD3 on a T cell, and to CD19 on a B cell (either a

cancer-causing B cell or a healthy B cell), this triggers the T cell to release its supply of cell-killing enzymes [84]. As a result, the B cell is destroyed.

As with any treatment that targets CD19, the destruction of healthy B cells as well as cancer-causing B cells means that the patients' ability to fight off infections is compromised. But, because CD19 isn't found on bone marrow stem cells, B cell numbers gradually get back to normal once treatment stops. Blinatumomab was licensed as a treatment of adult patients with ALL in the United States in 2014 and in Europe in 2015. The largest clinical trial with blinatumomab performed to date was the TOWER trial, which involved 405 adults with relapsed B cell ALL. In this trial, blinatumomab was compared to chemotherapy, and it improved survival times from a median of 4 months with chemotherapy to 7.7 months with blinatumomab. It also increased the complete remission rate from 16% to 34% [85].

Inotuzumab Ozogamicin

Inotuzumab ozogamicin (Besponsa) is an antibody-drug conjugate – an antibody against the CD22 protein, which has been chemically linked to ozogamicin – a derivative of a chemotherapy called calicheamicin. As with brentuximab vedotin, the antibody part of the treatment attaches to a cell surface protein (in this case, CD22) and the whole molecule (antibody plus chemotherapy) is drawn inside the cell. Ozogamicin is then released and kills the cell by causing breaks in its DNA [86].

CD22 is found on B cells that are maturing in the bone marrow. It is also found on the cancer cells of the vast majority of children and adults with ALL [86]. In a phase 3 clinical trial called INO-VATE ALL (NCT01564784),

---

[18] scFv – the antigen-binding segment of an antibody (Fv) constructed from a single chain (sc) of amino acids.

inotuzumab ozogamicin was compared to standard of care chemotherapy in 326 adults with relapsed ALL. Results for the first 218 patients showed that patients given inotuzumab ozogamicin were more likely to experience complete remission of their disease (80.7% vs. 29.4%). And, after two years, 23% of people in the inotuzumab ozogamicin group were alive, compared to 10% in the chemotherapy group [87]. Inotuzumab ozogamicin was licensed as a treatment for ALL in the United States and Europe in April 2017.

7.4 DRUGS THAT BLOCK B CELL RECEPTOR SIGNALING

The BCR has only recently become the subject of intensive research to create new cancer treatments. The first two drugs that block BCR signaling to be licensed as treatments were ibrutinib (Imbruvica) and idelalisib (Zydelig). Both these drugs received European and American approval as treatments for CLL and non-Hodgkin lymphoma (NHL) in 2013 and 2014. Since then, two more drugs, copanlisib (Aliqopa) and acalabrutinib (Calquence), have become licensed treatments (although as of December 2017, copanlisib was licensed in the United States but not in Europe).

An important point to remember when reading this section is that – as you might think – treatments that target BCR signaling are almost exclusively relevant to cancers that have developed from faulty B cells[19] and are irrelevant to cancers that are derived from T cells or other WBCs. However, as I mentioned earlier, the majority of hematological cancers diagnosed in the developed world are derived from B cells. Most trials of treatments

that target BCR signaling have involved people with either CLL or with a form of NHL in which BCR signaling is known to be active, such as follicular lymphoma or mantle cell lymphoma [23].

7.4.1 The BCR – What It Is and What It Does Normally

As you might recall from Section 7.2.1, BCRs are antibodies that are attached to the outer membrane of B cells (see Figure 7.3). Each B cell has about 100,000–200,000 identical BCRs anchored on its surface [88].

In order to understand why drugs that block BCR-controlled signaling pathways are now being used as cancer treatments, it's useful to know a few more facts about them:

- When a B cell's BCR connects with an antigen,[20] BCRs cluster together and trigger various signaling pathways inside the cell that involve many different kinases [23] (Figure 7.13).
- Unlike the growth factor receptors mentioned in Chapter 3, the BCR has no kinase activity of its own; it therefore cannot be blocked with a kinase inhibitor.
- Like the signaling pathways controlled by growth factor receptors, the signaling pathways activated by BCRs can cause B cells to grow, multiply, stay alive, and specialize (among other things).
- These signaling pathways involve proteins such as Ras, Raf, MEK, AKT, mTOR, and NFκB; these are many of the same proteins that cause cell growth, survival, and proliferation in solid tumors.
- The BCR also activates proteins that are vitally important only to WBCs, such as BTK and the δ (delta) form of PI3K (in solid tumors, it's more likely to be PI3Kα or PI3Kβ that is overactive).

---

[19] PI3Kδ inhibitors might also be useful for treating solid tumors.
[20] Remember that an antigen is anything that a BCR can connect with – usually it's a protein or other complex molecule on a pathogen's surface.

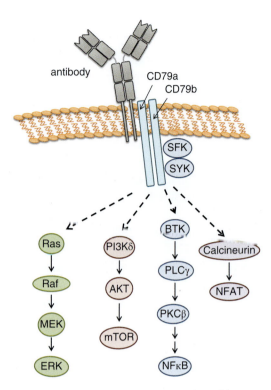

Figure 7.13 **Signaling pathways activated by the B cell receptor** [23]. When the BCR is activated by the presence of an antigen that it recognizes, it triggers the activation of various signaling pathways inside the cell. This activation is mediated via kinases (SFK and SYK) that associate with CD79a and CD79b. As well as being activated by antigens, low-level (tonic) activity of the BCR is necessary for cell survival.
Abbreviations: BCR – B cell receptor; mTOR – mammalian target of rapamycin; PI3K – phosphatidylinositol 3-kinase; ERK – extra-cellular-signal-regulated kinase; BTK – Bruton's tyrosine kinase; NFκB – nuclear factor-kappa-B; NFAT – nuclear factor of activated T cells; PKCβ – protein kinase C β; PLCγ – phospholipase Cγ; SFK – SRC family kinase

- As well as causing cell growth and proliferation in B cells that have connected with an antigen, mature B cells that haven't yet found an antigen they recognize (known as naïve B cells) also rely on their BCR. **They need a bit of tonic (i.e., low-level) BCR signaling to keep them alive** [89].

- And, as well as activating various signaling pathways, the **BCR is also involved in cell adhesion**; it helps B cells interact and connect with the cells around them [90].

7.4.2 How BCRs Signaling Goes Wrong in Hematological Cancers

As well as being essential for the survival and activation of healthy B cells, the BCR is also **essential for the survival of many B cell leukemias and lymphomas**. Sometimes, BCR signaling is overactive because of mutations in the cells' DNA. For example, the cancer cells of a type of NHL called "activated B cell-like diffuse large B cell lymphoma" (ABC DLBCL) contain mutations in the genes for CD79a or CD79b. In other cancers (such as CLL), the BCR is essentially normal, but it has become active, not in response to a pathogen, but instead in response to normal proteins on the surface of neighboring cells [23].

What scientists have now realized is that in each type and sub-type of B cell cancer, the BCR seems to play a slightly different role. For example, ABC DLBCL cells rely on BCR signaling for their survival. But in a germinal center B cell like DLBCL (GCB DLBCL), only a very low level of BCR signaling takes place, and blocking BCR signaling generally has no effect [23]. Table 7.5 briefly summarizes what we know about BCR signaling in various B cell cancers.

Scientists have created a variety of drugs that can block BCR signaling, such as BTK inhibitors, PI3Kδ inhibitors, pan-PI3K inhibitors, and SYK inhibitors.

7.4.3 BTK Inhibitors

BTK inhibitors, together with PI3K inhibitors, are changing the way that CLL and some forms of NHL are treated. Around the world, trials are taking place to discover how best to use these treatments to bring maximum benefit.

Table 7.5 BCR signaling in various B cell cancers.

Cancer type	Sub-type	Level and importance of BCR signaling to the cancer cells [28]
Non-Hodgkin lymphoma	ABC DLBCL	High level of BCR signaling due to a variety of gene mutations
	GCB DLBCL	Low-level activity or no activity; the cancer cells do not require BCR signaling for their survival
	Burkitt's lymphoma	Low-level (tonic) activity
	Follicular lymphoma	High level of BCR signaling; the cancer cells may be mistakenly responding to proteins (self-antigens) on the surface of neighboring cells
	Mantle cell lymphoma	High level of BCR signaling because various components of BCR signaling (such as Syk and BTK) are either mutated or overproduced
	Marginal zone lymphoma	High level of BCR signaling; could be caused by B cells responding inappropriately to pathogens, for example, viruses in their environment
B cell CLL		High level of BCR signaling; the cancer cells may be mistakenly responding to proteins (self-antigens) on the surface of neighboring cells
Hodgkin lymphoma		No BCR signaling
Multiple myeloma		BCR is not present on the cell surface [91]

About BTK

BTK is controlled by the BCR and is **an essential component of BCR signaling** [92]. In Figure 7.13, you can see that BTK is activated by kinases such as SFK (Src family kinases) and SYK. Once activated, BTK triggers the activity of other pathways and ultimately switches on the activity of NFκB, which is a powerful pro-survival protein (I haven't shown all the actions of BTK in Figure 7.13 as it gets far too complicated and confusing). As well as controlling the survival of B cells, BTK also affects cells' attachment to their neighbors and their ability to move between the blood and lymph tissues (lymph tissues include lymph nodes, spleen, and bone marrow) [91].

The Actions of BTK Inhibitors

Ibrutinib (Imbruvica) was the first BTK inhibitor developed. It is an irreversible inhibitor that chemically binds to an amino acid (a cysteine) that sits inside BTK's ATP-binding pocket (remember that BTK is a kinase and it

therefore needs ATP in order to phosphorylate its targets) [93]. When given to patients, two important things happen:

1. Firstly, ibrutinib has direct effects on BCR signaling in cancer cells, blocking NFκB activation and **encouraging the cells to die**.
2. Secondly, ibrutinib causes cancer cells in the patient's lymph nodes, spleen, and bone marrow to **detach from the cells around them and move into the blood**. In the blood, the cancer cells stop multiplying and start dying off [94].

Ibrutinib is a licensed treatment of people with mantle cell NHL,[21] marginal zone NHL (in the United States only), or CLL, due to the results of a series of phase 3 trials. For example, in the HELIOS trial, 578 patients with relapsed CLL were randomized to receive bendamustine + rituximab with or without ibrutinib. The addition of ibrutinib improved the response rate of patients from 24% to 79% [95]. Other trials have shown that ibrutinib is effective when used alone, and in combination with chemotherapy or CD20

---

[21] It's also licensed for people with Waldenstrom's macroglobulinaemia, a rare, slow-growing form of NHL.

antibodies [96]. It also has some activity against CLLs that contain mutations, such as *TP53* deletions and mutations, which cause resistance to chemotherapy and CD20 antibodies [97].

Ibruitnib is considered by doctors to be a very safe treatment, but it can cause side effects such as diarrhea that cause some patients to stop treatment [98]. Some of the side effects it causes are because it doesn't just inhibit BTK. It also blocks several other kinases such as the EGF receptor [99].

A second BTK inhibitor, acalabrutinib (Calquence) was approved as a treatment for mantle cell lymphoma in the United States in 2017. This approval was due to the results of a phase 2 trial involving just 124 patients, in which 81% of patients responded to acalabrutinib [100]. Acalabrutinib is currently being investigated in a range of phase 3 trials. In one trial (called ELEVATE CLL R/R), it is being directly compared to ibrutinib.

Many other irreversible BTK inhibitors are being developed, such as CC-292, BGB-3111, and ONO-4059 [101, 102].

Resistance to BTK Inhibitors

Not everyone who is given ibrutinib is helped by it. Also, some people whose cancer does respond, later develop resistance to it. Scientists have concluded that there are a variety of reasons for drug resistance, including:

1. **Mutations in BTK** (often affecting the cysteine amino acid that ibrutinib attaches to)
2. **Mutations in PLCγ** (a kinase activated by BTK)
3. **Overactive PI3K-AKT** signaling
4. Increased **NFκB activity** that is no longer dependent on BTK
5. Increased activity of **other signaling pathways** [103, 104]

There is some evidence that people with cancers that are resistant to a BTK inhibitor may benefit from a PI3K or Bcl-2 inhibitor such as idelalisib or venetoclax [96].

7.4.4 PI3K Delta Inhibitors

Like BTK inhibitors, PI3K delta (PI3Kδ) inhibitors are having a positive impact on the lives of people with CLL and some forms of NHL.

About PI3Kδ

PI3Kδ is **activated by the BCR** (see Figure 7.13). It is found in normal B cells, T cells, and NK cells, and it's also found in cancer-causing B cells [105]. The tonic, low-level activity of BCR signaling that keeps healthy B cells alive depends on PI3Kδ. It is also activated when BCRs respond to an antigen by triggering signaling pathways [23]. In addition to being activated by the BCR, PI3Kδ is also activated by other receptors found on the surface of WBCs, such as chemokine receptors.

When it is activated, PI3Kδ (like other forms of PI3K) converts phosphatidylinositol 4,5-bisphosphate (PIP$_2$)[22] into phosphatidylinositol 3,4,5-triphosphate (PIP$_3$). PIP$_3$ then activates AKT.

The Actions of PI3Kδ Inhibitors

Like BTK inhibitors, **PI3Kδ inhibitors can block BCR signaling**, and **they interfere with the cancer cells' ability to home to lymph nodes** and cause them to move into the blood [106]. These effects cause cancer cells to die. Unlike ibrutinib, idelalisib is a reversible inhibitor of its target.

Idelalisib (Zydelig) was the first selective PI3Kδ inhibitor to be licensed as a cancer treatment. In Europe, it is licensed in combination with rituximab or ofatumumab for

---

[22] PIP$_2$ is a small lipid molecule found in the cell membrane.

people with relapsed CLL who have already received prior treatment, and as a first-line treatment for people with CLL who have a 17p deletion or other *TP53* mutation[23] and who are ineligible to receive any other treatment [107]. It's used alone in the treatment of people with follicular NHL who have already received two other courses of treatment.

Idelalisib has not surprisingly been investigated in a range of phase 3 trials. For example, in a trial called "Study 116," it was given in combination with rituximab and compared to rituximab alone. The trial involved 220 people with relapsed CLL who were too unwell to receive chemotherapy. The results of the trial showed that the addition of idelalisib to rituximab improved response rates from 13% to 81% [108]. After one year, 66% of people who received idelalisib were still progression-free (i.e., their disease hadn't worsened) compared to 13% of the people who received rituximab alone [109].

In 2016, the results from three large clinical trials in which idelalisib was investigated in further groups of patients suggested that it can put patients at high risk of infections and autoimmune reactions [110]. The MHRA (Medicines and Healthcare Products Regulatory Agency) has since decided that idelalisib's benefits outweigh its drawbacks in the groups of patients for which it's already licensed [111]. However, some trials have been stopped [112].

In 2017, a second PI3K inhibitor, copanlisib (Aliqopa), was licensed as a treatment for follicular lymphoma in the United States. Copanlisib is a "pan-PI3K" inhibitor. That is, it blocks all four versions of PI3K, although it's better at blocking PI3Kα and PI3Kδ than

PI3Kβ or PI3Kγ [113](see Chapter 3, Figure 3.19 for more about the different forms of PI3K). The approval of copanlisib was due to the results of the Chronos-1 study, which involved 142 people with a variety of indolent lymphomas (such as follicular lymphoma or marginal zone lymphoma). Everyone in the trial had already received rituximab and chemotherapy. The overall response rate was 59.2%, but this was a single-arm trial, so there was no comparison with another treatment [114].

An important difference between copanlisib and idelalisib is that copanlisib is given as an infusion into the blood, whereas idelalisib is taken as a daily tablet. They also have different side effects and therefore might be appropriate for different groups of patients.

Other PI3Kδ inhibitors include duvelisib (which also blocks PI3Kγ), AMG319, INCB040093, INCB050465, and TGR-1202 [115].

In addition to their usefulness in B cell cancers, **PI3Kδ inhibitors are also in trials for solid tumors.** PI3Kδ inhibitors affect the activity of a variety of WBCs, including blocking the activity of regulatory T cells, which suppress immune responses. Scientists hope that PI3Kδ inhibitors might therefore encourage the patients' WBCs to attack their cancer cells [115].

Resistance to PI3Kδ Inhibitors

As with all targeted therapies, some patients do not respond to idelalisib treatment at the outset, and some that do respond later relapse. Scientists haven't yet discovered why this happens. Possibilities include increased activity of alternative PI3Ks (such as PI3Kα or PI3Kβ) or amplification[24] of the

---

[23] A 17p deletion and a *TP53* mutation are effectively the same thing – both faults affect the *TP53* gene and stop the p53 protein from doing its normal, cancer-suppressing job. When CLL cells contain a *TP53* mutation, it makes them particularly aggressive and difficult to treat.

[24] Gene amplification is when the cell accidently makes many copies of a gene and inserts them into its chromosomes.

MYC gene [104]. MYC is a powerful transcription factor[25] activated by many different signaling pathways; it is overactive in the majority of cancers [116] (see Chapter 1, Table 1.1 for more on MYC). There is evidence that people whose disease is resistant to idelalsisib might still benefit from another treatment such as ibrutinib or venetoclax [117].

7.4.5 SYK Inhibitors

SYK inhibitors haven't yet proved their worth as treatments for hematological cancers, but it's still early days.

About SYK

SYK (spleen tyrosine[26] kinase) is a tyrosine kinase found in the cytoplasm of WBCs. When BCR activity is triggered by the presence of an antigen, SYK then attaches to the CD79a and CD79b proteins. This attachment triggers phosphorylation of SYK, creating docking sites for other proteins. Some of those proteins are PI3Kδ, AKT, and PLCγ [118] (Figure 5.8 in Chapter 5 summarizes some of this information, but it wasn't possible to fit all the possible interactions of SYK into one diagram).

The Actions of SYK Inhibitors

As with BTK and PI3Kδ, SYK is involved both in the activation of various signaling pathways and with the attachment of B cells to their neighbors.

The first SYK inhibitor to be investigated in clinical trials was fostamatinib, but this drug is not particularly specific and caused lots of toxicities. A newer and more specific SYK inhibitor called entospletinib (GS-9973) looks more promising [118]. A range of other SYK inhibitors are in trials.

7.5 BCR-ABL INHIBITORS

Bcr-Abl inhibitors were some of the first targeted cancer treatments ever created. Over the past thirty years, thousands of people with CML have been treated with these drugs. In fact, because of Bcr-Abl inhibitors, the life expectancy of a person with CML is now approaching that of the general population [119].

7.5.1 About the Bcr-Abl Fusion Protein

The Bcr-Abl fusion protein is created when the t(9;22)(q34;q11) translocation occurs between chromosomes 9 and 22, fusing together the *ABL* gene (chromosome 9) with the *BCR* gene (chromosome 22). This forces the cell to make a Bcr-Abl fusion protein.

The t(9;22)(q34;q11) translocation was first discovered back in 1960 when American scientists working in Philadelphia noticed that the cancer cells of people with CML contained a minute version of chromosome 22. This mini chromosome was later called the "Philadelphia chromosome" [120].

The Bcr-Abl fusion protein is found in the cancer cells of virtually everyone with CML and in around 25% of people (mostly adults) with ALL.

The fusion protein contains virtually all of the Abl protein, which, when fused to Bcr, is a powerful, uncontrollable protein kinase. As with all kinases, Abl uses ATP as a source of phosphate, and it transfers phosphates from ATP onto tyrosine amino acids in many different target proteins (see Figure 7.14a). Through these targets, Bcr-Abl activates various signaling pathways that encourage cell survival and proliferation, including the Ras/Raf/MEK/ERK, PI3K/AKT/mTOR, and JAK/STAT pathways [121].

---

[25] See the Appendix if you want to learn what a transcription factor is.
[26] The one-letter abbreviation for tyrosine amino acid is Y – hence, the abbreviation SYK rather than STK for spleen tyrosine kinase.

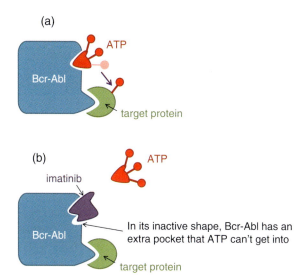

Figure 7.14 Imatinib blocks Bcr-Abl. (a) Bcr-Abl is in its active shape, and ATP has entered its ATP-binding pocket. Bcr-Abl removes a phosphate from ATP (which consequently becomes ADP) and transfers the phosphate onto a tyrosine amino acid in a target protein. **(b)** Imatinib can enter the ATP-binding site only when ATP is absent and Bcr-Abl is in its inactive shape (kinases cycle back and forth between their active and inactive shapes). When imatinib binds to Bcr-Abl, it traps it in its inactive shape and prevents ATP from entering. Without ATP, Bcr-Abl can't phosphorylate any of its targets.

7.5.2 The Actions of First-Generation Bcr-Abl Inhibitors

Imatinib (Glivec; Gleevec) was the first small molecule kinase inhibitor ever used as a cancer treatment. It is a "Type 2" kinase inhibitor (see Chapter 2, Section 2.3.2) which can attach to Bcr-Abl only when its ATP-binding site is empty (i.e., when ATP isn't there) and the kinase is in its inactive shape (see Figure 7.14b). When lodged in its ATP-binding site, imatinib prevents Bcr-Abl from phosphorylating target proteins.

The benefits of imatinib typically last for many years, particularly for people whose cancer is in the "chronic phase" (i.e., very slow growing) when their treatment starts. However, some patients' cancers do eventually become resistant. This typically happens because of cancer cells with additional mutations in their Bcr-Abl fusion gene.

Scientists have now discovered more than 50 different mutations affecting the kinase section of Bcr-Abl in the cancer cells of people whose disease has become resistant to imatinib. Many of these mutations trap the kinase is in its active shape. Imatinib, which can only bind to the inactive enzyme, can therefore no longer do its job [122].

7.5.3 Second- and Third-Generation Bcr-Abl Inhibitors

Second-generation Bcr-Abl inhibitors such as nilotinib (Tasigna) and dasatinib (Sprycel) have been designed to block many of the mutant versions of Bcr-Abl that imatinib can't block.

Nilotinib, like imatinib, can only bind to inactive Bcr-Abl, but it is 20 to 30 times better than imatinib at doing this. Dasatinib, however, can block Bcr-Abl when it's in a variety

Table 7.6   Bcr-Abl inhibitors licensed for use in the United States and United Kingdom.

Drug	Targets
Imatinib (Glivec; Gleevec)	Bcr-Abl, PDGF receptor, KIT
Nilotinib (Tasigna)	Bcr-Abl, PDGF receptor, KIT
Dasatinib (Sprycel)	Bcr-Abl, SRC-family kinases, KIT, PDGF receptor, ephrin receptor
Bosutinib (Bosulif)	Bcr-Abl, SRC-family kinases (SFKs)
Ponatinib (Iclusig)	Bcr-Abl (including the T315I mutant version of Bcr-Abl that isn't blocked by other licensed Bcr-Abl inhibitors), FLT3, RET, KIT, FGF receptors, PDGF receptors, VEGF receptors

Source: Information about the drugs listed was taken from: Quintas-Cardama A, Kantarjian H, Cortes J (2007). Flying under the radar: the new wave of BCR–ABL inhibitors. *Nature Reviews Drug Discovery* **6**: 834-848.

of different shapes [123]. Other Bcr-Abl inhibitors developed in recent years include bosutinib (Bosulif). Bosutinib is able to block both Bcr-Abl and a group of closely related kinases known as the SFKs.

One drawback of nilotinib, dasatinib, and bosutinib is that none of these drugs is able to block an important drug-resistant form of Bcr-Abl known as the T315I mutant (the 315th amino acid in the Bcr-Abl protein has changed from being a threonine to become an isoleucine). The only licensed drug able to block the T315I mutant is a third-generation Bcr-Abl inhibitor called ponatinib (Iclusig).

Together, these treatments have dramatically improved the survival of people with CML. We've also discovered more recently that sometimes ALL cells also contain the Bcr-Abl fusion protein and respond to the same treatments [124]. You can find a summary of licensed Bcr-Abl inhibitors in Table 7.6.

7.6 DRUGS THAT BLOCK THE PROTEASOME

Proteasome inhibitors and thalidomide and its derivatives (such as lenalidomide – see Section 7.7) are routinely used as treatments for multiple myeloma. They are also in trials for other hematological cancers and

bortezomib (a proteasome inhibitor) is licensed in Europe for mantle cell lymphoma (a form of NHL).

7.6.1 About the Proteasome

Proteasomes are hollow, cylindrical structures built from a number of separate proteins. They are found in the nucleus and cytoplasm of human cells. Their purpose is to break down proteins that have worn out, that haven't been made properly, or that the cell doesn't want [125]. The buildup of unwanted and broken proteins is toxic to cells. The proteasome is also responsible for the orderly and precise destruction of proteins such as cyclins during the cell cycle. This is essential to ensure that the cell grows and splits into two healthy "daughter" cells [125].

When a cell wants to destroy a protein, it first of all labels that protein with multiple copies of a small chemical called ubiquitin (this is a complicated process involving a variety of enzymes). The ubiquitins attached to the protein act as a signal telling the proteasome that the protein needs destroying. When it has taken hold of a protein, the proteasome then unravels the protein and feeds it through its cylindrical core. This core has many enzyme sites which chop up the protein and release its amino acids for re-use (see Figure 7.15).

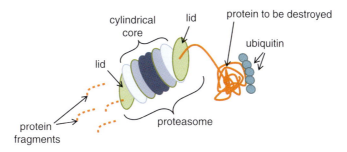

Figure 7.15 Protein destruction by a proteasome. Proteasomes destroy proteins that have been labeled with multiple copies of a chemical called ubiquitin. The labeled protein attaches to one of the proteasome's "lids." The proteasome then unfolds the protein and feeds it through its hollow, cylindrical core. Within this core are enzyme sites that chop up the protein.

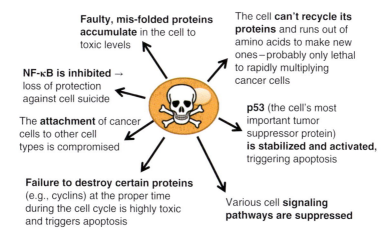

Figure 7.16 Potential reasons why proteasome inhibitors kill cancer cells. The relative importance and impact of each of these mechanisms is still unknown.

7.6.2 The Actions of Proteasome Inhibitors

Proteasome inhibitors such as bortezomib (Velcade), carfilzomib (Kyprolis), ixazomib (Ninlaro), marizomib, and oprozomib, all work by blocking some of the proteasome's internal enzyme sites. Bortezomib, the first proteasome inhibitor ever tested in clinical trials, is a reversible inhibitor, whereas carfilzomib and oprozomib are irreversible inhibitors. Ixazomib (another reversible inhibitor) and oprozomib can both be given in tablet form, whereas bortezomib, carfilzomib, and marizomib have to be given by intravenous infusion or subcutaneous injection [126, 127].

The precise reason why proteasome inhibitors kill cancer cells is still controversial. However, they are known to have a variety of impacts on cells (summarized in Figure 7.16). One of the earliest mechanisms to be discovered was that blocking the proteasome indirectly causes inhibition of NFκB [128]. NFκB protects cells (particularly cancer cells) against apoptosis.[27] When the proteasome is blocked,

---

[27] Apoptosis is the orderly process through which our cells self-destruct when they are old, faulty, or no longer needed.

an inhibitor of the NFκB pathway (called IκB) can no longer be broken down, and instead it accumulates in the cell. IκB blocks NFκB and removes the cell's protection against apoptosis [128].

Other potential mechanisms of action of proteasome inhibitors include [128]:

- Causing the toxic accumulation of misfolded and broken proteins
- Causing the accumulation of cyclins at inappropriate stages of the cell cycle
- Causing the accumulation of p53, a powerful tumor suppressor protein able to trigger apoptosis

It is worth noting that, unlike BTK inhibitors or PI3K inhibitors, proteasome inhibitors weren't deliberately created as cancer treatments. In fact, prior to being tested for cancer, bortezomib was first explored as a treatment to prevent muscle wasting, and later as an anti-inflammatory [129]. Hence, what we know now about proteasome inhibitors' mechanisms of action has been pieced together after the completion of clinical trials proving them to be effective.

Over the years, huge numbers of patients have taken part in clinical trials investigating the usefulness of proteasome inhibitors against multiple myeloma. Some of the most recent trials have explored the usefulness of carflizomab and ixazomib.

For example, in the ASPIRE phase 3 trial, carflizomib was combined with dexamethasone (dex) and lenalidomide (len), and compared against dex plus len alone. This trial involved 792 patients, most of whom had received at least two other courses of treatment, often including bortezomib. In the trial, median PFS was 26.3 months with the addition of carfilzomib, and 17.6 months without [130]. A second trial, ENDEAVOR, compared dex + carfilzomib to dex + bortezomib. Median PFS was 18.7 months with carfilzomib versus 9.4 months with bortezomib [131].

The largest ixazomib trial completed to date is the TOURMALINE-MM1 phase 3 trial, which involved 722 people with relapsed multiple myeloma. As in the ASPIRE trial, ixazomib was given in combination with dex + len and compared to dex + len alone. Median PFS was 20.6 months with ixazomib and 14.7 months without [132].

7.6.3 Combining Proteasome Inhibitors with HDAC Inhibitors

One of reasons why proteasome inhibitors kill myeloma cells is because they cause the toxic accumulation of faulty, mis-folded, and broken proteins. However, cancer cells sometimes survive this by bundling all the faulty proteins into a compartment called an aggresome, where they are then destroyed. A protein called HDAC6 (histone deacetylase 6) is thought to help cells transport faulty proteins into these aggresomes [133]. HDAC inhibitors, such as panobinostat (Farydak) and vorinostat (Zolinza), block the creation of aggresomes and increase the anti-cancer effects of proteasome inhibitors [134].

However, although this all sounds very neat, it's important to know that there are at least 18 different HDAC proteins in human cells, and they perform a range of different functions. One of their most well-known actions is to control gene transcription (and hence the production of proteins) by controlling the accessibility of genes to transcription factors. So adding an HDAC inhibitor to a cancer patient's treatment is likely to have a range of different impacts on both cancer cells and healthy cells. In fact, HDAC inhibitors have at least six different mechanisms of action against multiple myeloma cells that have nothing to do with aggresomes [135]. Despite this complexity, panobinostat in combination with a proteasome inhibitor is a licensed combination in the United States and Europe.

The approval of panobinostat was due to the results from a subgroup of patients who took part in the PANORAMA-1 study. This subgroup of 193 patients had received at least two previous courses of treatment for their disease. The addition of panobinostat to a combination of bortezomib and dex improved patients' median PFS from 5.8 months to 10.6 months, and the response rate from 41% to 59%. However, 36% of patients experienced side effects that caused them to discontinue treatment with panobinostat [136].

7.7 THALIDOMIDE AND ITS DERIVATIVES

Like proteasome inhibitors, thalidomide and its derivatives lenalidomide (Revlimid) and pomalidomide (Imnovid; Pomalyst) are primarily used as treatments for multiple myeloma. Lenalidomide is also given to people with myelodysplastic syndromes,[28] and it's licensed for some people with mantle cell lymphoma.

Thalidomide, lenalidomide, and pomalidomide are often described as "immunomodulatory drugs" (IMiDs) because of their impact on the immune system. However, this term can be confusing as it sometimes gets used to describe other treatments (such as the antibodies that block checkpoint proteins on the surface of T cells – see Chapter 5, Section 5.3).

As with the proteasome inhibitors, thalidomide was not deliberately created to be a cancer treatment. In fact, it is famous for being the treatment for morning sickness that caused thousands of women to give birth to children with deformities in the early 1960s. It was only in the late 1990s that

doctors began testing thalidomide as a treatment for cancer.

Many different mechanisms of action have been discovered for thalidomide (summarized in Figure 7.17) including [137]:

1. Acting as an anti-inflammatory agent by blocking the release of TFNα by myeloid WBCs
2. Boosting the cancer-fighting activity of several different types of lymphoid WBCs (e.g., dendritic cells, cytotoxic T cells, and NK cells), and blocking the immune-suppressing effects of regulatory T cells (Tregs)
3. Blocking angiogenesis by disrupting the interaction between multiple myeloma cells and bone cells
4. Preventing multiple myeloma cells from proliferating and triggering them to undergo apoptosis

However, do be aware that the full mechanism of action of thalidomide is unknown, and there are many other postulated mechanisms outside of the four I've described here.

7.7.1 Thalidomide Derivatives

Thalidomide can be a helpful treatment for people with multiple myeloma (for an over-review of many different clinical trials, see [138]). But, as with virtually all treatments, it has limitations in terms of its effectiveness and side effects. Scientists have therefore tried to improve its properties by tweaking its chemical structure. By doing this, they created two new drugs, lenalidomide and pomalidomide, which have a very similar structure to that of thalidomide. Scientists believe that these two, newer drugs cause less severe side effects than thalidomide while also being more potent at blocking TNFα release and at activating T cells [137].

---

[28] Myelodysplastic syndromes are blood disorders that cause a drop in the number of healthy white blood cells.

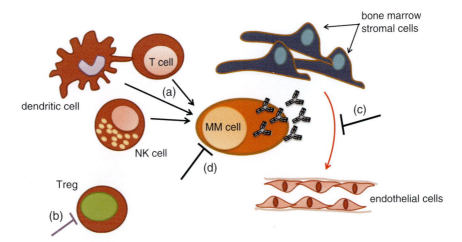

Figure 7.17 **Mechanisms of action of immunomodulatory drugs (IMiDs). (a)** IMiDs increase activity of cancer-fighting white blood cells: dendritic cells, T cells, and NK cells. **(b)** IMiDs suppress the activity of regulatory T cells. **(c)** IMiDs block angiogenesis by preventing multiple myeloma cells from triggering the release of VEGF by bone marrow stromal cells. **(d)** IMiDs can directly suppress proliferation and trigger multiple myeloma cell death.
Abbreviations: IMiDs – immunomodulatory drugs; NK – natural killer; Treg – regulatory T cell; VEGF – vascular endothelial growth factor

There have a few studies in which thalidomide and lenalidomide have been compared head to head (see [139] and [140] for two examples]. In several hospitals around the world, doctors have also looked back at their patients and compared the outcomes of people given thalidomide with those given lenalidomide [141]. In general, these researchers have concluded that the survival times of the two sets of patients are similar, but that lenalidomide does indeed cause less severe side effects. Various trials have shown that pomalidomide can be helpful for people whose disease is resistant to lenalidomide [142].

7.8 JAK2 INHIBITORS

In Chapter 3, I described the JAK-STAT signaling pathway and mentioned that it is overactive in some cancers. In particular, one of the four versions of JAK, called JAK2, is mutated in a high proportion of blood cancers known as the myeloproliferative neoplasms (MPNs).

7.8.1 About JAK-STAT Signaling

Just to recap: the JAK-STAT pathway (illustrated in Chapter 3, Figure 3.20 and described in Chapter 3, Section 3.9.1) is triggered by a range of signaling proteins such as cytokines and growth factors. These signaling proteins attach to receptors on the cell surface, which then trigger the activity of JAK and of other signaling pathways such as Ras/Raf/MEK/ERK and PI3K/AKT/mTOR. Each receptor is wired up in a slightly different way, and has a different ability to activate each pathway [143]. The receptors most able to trigger JAK-STAT activity are the cytokine receptors found on the surface of WBCs.

JAK is a kinase, and once it has been activated, it phosphorylates transcription factors known as STATs. These then pair up and move into the cell's nucleus. In the nucleus, STATs switch on the production of proteins that cause the cell to proliferate and help it to survive.

Mutated forms of JAK2 found in MPN cells cause them to grow and multiply. In recent years, scientists have concluded that all MPNs, even those in which JAK2 is normal, are driven by excessive JAK-STAT pathway activity [144].

For more about the JAK-STAT pathway and JAK-STAT inhibitors, see Chapter 3, Section 3.9.3.

7.8.2 Uses of JAK2 Inhibitors

Ruxolitinib (Jakafi; Jakavi) has been the subject of numerous clinical trials and is licensed in Europe and the United States to treat people with myelofibrosis and polycythaemia vera. Ruxolitinib and other JAK inhibitors are also in trials for various types of chronic and acute leukemia and for a variety of solid tumors [145, 146].

The benefits of ruxolitinib first became apparent when it was given to people with myelofibrosis in the COMFORT I and COMFORT II trials. In these trials, it became clear that ruxolitinib can reduce the size of people's spleens (people with myelofibrisos and other MPNs commonly have an enlarged spleen) and improve their symptoms and quality of life. It also improves survival times [147, 148].

Approval for ruxolitinib against polycythemia vera was based on the RESPONSE trial, in which ruxolitinib was compared to "best available therapy" in 222 patients. Treatment with ruxolitinib again shrank people's spleens and improved their symptoms and quality of life. Ruxolitinib also helped keep their red blood cells at normal levels. Many people experienced long-term control of their disease [149, 150].

7.9 BCL-2 INHIBITORS

Bcl-2 is a powerful protein that can protect cells from undergoing apoptosis (i.e., it protects them from death). Bcl-2 is not a kinase, and it's not on the cell surface; so it can't be blocked with a kinase inhibitor or a monoclonal antibody. Instead, scientists have created a variety of molecules that either prevent the Bcl-2 protein from being made or that bind to and block the Bcl-2 protein.

Bcl-2 inhibitors might be useful against a wide range of cancers, but so far most trials have involved patients with CLL. The first Bcl-2 inhibitor to be approved for use is a drug called venetoclax (Venclyxto; Venclexta), which was approved for the treatment for people with CLL in both Europe and the United States in 2016.

7.9.1 Bcl-2 Protects Cancer Cells from Apoptosis

One of the fundamental properties of cancer cells is that they contain DNA damage. This damage would normally activate proteins such as Bax, Bid, and Bak, which trigger the release of cytochrome C from the cells' mitochondria. Cytochrome C activates caspase proteins that trigger apoptosis [151] (Figure 7.18). Cancer cells often avoid death by producing high levels of apoptosis-suppressing proteins such as Bcl-2 and its close relatives Mcl-1 and Bcl-x$_L$. These proteins block Bax, Bid, and Bak (see Figure 7.19a), and they therefore prevent cytochrome C release.

Bcl-2 was first discovered in follicular lymphoma cells, in which a chromosome translocation causes massive overproduction of Bcl-2. The cells of CLL, multiple myeloma, diffuse large B cell lymphoma, mantle cell lymphoma, ALL, and some solid tumors also contain high levels of Bcl-2 [152, 153]. In some cancers, it is not Bcl-2 which is at fault but another part of the apoptosis-triggering machinery, such as overproduction of Mcl-1, or a lack of Bax or Bak [153].

7.9.2 Mechanism of Action of Bcl-2 Inhibitors

Scientists have tried various approaches to block Bcl-2. The approach that has so far proved most useful is to create drugs that

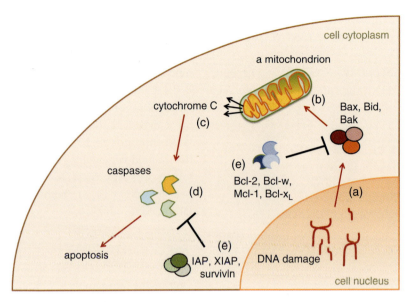

Figure 7.18 **Bcl-2 protects cells from apoptosis. (a)** When a cell's DNA becomes damaged or it detects the presence of lots of mis-folded proteins or another problem, the cell activates apoptosis-promoting proteins such as Bax, Bid, and Bak. **(b)** These pro-apoptosis proteins cause pores to form in the outer membrane of mitochondria. **(c)** A chemical called cytochrome C exits the mitochondria through the newly formed pores. **(d)** Cytochrome C triggers the activity of numerous caspase enzymes, which destroy many of the cell's proteins, leading to apoptosis. **(e)** Apoptosis can be prevented by proteins (such as Bcl-2) that block the activity of pro-apoptosis proteins, or by proteins (such as IAP) that block the activity of caspases.
Abbreviations: IAP – inhibitor of apoptosis

directly interact with Bcl-2 and prevent it from blocking apoptosis. These drugs are known as "BH3 mimetics", because they mimic the BH3 domain[29] found in naturally occuring "BH3-only" proteins. BH3-only proteins normally trigger apoptosis by using their BH3 domain to block Bcl-2 and other proteins like it (Figure 7.19b). Our cells trigger the activity of BH3-only proteins when they decide to die. So, drugs that mimic the shape of the BH3 domain can also block Bcl-2 and trigger cell death (Figure 7.19c).

Confusingly, all the proteins I've mentioned when talking about Bcl-2 inhibitors, plus a few extras (Bcl-2, Bcl-w, Mcl-1, Bcl-x_L, Bax, Bid, Bak, Bim, Puma, Bad, Noxa, Bid, and Bik) are part of the same family of proteins (and, in

fact, all of them have BH3 domains). There are at least 16 family members in human cells, some of which trigger apoptosis and some which prevent it [152, 153]. It's taken scientists several decades to work out the details of this family of proteins and to use this knowledge to kill cancer cells.

7.9.3 Uses of Bcl-2 Inhibitors

Several BH3 mimetics have been evaluated in clinical trials. As I write this, venetoclax is the furthest through development and was given FDA approval in April 2016 and EU approval in December 2016 for people with CLL. Two other drugs, obatoclax and navitoclax, were dropped because of toxicities – these drugs block Bcl-x_L as well as Bcl-2, and

---

[29] Its full name is the Bcl-2 homology domain-3.

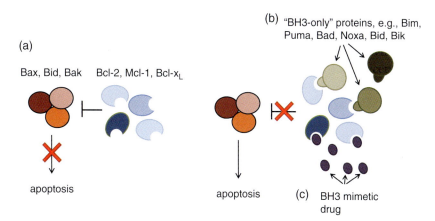

Figure 7.19 Mechanism of action of BH3-mimetic drugs. **(a)** Bcl-2, Mcl-1, and Bcl-x$_L$ block apoptosis by preventing the activation of Bax, Bid, and Bak. **(b)** DNA damage and other stress signals activate "BH3-only" proteins, which block Bcl-2, Mcl-1, and Bcl-x$_L$ and thereby allow apoptosis to take place. **(c)** Drugs that mimic BH3 also block Bcl-2, Mcl-1, and Bcl-x$_L$ and trigger apoptosis.

they therefore kill the body's platelets, which need Bcl-x$_L$ for survival. Venetoclax does not block Bcl-x$_L$ and therefore does not cause the same problem [154].

Venetoclax is licensed for people with CLL whose disease is resistant to BCR signaling inhibitors. It's also licensed for people whose CLL is predicted to be particularly aggressive because the cancer cells have a 17p deletion or *TP53* mutation (17p is the location of the *TP53* gene, so both of these mutations cause loss of the normal p53 tumour suppressor protein). Trials are also under way in other hematological cancers (including B cell lymphomas, multiple myeloma, and AML).

Unusually, the approvals of venetoclax in Europe and the United States were based on the results of phase 1 and phase 2 trials. One phase 2, single-arm study involved 107 people with CLL whose cancer cells contained deletion of *TP53*. In this trial, venetoclax brought about a response in 85 patients (79.4%) [155]. All the patients in the trial had relapsed or treatment-resistant disease, and

because of their *TP53* deletion, would have been unlikely to benefit from standard treatments such as chemotherapy combined with rituximab [156]. Results from phase 3 trials were just beginning to emerge in December 2017.

7.10 FLT3 AND KIT INHIBITORS

FLT3 and KIT are tantalizing drug targets for AML. They are growth factor receptors found on the cell surface that, like other growth factor receptors, control signaling pathways involving Ras, PI3K, and JAK proteins (Figure 7.20).Both receptors are found on the surface of very immature WBCs (known as primitive hematopoietic progenitor cells) in the bone marrow and are necessary for normal hematopoiesis [157].[30]

Mutation and over-expression of KIT and FLT3 are common in AML. In addition, the mutation and overproduction of these proteins is linked to poor survival times and a high risk of relapse [158, 159]. FLT3 and KIT

---

[30] Hematopoiesis is a process that takes place in our bone marrow in which hematopoietic stem cells multiply to give rise to all our blood cells and other components of the blood – shown in Chapter 5, Figure 5.1.

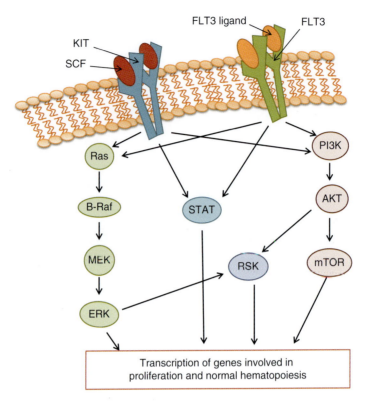

Figure 7.20 Signaling pathways controlled by FLT3 and KIT. Like the EGF receptor and other growth factor receptors, activation of FLT3 and KIT by their ligands leads to activation of various signaling pathways. **Abbreviations:** SCF – stem cell factor; FLT3 – FMS-like tyrosine kinase 3; STAT – signal transducer and activator of transcription; mTOR – mammalian target of rapamycin; PI3K – phosphatidylinositol 3-kinase; ERK – extracellular-signal-regulated kinase; RSK – p90 ribosomal S6 kinase

inhibitors have been developed and tested in trials. Currently, FLT3 inhibitors look to be the more promising and the first one, midostaurin (Rydapt), was licensed by the FDA in the United States in April 2017 and in Europe in September 2017.

7.10.1 FLT3 Mutations in AML

FLT3 responds to the presence of a growth factor called FLT3 ligand. Mutant versions of FLT3, which activate signaling pathways even when no FLT3 ligand is present, are found in the cancer cells of about 30% of people with AML [159]. The most common sort of mutation (found in around 23% of AML cases) is an internal tandem duplication (ITD) (Figure 7.21). ITDs occur when

part of the FLT3 gene is accidently duplicated and then reinserted back into the gene [160]. Point mutations affecting just one amino acid in the kinase domain of FLT3 are found in a further 7% of AML patients [159]. In addition, wild-type (i.e., normal, unmutated FLT3) is overproduced in 70%–100% of AML patients [161].

7.10.2 FLT3 Inhibitors

Because FLT3 is a growth factor receptor and therefore has kinase activity, it is possible to target it with kinase inhibitors. The first FLT3 inhibitors tested in trials, such as sorafenib, sunitinib, lestaurtinib, and midostaurin, block a wide range of different kinases [162]. These relatively nonspecific kinases inhibitors have

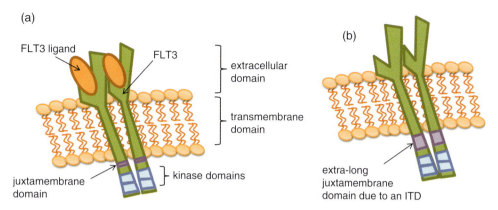

Figure 7.21 The structure of FLT3 showing the impact of internal tandem duplications. **(a)** The normal FLT3 protein is a growth factor receptor that responds to the presence of FLT3 ligand. FLT3 contains various different regions or "domains". The extracellular domain protrudes out of the cell and is where FLT3 ligand binds. The transmembrane domain spans the cell membrane. The juxtamembrane domain is just inside the cell, close to the membrane, and the protein's two kinase domains are inside the cell and responsible for activating signaling pathways. **(b)** When the *FLT3* gene is affected by mutations known as internal tandem duplications (ITDs), the FLT3 protein has a longer juxtamembrane domain. This change in the protein's shape causes its kinase domains to be constantly active.
Abbreviations: FLT3 – FMS-like tyrosine kinase

often given fairly modest benefits and cause lots of toxicities [163]. However, midostaurin became a licensed treatment in the United States and Europe in 2017 thanks to the results of the CALGB10603 (RATIFY) study involving over 700 patients. In this study, the median overall survival was 74.7 months in the group of patients given midostaurin compared to 25.6 months in patients give placebo. The proportion of people still alive after four years was 51.4% versus 44.3% [164].

Newer drugs such as quizartinib (AC220), crenolanib, gilteritinib (ASP2215), and PLX3397 have been designed to be much more selective FLT3 inhibitors. Trials with these agents report response rates of around 50%–60% in patients with FLT3-mutated AML [162], and the results of a phase 3 trial of quizartinib in AML [165], due in 2018, are hotly anticipated [166].

7.10.3 KIT Inhibitors

KIT inhibitors have a well-established role in the treatment of gastrointestinal stromal tumors (in which *KIT* gene mutations are common [167]). *KIT mutations are also present in some AMLs* [168, 169] and in mastocytosis – a disease of mast cells.[31] Most *KIT* mutations in AML cells affect KIT's activation loop, which controls the protein's kinase activity, or the extracellular domain [168].

Various KIT inhibitors have been tested in patients with AML, including imatinib and dasatinib [163, 169]. As well as blocking KIT, imatanib and dasatinib block a range of other kinases such as Bcr-Abl, PDGFR, and TEL. Thus far the trials have been relatively small and the results have been difficult to interpret [170, 171]. Other kinase inhibitors able to block KIT include nilotinib, sunitinib, pazopanib, and quizartinib. Again, all of these

---

[31] Mast cells are white blood cells found in the skin, stomach, and lungs – they are filled with histamine and are responsible for many of the symptoms of allergic reactions. Mastocytosis is a disease in which there are too many mast cells.

drugs block multiple kinases. It's going to be a few more years before we know whether KIT inhibitors have a future as treatments for AML.

7.11 IDH2 INHIBITORS

Mutations affecting two genes that code for IDH enzymes have been found in the cancer cells of about 12% of people with AML [172, 173]. IDH enzymes are involved in cell metabolism (the creation of energy for the cell). Mutant IDH enzymes found in AML cells produce high levels of a chemical called beta-hydroxygutarate (2-HG), which can prevent immature myeloid white blood cells from maturing properly [171].

Enasidenib (Idhifa) is the first IDH2 inhibitor to be licensed as a treatment for cancer. It was approved for people with IDH2-mutated AML in August 2017 in the United States. The approval was based on a single-arm study called AG221-C-001, in which 23% of 199 people given enasidenib had a complete remission [174]. A phase 3 trial (IDHENTIFY) involving 316 people with IDH2-mutated AML is due to report its findings in 2020.

7.12 CAR-MODIFIED T CELL THERAPY

I described CAR T cell therapy in detail in Chapter 5, Section 5.4.2. I also included brief results from two trials that led to the approval of tisagenlecleucel (Kymriah) and axicabtagene ciloleucel (Yescarta). Both of these treatments involve genetically modifying some of the patient's T cells so that they target cells which produce CD19. Tisagenlecleucel is licensed for children and young adults with ALL, whereas axicabtagene ciloleucel is licensed for adults with

various aggressive forms of NHL. A huge number of other CAR T cell approaches are being developed.

7.13 FINAL THOUGHTS

In this chapter, I have described a range of targeted therapies that have been, or are being developed, for the treatment of leukemias, lymphomas, and multiple myeloma. Many of these treatments build on decades of in-depth scientific studies on the nature of cancer cells – such as BTK, PI3Kδ, and Bcl-2 inhibitors. Others represent gradual improvements on treatments that have already been in use for many years such as some of the new anti-CD20 antibodies. Yet others owe their use to serendipity and lateral thinking, such as thalidomide derivatives and proteasome inhibitors.

However, although I've described lots of exciting developments and new treatments, there are some forms of hematological cancer where we've made very little progress. For example, we've seen relatively little progress in improving the survival times of adults with acute leukemias.

In addition, although we've seen lots of new treatments created for CLL, B cell NHL, and even multiple myeloma, these treatments are generally extending survival times rather than offering the possibility of a cure.

Inevitably, there are some licensed treatments that I've missed out of this chapter. Some are licensed for cancers that are extremely rare (e.g., acute promyelocytic leukemia and hairy cell leukemia) or that come in a range of equally rare forms (e.g., T cell lymphomas). With these cancers, I took the decision that the treatments for them are too niche to warrant including in a book aimed at a broad range of readers. I apologize if you were hoping to learn about a treatment that I haven't covered.

REFERENCES

1 Sompayrac LM (2015). How the Immune System Works (The How it Works Series) Paperback–Oct 23, 2015. https://www.amazon.co.uk/How-Immune-System-Works/dp/1118997778/ref=dp_ob_title_bk [Accessed January 5, 2018].

2 Murphy K, Weaver C (2016). *Janeway's Immunobiology*. New York: Garland Science; 9 edition. http://www.garlandscience.com/product/isbn/9780815345510 [Accessed January 5, 2018].

3 Jamieson CHM et al. (2008). Miscreant myeloproliferative disorder stem cells. *Leukemia* **22**: 2011–2019.

4 Cammenga J (2005). Gatekeeper pathways and cellular background in the pathogenesis and therapy of AML. *Leukemia* **19**: 1719–1728.

5 Inaba H et al. (2013). Acute lymphoblastic leukaemia. *Lancet* **381**(9881): 1943–1955.

6 Kuppers R (2005). Mechanisms of B-cell lymphoma pathogenesis. *Nat Rev Cancer* **5**: 251–262.

7 Du MQ and Isaccson PG (2002). Gastric MALT lymphoma: From aetiology to treatment. *Lancet Oncol* **3**(2): 97–104.

8 Information taken from two parts of the the Cancer Research UK website: The "About Cancer" section http://www.cancerresearchuk.org/about-cancer/ and the "Cancer Statistics for the UK" section: http://www.cancerresearchuk.org/health-professional/cancer-statistics [Accessed January 5, 2018].

9 Estimates of survival times for people with various types of non-Hodgkin lymphoma are taken from the Haematological Malignancy Research Network: https://www.hmrn.org/statistics/quick [Accessed January 5, 2018].

10 Larkin K, Blum W (2014). Novel Therapies in AML: Reason for Hope or Just Hype? *Am Soc Clin Oncol Educ Book*. 2014: e341–51.

11 Ehninger et al. (2014). Distribution and levels of cell surface expression of CD33 and CD123 in acute myeloid leukemia. *Blood Cancer J* **13**(4): e218.

12 Hoelzer D (2015). Personalized medicine in adult acute lymphoblastic leukemia. *Haematologica* **100**(7): 855–858.

13 Bower H et al. (2016). Life expectancy of patients with chronic Myeloid Leukemia approaches the life expectancy of the general population. *J Clin Oncol* **34**(24): 2851–2857.

14 Puiggros A et al. (2014). Genetic abnormalities in chronic lymphocytic leukemia: Where we are and where we go. *BioMed Res Int* **2014**: 435983.

15 Kipps J et al. (2017). Chronic lymphocytic leukaemia. *Nat Rev Dis Primers* **19**(3): 16096.

16 For a nice overview of CLL features that determine its aggressiveness see: CLL Support Association. Making sense of prognostic factors in CLL – Professor Andrew Pettitt – circa 2006. [online] Available at: https://www.cllsupport.org.uk/making-sense-prognostic-factors-cll-professor-andrew-pettitt-circa-2006 [Accessed January 4, 2018].

17 Diefenbach C and Advani R (2014). Customized targeted therapy in Hodgkin lymphoma: Hype or hope? *Hematol Oncol Clin North Am* **28**(1): 105–122.

18 Morgan GJ et al. (2012). The genetic architecture of multiple myeloma. *Nat Rev Cancer* **12**: 335–348.

19 Data from Haematological Malignancy Research Network:: Incidence and Survival. [online] Available at: www.hmrn.org/Statistics/quick [Accessed January 5, 2018].

20 Cammenga J (2005). Gatekeeper pathways and cellular background in the pathogenesis and therapy of AML. *Leukemia* **19**: 1719–1728.

21 Inaba H et al. (2013). Acute lymphoblastic leukaemia. *Lancet* **381**: 1943–1955.

22 Seifert M et al. (2012). Cellular origin and pathophysiology of chronic lymphocytic leukemia. *JEM* **209**(12): 2183.

23 Young RM, Staudt LM (2013). Targeting pathological B cell receptor signalling in lymphoid malignancies. *Nat Rev Drug Discov* **12**: 229–243.

24 de Leval L, Gualard P (2014). Cellular origin of T-cell lymphomas. *Blood* **123**(19): 2909–2910.

25 Rowley JD (2008). Chromosomal translocations: Revisited yet again. *Blood* **112**: 2183.

26 Baliakas P et al. (2014). Chromosomal translocations and karyotype complexity in chronic lymphocytic leukemia: A systematic reappraisal of classic cytogenetic data. *Am J Hematol*. **89**(3): 249–255.

27 For more about chromosomes and the way chromosome locations are written down, see: Genetics Home Reference (2017). How do geneticists indicate the location of a gene? [online] Available at: https://ghr.nlm.nih.gov/primer/howgeneswork/genelocation [Accessed January 5, 2018].

28 Rossi D and Gaidano G (2012). Molecular genetics of high-risk chronic lymphocytic leukemia. *Expert Rev Hematol* **5**(6): 593–602.

29 Hull EE et al. (2016). HDAC inhibitors as epigenetic regulators of the immune system: Impacts on cancer therapy and inflammatory diseases. *Biomed Res Int* **2016**: 8797206.

30 My sources of information are: The emc (electronic medicines compendium) http://www.medicines.org.uk/emc/; the National Cancer Institute list of cancer drugs http://www.cancer.gov/about-cancer/treatment/drugs; the European Medicines Agency http://www.ema.europa.eu/ema/

31 Humanized and fully human antibodies aren't necessarily better than mouse or chimeric. For a discussion, see: Getts DR, Getts MT, McCarthy DP et al. (2010). Have we overestimated the benefit of human(ized) antibodies? *MAbs* **2**(6): 682–694.

32 For more about the general properties of mAb treatments, see the Cancer Research UK website: http://www.cancerresearchuk.org/about-cancer/cancers-in-general/treatment/biological/types/about-monoclonal-antibodies [Accessed January 5, 2018].

33 Katz BZ, Herishanu Y (2014). Therapeutic targeting of CD19 in hematological malignancies: Past, present, future and beyond. *Leuk Lymphoma* **55**(5): 999–1006.

34 Hammer O (2012). CD19 as an attractive target for antibody-based therapy. *MAbs* **4**(5): 571–577.

35 Maloney DG (2012). Anti-CD20 antibody therapy for B-cell lymphomas. *N Engl J Med* **366**: 2008–2016.

36 Tu X, LaVallee T, Lechleider R (2011). CD22 as a target for cancer therapy. *J Exp Ther Oncol* **9**(3): 241–248.

37 Kreitman RJ & Pastan I (2011). Antibody Fusion Proteins: Anti-CD22 Recombinant Immunotoxin Moxetumomab Pasudotox. *Clin Cancer Res* **17**: 6398.

38 Waldmann TZ (2007). Daclizumab (anti-Tac, Zenapax) in the treatment of leukemia/lymphoma. *Oncogene* **26**: 3699–3703.

39 Coiffier B, Federico M, Caballero D (2014). Therapeutic options in relapsed or refractory peripheral T-cell lymphoma. *Cancer Treatment Rev* **40**(9): 1080–1088.

40 Schirrmann T, Steinwand M, Wezler X et al. (2014). CD30 as a therapeutic target for lymphoma. *BioDrugs* **28**(2): 181–209.

41 Hu S et al. (2013). CD30 expression defines a novel subgroup of diffuse large B-cell lymphoma with favorable prognosis and distinct gene expression signature: A report from the International DLBCL Rituximab-CHOP Consortium Program Study. *Blood* **121**(14): 2715–2724.

42 Loke J, Khan JN, Wilson JS (2015). Mylotarg has potent anti-leukaemic effect: A systematic review and meta-analysis of anti-CD33 antibody treatment in acute myeloid leukaemia. *Ann Hematol* **94**(3): 361–373.

43 Kenderian SS, Ruella M, Shestova O (2015). CD33-specific chimeric antigen receptor T cells exhibit potent preclinical activity against human acute myeloid leukemia. *Leukemia* **29**(8): 1637–1647.

44 Phipps C, Chen Y, Gopalakrishnan S (2015). Daratumumab and its potential in the treatment of multiple myeloma: Overview of the preclinical and clinical development. *Ther Adv Hematol* **6**(3): 120–127.

45 Van de Donk N et al. (2016). Monoclonal antibodies targeting CD38 in hematological malignancies and beyond. *Immunol Rev* **270**(1): 95–112.

46 Alinari L, Lapalombella R, Andritsos L et al. (2007). Alemtuzumab (Campath-1H) in the treatment of chronic lymphocytic leukemia. *Oncogene* **26**: 3644–3653.

47 Jaglowski SM, Alinari L, Lapalombella R (2010). The clinical application of monoclonal antibodies in chronic lymphocytic leukemia. *Blood* **116**(19): 3705–3714.

48 Tobinai K, Takahashi T, Akinaga S (2012). Targeting chemokine receptor CCR4 in adult T-cell leukemia-lymphoma and other T-cell lymphomas. *Curr Hematol Malig Rep* **7**(3): 235–240.

49 Lonial S, Dimopoulos M, Palumbo A et al. (2015). Elotuzumab therapy for relapsed or refractory multiple myeloma. *N Engl J Med* **373**(7): 621–631.

50 For a review, see: Lim SH, Levy R (2014). Translational medicine in action: Anti-CD20 therapy in lymphoma. *J Immunol* **193**(4): 1519–1524.

51 Weiner GJ (2010). Rituximab: Mechanism of action. *Semin Haematol* **47**(2): 115–123.

52 Summarized along with a helpful description of the complement pathway in: Zhou X, Hu W, Qin X (2008). The role of complement in the mechanism of action of Rituximab for B-cell lymphoma: Implications for therapy. *The Oncologist* **13**(9): 954–966.

53 For a review of lots of different approaches to building better antibody-based treatments, see: Weiner GJ (2015). Building better monoclonal antibody-based therapeutics. *Nat Rev Cancer* **15**: 361–370.

54 For an interesting description of why Bexxar failed to become a widely used treatment, see: Timmerman L (2013). Why Good Drugs Sometimes Fail: The Bexxar Story. Xconomy website. [online] Available at:http://www.xconomy.com/national/2013/08/26/why-good-drugs-sometimes-fail-in-the-market-the-bexxar-story/ [Accessed January 5, 2018].

55 Reviewed in: Larson SM, Carrasquillo JA, Cheung NK et al. (2015). Radioimmunotherapy of human tumours. *Nat Rev Cancer* **15**: 347–360.

56 Harding FA et al. (2010). The immunogenicity of humanized and fully human antibodies. *Mabs* **2**(3): 256–265.

57 Castillo F, Milani C, Mendez-Allwood D (2009). Ofatumumab, a second-generation anti-CD20 monoclonal antibody, for the treatment of lymphoproliferative and autoimmune disorders. *Expert Opin Investig Drugs* **18**(4): 491–500.

58 For an overview, see: Weiner GJ (2015). Building better monoclonal antibody-based therapeutics. *Nat Rev Cancer* **15**: 361–370.

59 Illidge T, Klein C, Sehn LH (2015). Obinutuzumab in hematologic malignancies: Lessons learned to date. *Cancer Treat Rev* **41**(9): 784–792.

60 Goede V et al. (2014). Obinutuzumab plus chlorambucil in patients with CLL and coexisting conditions. *N Engl J Med* **370**: 1101–1110.

61 Sehn LH et al. (2016). Obinutuzumab plus bendamustine versus bendamustine monotherapy in patients with rituximab-refractory indolent non-Hodgkin lymphoma (GADOLIN): A randomised, controlled, open-label, multicentre, phase 3 trial. *Lancet Oncol* **17**(8): 1081–1093.

62 Sehn LH et al. (2015). Randomized Phase II Trial Comparing Obinutuzumab (GA101) With Rituximab in Patients With Relapsed CD20+ Indolent B-Cell Non-Hodgkin Lymphoma: Final Analysis of the GAUSS Study. *J Clin Oncol* **33**(30): 3467–3474.

63 van Imhoff GW et al. (2017). Ofatumumab versus Rituximab salvage chemoimmunotherapy in relapsed or refractory diffuse large B-cell lymphoma: The ORCHARRD Study. *J Clin Oncol* **35**(5): 544–551.

64 For a write-up on this, and a list of biosimilar versions of rituximab in trials, see: GaBi online, Biosimilars of rituximab (2015). [online] Available at:: http://www.gabionline.net/Biosimilars/General/Biosimilars-of-rituximab [Accessed January 5, 2018].

65 European Medicines Agency (2017). Truxima. [online] Available at: http://www.ema.europa.eu/ema/index.jsp?curl=pages/medicines/human/medicines/004112/human_med_002077.jsp&mid=WC0b01ac058001d124 [Accessed January 5, 2018].

66 European Medicines Agency (2017). Meeting highlights from the Committee for Medicinal Products for Human Use (CHMP) April 18–21, 2017. [online] Available at: http://www.ema.europa.eu/ema/index.jsp?curl=pages/news_and_events/news/2017/04/news_detail_002732.jsp&mid=WC0b01ac058004d5c1 [Accessed January 5, 2018].

67 Magen H, Muchtar E (2016). Elotuzumab: The first approved monoclonal antibody for multiple myeloma treatment. *Ther Adv Hematol* **7**(4): 187–195.

68 Veilette A, Guo H. (2013). *Crit Rev Onc Hematol* **88**: 168–177.

69 Zhang K et al. (2017). Magic year for multiple myeloma therapeutics: Key takeaways from the ASH 2015 annual meeting. *Oncotarget* **8**(6): 10748–10759.

70 Lonial S et al. (2015). Elotuzumab therapy for relapsed or refractory multiple myeloma. *N Engl J Med* **373**(7): 621–631.

71 van de Donk NWCJ et al. (2016). Clinical efficacy and management of monoclonal antibodies targeting CD38 and SLAMF7 in multiple myeloma. *Blood* **127**: 681–695.

72 Sanchez L (2016). Daratumumab: A first-in-class CD38 monoclonal antibody for the treatment of multiple myeloma. *J Hematol Oncol* **9**: 51.

73 Palumbo A et al. (2016). Daratumumab, Bortezomib, and Dexamethasone for Multiple Myeloma. *N Engl J Med* **375**(8): 754–766.

74 Dimopoulos MA et al. (2016). Daratumumab, lenalidomide, and dexamethasone for multiple myeloma. *N Engl J Med* **375**(14): 1319–1331.

75 Graf SA, Gopal AK (2014). Treatment of relapsed classical Hodgkin lymphoma in the brentuximab vedotin era. *Hematology Am Soc Hematol Educ Program* **2014**(1): 151–157.

76 Younes A et al. (2012). Results of a pivotal phase II study of brentuximab vedotin for patients with relapsed or refractory Hodgkin's lymphoma. *J Clin Oncol* **30**(18): 2183–2189.

77 Moskowitz CH et al. (2015). Brentuximab vedotin as consolidation therapy after autologous stem-cell transplantation in patients with Hodgkin's lymphoma at risk of relapse or progression (AETHERA): A randomised, double-blind, placebo-controlled, phase 3 trial. *Lancet* **385**: 1853–1862.

78 Peggs KS (2015). Recent advances in antibody-based therapies for Hodgkin Lymphoma. *Br J Haematol* **171**: 171–178.

79 Galanina N et al. (2017). Emerging role of checkpoint blockade therapy in lymphoma. *Ther Adv Hematol* **8**(2): 81–90.

80 FDA (2016). Nivolumab (Opdivo) for Hodgkin Lymphoma. [Online] Available at: https://www.fda.gov/Drugs/InformationOnDrugs/ApprovedDrugs/ucm501412.htm [accessed January 5, 2018].

81 Goodman A et al. (2017). PD-1-PD-L1 immune-checkpoint blockade in B-cell lymphomas. *Nat Rev Clin Oncol* **14**(4): 203–220.

82 Gniadek TJ et al. (2017). Heterogeneous expression of PD-L1 in pulmonary squamous cell carcinoma and adenocarcinoma: Implications for assessment by small biopsy. *Modern Pathol* **30**: 530–538.

83 Green LM (2016). Nivolumab-Brentuximab Vedotin combo active and safe in relapsed Hodgkin lymphoma. OncLive [online] Available at: http://www.onclive.com/conference-coverage/ash-2016/nivolumabbrentuximab-vedotin-combo-active-and-safe-in-relapsed-hodgkin-lymphoma [Accessed January 5, 2018].

84 Jabbour E et al. (2015). Monoclonal antibodies in acute lymphoblastic leukemia. *Blood* **125**(26): 4010–4016.

85 Kantarjian H et al. (2017). Blinatumomab versus chemotherapy for advanced acute lymphoblastic leukemia. *N Engl J Med* **376**(9): 836–847.

86 Thota S, Advani A (2017). Inotuzumab ozogamicin in relapsed B-cell acute lymphoblastic leukemia. *Eur J Haematol* **98**(5): 425–434.

87 Kantarjian HM et al. (2016). Inotuzumab ozogamicin versus standard therapy for acute lymphoblastic leukemia. *N Engl J Med* **375**: 740–753.

88 Yang J, Reth M (2016). Receptor dissociation and B-cell activation. *Curr Top Microbiol Immunol* **393**: 27–43.

89 Kraus M, Alimzhanov MB, Rajewsky N et al. (2004). Survival of resting mature B lymphocytes depends on BCR signaling via the Igα/β heterodimer. *Cell* **117**: 787–800.

90 Reviewed in: Woyach JA, Johnson AJ, Byrd JC (2012). The B-cell receptor signaling pathway as a therapeutic target in CLL. *Blood* **120**(6): 1175–1184.

91 Hendricks RW, Yuvaraj S, Kil LP (2014). Targeting Bruton's tyrosine kinase in B cell malignancies. *Nat Rev Cancer* **14**: 219–232.

92 Reviewed in: Aalipour A, Advani RH (2014). Bruton's tyrosine kinase inhibitors and their clinical potential in the treatment of B-cell malignancies: Focus on ibrutinib. *Ther Adv Hematol* **5**(4): 121–133.

93 Honigberg LA et al. (2010). The Bruton tyrosine kinase inhibitor PCI-32765 blocks B-cell activation and is efficacious in models of autoimmune disease and B-cell malignancy. *PNAS* **107**(29): 13075–13080.

94 Described in more detail in: Wiestner A (2015). The role of B-cell receptor inhibitors in the treatment of patients with chronic lymphocytic leukemia. *Haematologica* **100**(12): 1495–1507.

95 Chanan-Kahn A et al. (2016). Ibrutinib combined with bendamustine and rituximab compared with placebo, bendamustine, and rituximab for previously treated chronic lymphocytic leukaemia or small lymphocytic lymphoma (HELIOS): A randomised, double-blind, phase 3 study. *Lancet Oncol* **17**(2): 200–211.

96 Reviewed in: Bose P, Gandhi V (2017). Recent therapeutic advances in chronic lymphocytic leukemia. *F1000Research* **6**: 1924.

97 O'Brien S et al. (2016). Ibrutinib for patients with relapsed or refractory chronic lymphocytic leukaemia with 17p deletion (RESONATE-17): A phase 2, open-label, multicentre study. *Lancet Oncol* **17**(10): 1409–1418.

98 Falchi L et al. (2016). BCR signaling inhibitors: An overview of toxicities associated with Ibrutinib and Idelalisib in patients with chronic lymphocytic leukemia. *Mediterr J Hematol Infect Dis* **8**(1): e2016011.

99 Reviewed in: Byrd JC et al. (2015). Acalabrutinib (ACP-196) in Relapsed chronic lymphocytic leukemia. *N Engl J Med* **374**: 323–332.

100 Wang M et al. (2017). Acalabrutinib in relapsed or refractory mantle cell lymphoma (ACE-LY-004): A single-arm, multicentre, phase 2 trial. *Lancet* 2017 Dec 11. pii: S0140-6736(17)33108-2. [Epub ahead of print].

101 For a longer list of BTK inhibitors in development, see: Akinleye A et al. (2013). Ibrutinib and novel BTK inhibitors in clinical development. *J Hematol Oncol* **6**: 59.

102 Cheah CY, Fowler NH, Wang ML (2016). Breakthrough therapies in B-cell non-Hodgkin lymphoma. *Ann Oncol* **27**(5): 778–787.

103 For a detailed overview of the topic of BTK resistance, see: Zhang SQ et al. (2015). Mechanisms of ibrutinib resistance in chronic lymphocytic leukaemia and non-Hodgkin lymphoma. *Br J Haematol* **170**: 445–456.

104 Woyach JA, Johnson AJ (2015). Targeted therapies in CLL: Mechanisms of resistance and strategies for management. *Blood* **126**(4): 471–477.

105 Maffei R et al. (2015). Targeting neoplastic B cells and harnessing microenvironment: The "double face" of ibrutinib and idelalisib. *J Hematol Oncol* **8**: 60.

106 Blunt MD, Steele AJ (2015). Pharmacological targeting of PI3K isoforms as a therapeutic strategy in chronic lymphocytic leukaemia. *Leuk Res Rep* **4**(2): 60–63.

107 For full details, refer to the emc: Zydelig (idelalisib) 100mg. Therapeutic indications. Emc [online]. Available at: http://www.medicines.org.uk/emc/medicine/29202#INDICATIONS [Accessed January 5, 2018].

108 Furman RR et al. (2014). Idelalisib and rituximab in relapsed chronic lymphocytic leukemia. *N Engl J Med* **370**(11): 997–1007.

109 Sharman J et al. (2014). Second interim analysis of a phase 3 study of idelalisib (ZYDELIG®) plus rituximab (R) for relapsed chronic lymphocytic leukemia (CLL): Efficacy analysis in patient subpopulations with del(17p) and other adverse prognostic factors. *Blood* **124**: 330.

110 CancerNetwork (2017). PI3K Inhibitors: Understanding Toxicity Mechanisms and Management. [online]. Available at: http://www.cancernetwork.com/oncology-journal/pi3k-inhibitors-understanding-toxicity-mechanisms-and-management [Accessed January 5, 2018].

111 Medicines and Healthcare products Regulatory Agency (2016). Idelalisib (Zydelig): Updated Indications and Advice on Minimising the Risk of Infection. Gov.uk website [online]. Available at: https://www.gov.uk/drug-safety-update/idelalisib-zydelig-updated-indications-and-advice-on-minimising-the-risk-of-infection [Accessed January 5, 2018].

112 Lowes R (2016). Gilead Stops Six Trials Adding Idelalisib to Other Drugs. Medscape website [online]. Available at: https://www.medscape.com/viewarticle/860372 [Accessed January 5, 2018].

113 Liu N et al. (2013). BAY 80-6946 is a highly selective intravenous PI3K inhibitor with potent p110α and p110δ activities in tumor cell lines and xenograft model. *Mol Cancer Ther* **12**: 2319–2330.

114 Dreyling M et al. (2017). CT149 – Copanlisib in patients with relapsed or refractory indolent B-cell lymphoma: Primary results of the pivotal Chronos-1 study. CT149. Presented at the 2017 AACR Annual Meeting, April 4, 2017; Washington, DC.

115　Stark AK et al. (2015). PI3K inhibitors in inflammation, autoimmunity and cancer. *Curr Opin Pharmacol* **23**: 82–91.

116　Tansey WP (2014). Mammalian MYC proteins and cancer. *New J Sci* **2014**: 757534.

117　Mato AR et al. (2017). Optimal sequencing of ibrutinib, idelalisib, and venetoclax in chronic lymphocytic leukemia: Results from a multicenter study of 683 patients. *Ann Oncol* **28**(5): 1050–1056.

118　Sharman J et al. (2015). An open-label phase 2 trial of entospletinib (GS-9973), a selective spleen tyrosine kinase inhibitor, in chronic lymphocytic leukemia. *Blood* **125**(15): 2336–2343.

119　Bower H et al. (2016). Life expectancy of patients with chronic myeloid leukemia approaches the life expectancy of the general population. *J Clin Oncol* **34**(24): 2851–2857.

120　Nowell PC (2007). Discovery of the Philadelphia chromosome: A personal perspective. *J Clin Invest* **117**(8): 2033–2035.

121　Cilloni D, Saglio G (2012). Molecular pathways: BCR-ABL. *Clin Cancer Res* **18**: 930.

122　Quintas-Cardama A, Kantarjian H, Cortes J (2007). Flying under the radar: The new wave of BCR–ABL inhibitors. *Nat Rev Drug Discov* **6**: 834–848.

123　Shah NP, Tran C, Lee FY et al. (2004). Overriding imatinib resistance with a novel ABL kinase inhibitor. *Science* **305**(5682): 399–401.

124　You can find an overview of this topic in: Maino E, Sancetta R, Viero P (2014). Current and future management of Ph/BCR-ABL positive ALL. *Expert Rev Anticancer Ther* **14**(6): 723–740.

125　Navon A, Ciechanover A (2009). The 26 S Proteasome: From basic mechanisms to drug targeting. *J Biol Chem* **284**: 33713–33718.

126　For a concise review of proteasome inhibitors, see: Moreau P (2014). Oral therapy for multiple myeloma: Ixazomib arriving soon. *Blood* **124**(7): 986–987.

127　Teicher BA, Tomaszewski JE (2015). Proteasome inhibitors. *Biochem Pharmacol* **96**(1): 1–9.

128　For a summary of many potential mechanisms of action of proteasome inhibitors, see: Crawford LJ, Walker B, Irvine AE (2011). Proteasome inhibitors in cancer therapy. *J Cell Commun Signal* **5**: 101–110.

129　Sanchez-Serrano I (2006). Success in translational research: Lessons from the development of bortezomib. *Nat Rev Drug Discov* **5**: 107–114.

130　Stewart AK et al. (2015). Carfilzomib, lenalidomide, and dexamethasone for relapsed multiple myeloma. *N Engl J Med* **372**: 142–152.

131　Dimopoulos MA et al. (2016). Carfilzomib and dexamethasone versus bortezomib and dexamethasone for patients with relapsed or refractory multiple myeloma (ENDEAVOR): A randomised, phase 3, open-label, multicentre study. *Lancet Oncol.* **17**(1): 27–38.

132　Moreau P et al. (2016). Oral Ixazomib, lenalidomide, and dexamethasone for multiple myeloma. *N Engl J Med* **374**(17): 1621–1634.

133　Hideshima T, Richardson PG, Anderson KC (2011). Mechanism of action of proteasome inhibitors and deacetylase inhibitors and the biological basis of synergy in multiple myeloma. *Mol Cancer Therapeutics* **10**(11): 2034–2042.

134　Richardson PG et al. (2013). PANORAMA 2: Panobinostat in combination with bortezomib and dexamethasone in patients with relapsed and bortezomib-refractory myeloma. *Blood* **122**: 2331–2337.

135　Tandon N, Ramakrishnan V, Kumar SK (2016). Clinical use and applications of histone deacetylase inhibitors in multiple myeloma. *Clin Pharmacol* **8**: 35–44.

136　Raedler LA (2016). Farydak (Panobinostat): First HDAC Inhibitor Approved for Patients with Relapsed Multiple Myeloma. *Am Health Drug Benefits* **9**(Spec Feature): 84–87.

137　Quach H et al. (2010). Mechanism of action of immunomodulatory drugs (IMiDS) in multiple myeloma. *Leukemia* **24**: 22–32.

138　Palumbo A et al. (2008). Thalidomide for the treatment of multiple myeloma: 10 years later. *Blood* **111**: 3968–3977.

139　Stewart AK et al. (2015). Melphalan, prednisone, and thalidomide vs melphalan, prednisone, and lenalidomide (ECOG E1A06) in untreated multiple myeloma. *Blood* **126**(11): 1294–1301.

140　Melphalan, prednisone, and lenalidomide versus melphalan, prednisone, and thalidomide) in untreated multiple myeloma. *Blood* **127**(9): 1109–1116.

141 Luo J et al. (2017). Comparative effectiveness and safety of thalidomide and lenalidomide in patients with multiple myeloma in the United States of America: A population-based cohort study. *Eur J Cancer* **70**: 22–33.

142 Holstein SA, McCarthy PL (2017). Immunomodulatory drugs in multiple myeloma: Mechanisms of action and clinical experience. *Drugs* **77**(5): 505–520.

143 Vainchenker W, Constantinescu SN (2013). JAK/STAT signaling in hematological malignancies. *Oncogene* **32**: 2601–2613.

144 Skoda RC et al. (2015) Pathogenesis of myeloproliferative neoplasms. *Exp Hematol* **43**: 599–608.

145 Springuel L, Renauld J-C, Knoops L (2015). JAK kinase targeting in hematologic malignancies: A sinuous pathway from identification of genetic alterations towards clinical indications. *Haematologica* **100**: 1240–1253.

146 Thomas SJ et al. (2015). The role of JAK/STAT signalling in the pathogenesis, prognosis and treatment of solid tumours. *BJC* **113**: 365–371.

147 Verstovsek S et al. (2012). A double-blind, placebo-controlled trial of ruxolitinib for myelofibrosis. *N Engl J Med* **366**(9): 799–807.

148 Cervantes F et al. (2013). Three-year efficacy, safety, and survival findings from COMFORT-II, a phase 3 study comparing ruxolitinib with best available therapy for myelofibrosis. *Blood* **122**: 4047–4053.

149 Vannucchi AM et al. (2015). Ruxolitinib versus standard therapy for the treatment of polycythemia vera. *N Engl J Med* **372**(5): 426–435.

150 Vertovsek S et al. (2016). Ruxolitinib versus best available therapy in patients with polycythemia vera: 80-week follow-up from the RESPONSE trial. *Haematologica* **101**(7): 821–829.

151 For a detailed overview of apoptosis, see: Elmore S (2007). Apoptosis: A review of programmed cell death. *Toxicol Pathol* **35**(4): 495–516.

152 Anderson MA, Huang D, Roberts A (2014). Targeting BCL2 for the treatment of lymphoid malignancies. *Semin Hematol* **51**: 219–227.

153 Delbridge ARD, Strasser A (2015). The BCL-2 protein family, BH3-mimetics and cancer therapy. *Cell Death Differentiation* **22**: 1071–1080.

154 Delbridge ARD et al. (2016). Thirty years of BCL-2: Translating cell death discoveries into novel cancer therapies. *Nat Rev Cancer* **16**(2): 99–109.

155 Stilgenbauer S et al. (2016). Venetoclax in relapsed or refractory chronic lymphocytic leukaemia with 17p deletion: A multicentre, open-label, phase 2 study. *Lancet Oncol* **17**(6): 768–778.

156 Rossi D et al. (2015). Molecular prediction of durable remission after first-line fludarabine-cyclophosphamide-rituximab in chronic lymphocytic leukemia. *Blood* **126**: 1921–1924.

157 Lyman SD et al. (1994). The flt3 ligand: A hematopoietic stem cell factor whose activities are distinct from steel factor. *Stem Cells* **12** Suppl 1: 99–107.

158 Paschka P, Dohner K (2013). Core-binding factor acute myeloid leukemia: Can we improve on HiDAC consolidation? *Hematology Am Soc Hematol Educ Program* **2013**: 209–219.

159 Wander SA, Levis MJ, Fathi AT (2014). The evolving role of FLT3 inhibitors in acute myeloid leukemia: Quizartinib and beyond. *Ther Adv Hematol* **5**(3): 65–77.

160 Stirewalt DL, Radich JP. The role of FLT3 in haematopoietic malignancies. *Nat Rev Cancer* **3**: 650–655.

161 Gilliland G, Griffin JD (2002). The roles of FLT3 in hematopoiesis and leukemia. *Blood* **100**(5): 1532–1542.

162 For a helpful discussion of early trials with FLT3 inhibitors, see: Lancet JE (2015). FLT3 Inhibitors for Acute Myeloid Leukemia. *Clin Adv Hematol Oncol* **13**(9): 573–575.

163 Larkin K, Blum W (2014). Novel therapies in AML: Reason for hope or just hype? *Am Soc Clin Oncol Educ Book* 2014: e341–51.

164 Stone RM et al. (2017). Midostaurin plus chemotherapy for acute myeloid leukemia with a *FLT3* mutation. *N Engl J Med* **377**: 454–464.

165 For details of the trial, search for NCT02039726 on the ClinicalTrials.gov website: https://clinicaltrials.gov/ct2/show/NCT02039726?term=NCT02039726&rank=1 [accessed January 5, 2018].

166 For a discussion of the possible results see: OncLive (2017). Expert Discusses Promise of

Quizartinib in AML. [online] Available at: http://www.onclive.com/web-exclusives/ expert-discusses-promise-of-quizartinib-in-aml [accessed January 5, 2018].

167 Xu Z et al. (2014). Frequent KIT Mutations in Human Gastrointestinal Stromal Tumors. *Scientific Reports* **4**: 5907.

168 Paschka P, Dohner K (2013). Core-binding factor acute myeloid leukemia: Can we improve on HiDAC consolidation? *Hematology Am Soc Hematol Educ Program* **2013**: 209–219.

169 Coombs CC, Tallman MS, Levine RL (2015). Molecular therapy for acute myeloid leukaemia. *Nat Rev Clin Oncol* **13**(5): 305–318.

170 For an example of a trial, see: Marcucci G et al. (2014). Adding *KIT* Inhibitor Dasatinib (DAS) to Chemotherapy Overcomes the Negative Impact of KIT Mutation/over-Expression in Core Binding Factor (CBF) Acute Myeloid Leukemia (AML): Results from CALGB 10801 (Alliance). Oral presentation at the *56th Annual Meeting and Exposition of the American Society of Hematology.* San Francisco, California.

171 Medinger M et al. (2016). Novel prognostic and therapeutic mutations in acute myeloid leukemia. *Cancer Genomics Proteomics* **13**(5): 317–330.

172 Reitman Z, Yan H (2010). Isocitrate dehydrogenase 1 and 2 Mutations in cancer: Alterations at a crossroads of cellular metabolism. *J Natl Cancer Inst* **102**(13): 932–941.

173 Stein EM (2018). Enasidenib, a targeted inhibitor of mutant IDH2 proteins for treatment of relapsed or refractory acute myeloid leukemia. *Future Oncol* **14**(1): 23–40.

174 U.S. Food and Drug Administration (2017). FDA Granted Regular Approval to Enasidenib for the Treatment of Relapsed or Refractory AML. [online] Available at: https://www.fda. gov/Drugs/InformationOnDrugs/ ApprovedDrugs/ucm569482.htm [Accessed January 5, 2018].

Appendix

A INFORMATION ON CELLS, DNA, GENES, AND CHROMOSOMES

Stated Clearly www.statedclearly.com

- An animation-led US website that explains various scientific concepts.
- Their video *What Is DNA and How Does It Work?* is a fantastic starting point for anyone confused about what DNA is and how it contains the instructions for making living things.

The "yourgenome" website www.yourgenome.org

- From the UK Wellcome Genome Campus.
- I recommend the "In the Cell" section, which includes a great video, *From DNA to Protein*, as well as pages such as: "What Is DNA?" "What is a Gene?" and "What is a Cell?"
- It includes articles, animations, and activities.

The New Genetics https://publications.nigms.nih.gov/thenewgenetics/index.html

- From the US National Institute of General Medical Sciences.

- It includes a section called "How Genes Work" – an easy-to-read but relatively in-depth overview of how the information in DNA is copied and used to make proteins.

The Khan Academy www.khanacademy.org/science/biology

- A US organization offering global online education.
- Contains a wealth of information (mostly overviews and videos) on a huge range of subjects.
- Includes "Structure of a Cell," "Cell Signaling," "DNA as the Genetic Material," "Central Dogma (DNA to RNA to Protein)," and "Gene Regulation."

Scitable www.nature.com/scitable/topics

- A free online teaching portal from Nature Education.
- For those of you who want more science!
- Contains detailed but fairly straightforward articles with many illustrations.
- I recommend their ebooks *Cell Biology* and *Essentials of Genetics*.

A Beginner's Guide to Targeted Cancer Treatments, First Edition. Elaine Vickers.
© 2018 John Wiley & Sons Ltd. Published 2018 by John Wiley & Sons Ltd.

Glossary of Terms

Acute lymphoblastic leukemia (ALL) An aggressive form of leukemia that is most common in children. It develops from immature white blood cells called lymphocytes in the bone marrow.

Acute myeloid leukemia (AML) An aggressive form of leukemia that is most common in adults aged over 65. It develops from immature white blood cells (granulocytes or monocytes) in the bone marrow.

ADCC (antibody-dependent cell-mediated cytotoxicity) The process by which a white blood cell (such as a macrophage or natural killer cell) binds to an antibody attached to a protein on the surface of a cell and then kills the cell.

Aerobic glycolysis The fermentation of glucose to create lactate and produce energy in the form of ATP. Cancer cells preferentially use this process to create ATP even when they have sufficient oxygen to perform normal respiration.

Adoptive cell transfer A form of immunotherapy in which modified cells are transferred into a patient. It includes immunotherapies in which T cells or dendritic cells are removed from a patient's blood, modified, and then returned.

Adjuvant treatment A treatment that is given together with, or following, another treatment. It commonly refers to giving a patient chemotherapy soon after surgery.

Adrenal glands Glands that sit on top of our kidneys and produce a range of hormones.

Allele Different versions of the same gene are called alleles. We are born with two alleles of each gene in our genome, one from each parent.

Amino acids These are small chemical compounds mostly made from carbon, oxygen, hydrogen, and nitrogen. They are attached to one another by ribosomes to create proteins. There are 20 common amino acids. The number, order, and physical and chemical characteristics of the amino acids that make up a protein determine its shape, function, and other properties.

Amplification (of a gene) Describes the fact that a cell has accidentally made extra copies of a gene.

Anaplastic lymphoma kinase (ALK) A growth factor receptor that in humans is encoded by the *ALK* gene.

Androgen receptors Part of a family of intracellular receptors that respond to hormones. Androgen receptors are activated

A Beginner's Guide to Targeted Cancer Treatments, First Edition. Elaine Vickers.
© 2018 John Wiley & Sons Ltd. Published 2018 by John Wiley & Sons Ltd.

by testosterone and dihydrotestosterone, and they are important in driving the growth and survival of almost all prostate cancers.

Aneuploid A word used to describe cells that contain the wrong number of chromosomes. Cancer cells are often aneuploid. Normal cells contain two copies of each of its 22 chromosomes, plus two X chromosomes or an X and a Y (46 in total).

Angiogenesis The development of a new blood vessel from a pre-existing blood vessel.

Angiogenesis inhibitors Treatments that block angiogenesis, usually by interfering with VEGF or VEGF receptors.

Antibody A large, Y-shaped protein produced by B cells in response to an infection. They circulate in the blood and attach precisely to their target, after which they attract complement proteins and white blood cells such as macrophages and natural killer cells. They can also be manufactured by living cells in a laboratory and used as cancer treatments.

Antibody–drug conjugate An antibody to which a toxic compound (such as chemotherapy) has been attached. The aim is that the antibody attaches to its target on the surface of a cancer cell, and then gets drawn inside the cell and delivers the drug, which kills the cell.

Antigen A protein or other molecule to which an antibody or T cell can attach. It could be a protein or other molecule found on the surface of a cancer cell, bacterium, or virus.

Adipocytes Specialized cells that store energy as fat (lipid). Also known as lipocytes and fat cells.

APOBEC enzymes A family of enzymes that protect our cells from viruses by chopping up their DNA. When inappropriately activated in human cells, they add to the DNA mutations in that cell. Cancer cells often contain patterns of DNA mutations that are caused by overactive APOBEC enzymes.

Apoptosis Also called "programmed cell death." A very precise, orderly, and tightly controlled process through which a cell self-destructs. It can be triggered when a cell's DNA is damaged or when so-called "death receptors" on its surface are triggered.

ATP (adenosine tri-phosphate) A chemical compound produced from the breakdown of glucose from our food. It contains high-energy chemical bonds, and it is used as the source of energy for every chemical reaction and energy-dependent process in our body.

Basket trial A clinical trial in which patients with different types of cancer are entered into a single trial because their cancers share a common feature, such as the presence of a particular DNA mutation.

Basement membrane A thin, fibrous layer of proteins that lies immediately underneath every sheet of epithelial cells in our body. It can also surround cells or separate two sheets of cells from one another. It provides structural support, limits contact between different cell types, and acts as a sieve. Also called the basal lamina.

B cells (B lymphocytes) Specialized white blood cells made in the bone marrow that have B cell receptors (BCRs) on their surface. They use their BCRs to detect infections. If they recognize an infection, they may release their BCRs (now called antibodies) into the blood. An antibody-producing B cell is called a plasma cell.

B cell receptor (BCR) BCRs are receptor proteins found on the surface of B cells. BCRs are constructed from immunoglobulin (Ig)/antibody genes. These genes are rearranged and pieced together by each B cell to create a unique BCR.

Bcl-2 inhibitors Drugs that inhibit Bcl-2 (B cell lymphoma 2), a protein protects our cells from death by apoptosis. So far they have successfully been used to treat chronic lymphocytic leukemia.

B-Raf inhibitor These drugs are most commonly used to treat people whose metastatic melanoma has a mutation in the *BRAF* gene. B-Raf is made from the *BRAF* gene, and it is a component of the MAP kinase (MAPK) signaling pathway.

Bcr-Abl A fusion protein made from two proteins called Bcr and Abl. This fusion protein is caused by a translocation between chromosomes 9 and 22, which is found in the cells of people with chronic myeloid leukemia (CML). The same translocation is sometimes found in acute lymphoblastic leukemia (ALL).

Biological agents Sometimes used as a term to refer to targeted treatments or immunotherapies, but has various meanings depending on the user.

Biomarker Something biological (such as the presence or absence of a particular gene mutation) that can be measured and evaluated to give useful information, such as how aggressive a cancer is or whether a patient is likely to benefit from a particular treatment.

Biopsy A small part of a tumor removed using needles or during surgery for later analysis.

Biosimilar A treatment that is a copy of a protein-based treatment such as a monoclonal antibody. They are called biosimilar rather than generic treatments because they are highly complex molecules made by living cells, and they may not be biologically identical to the original.

Blood brain barrier Refers to the fact that in our brain the cells lining the blood vessels (called endothelial cells) are slightly different, less permeable, and closer together than in the rest of the body. Thus, the brain is protected from many toxins and drugs that might be present in the blood.

BRCA1 and BRCA2 Two proteins made from the *BRCA1* and *BRCA2* genes. These proteins are both involved in a DNA repair process called homologous recombination (HR), and loss or suppression of either gene results in the cell being unable to perform HR. Many different inherited mutations in either *BRCA1* or *BRCA2* cause women to have a high risk of breast and ovarian cancer.

BTK (Bruton's tyrosine kinase) A kinase that plays a crucial role in B cell development and activation.

Cancer growth blockers Sometimes used as a term for treatments that block cell communication pathways.

Cancer growth inhibitors Sometimes used as a term for treatments that block cell communication pathways.

Cancer stem cell A cancer cell that has some of the properties of a normal stem cell; that is, it can both self-renew and give rise to other cancer cell types.

CAR-T cells T cells that are genetically engineered to produce special receptors on their surface called chimeric antigen receptors (CARs). CARs are proteins that allow the T cells to recognize a specific protein on tumor cells.

Carcinogen Anything that causes cancer is called a carcinogen.

Carcinoma A cancer that has developed from faulty epithelial cells.

Catalyst Something that causes the rate of a chemical reaction to increase. Enzymes are specialized proteins that act as catalysts in living cells.

CD (cluster of differentiation) antigen CD antigen is a general name used for the proteins and other molecules found on the surface of cells, particularly white blood cells.

CDC (complement-mediated cytotoxicity) When the complement protein C1q binds to an antibody attached to a protein on the surface of a cell, further complement proteins attach to C1q, forming a "membrane attack complex" which kills the cell.

Cell cycle The ordered and tightly controlled process a cell goes through each time it divides. Involves four phases: G1, S, G2, and mitosis.

Cell cycle checkpoints Times within the cell cycle when a cell halts the cell cycle and checks that everything is progressing properly.

Cell division The process by which a cell splits in two to create two cells.

Cell signaling The processes through which cells communicate with one another. Often involves receptors on the cell surface that can trigger the activity of cell signaling pathways within the cell.

Checkpoint protein A group of proteins found on the surface of white blood cells such as T cells. The checkpoint proteins on T cells are used by our body to control their level of activity. Examples include PD-1 and CTLA-4.

Checkpoint inhibitor A drug that blocks the activation of checkpoint proteins on T cells. Their purpose is to increase the activity of cancer-fighting T cells and hence destroy a tumor.

Chemotherapy Could refer to any drug used to treat cancer. However, chemotherapy is generally a term used to describe drugs that kill rapidly multiplying cells. Many of these drugs have been developed from natural chemicals extracted from plants or from mustard gases used in warfare. They generally cause side effects due to the destruction of healthy cells in the gut, immune system, and hair follicles (i.e., vomiting, vulnerability to infections, and hair loss).

Chimeric A chimeric protein contains bits of protein from more than one organism. For example, some monoclonal antibodies are chimeric as they are made of both mouse and human protein.

Chromosome A structure made from tightly coiled and packaged DNA, which is wrapped around histone proteins. Chromosomes are used to store the DNA in our cells safely. They have to be uncoiled for the chromosome to be duplicated or for genes to be transcribed to make proteins.

Chronic lymphocytic leukemia (CLL) A type of blood cancer that develops from mature lymphocytes. The majority are derived from B cells.

Chronic myeloid leukemia (CML) A blood cancer that develops from immature granulocyte white blood cells in the bone marrow.

Circulating tumor DNA (ctDNA) DNA that has escaped from a cancer and is circulating freely in the blood of a patient – also called circulating free DNA. ctDNA can be purified and used to detect DNA mutations in cancer cells or used to predict cancer recurrence or resistance to treatment.

Codon Ribosomes "read" mRNA three bases at a time. Each three base pair grouping is called a codon. Each codon (e.g., CAA, AUU, or GCU) instructs the ribosome to add a particular amino acid (e.g., glutamine, isoleucine, or alanine) to the protein it is constructing.

Combination therapy The use of two or more treatments that are given together to people with cancer. Often refers to a combination of two or more chemotherapies.

Complement proteins A complex system of proteins found in our blood that form part of our immune system. They work together to kill invaders and send signals to white blood cells.

Conjugated antibody An antibody that has been fused to something else such as a chemotherapy or radioactive particle.

Constant region The back-end of an antibody (also called the Fc). It is the part of the antibody that attracts white blood cells that have Fc receptors on their surface such as macrophages and natural killer cells.

Cross-talk When a protein or other molecule involved in a signaling pathway also influences the activity of another signaling pathway.

Cyclins A set of proteins that are manufactured and destroyed at precise points during the cell cycle and that control cyclin-dependent kinases (CDKs).

Cyclin-dependent kinase (CDK) A set of proteins that regulate the progression of a cell through the cell cycle by phosphorylating a protein called RB (retinoblastoma protein). They are controlled by cyclins.

Cytokines Similar to growth factors but largely secreted by cells of the immune system. Include chemokines and interleukins.

Cytoplasm The fluid that fills a cell and is enclosed by the cell membrane. It contains thousands of proteins alongside many different structures and compartments.

Cytotoxic Something that is toxic to living cells.

Dendritic cell A type of white blood cell. Millions of these cells patrol the body looking for infections and other problems. They display on their surface fragments of proteins they have found, and they look for T cells and B cells that recognize these fragments and can respond to the infection. They can also display fragments from cancer proteins and initiate a cancer-fighting immune response.

Desmoplasia Refers to the accumulation of fibrous proteins within the tumor microenvironment. It can act as a physical barrier that prevents cancer treatments from moving freely within a tumor and is a major cause of treatment resistance in pancreatic cancer in particular.

Diagnostic biomarker A biomarker that can be used to diagnose a particular type or sub-type of cancer.

Dimer When two identical (or closely related) proteins pair up, they create a dimer.

Dimerization When two proteins bump into one another and stick together to form a dimer, for example, when two epidermal growth factor (EGF) receptors are bound to EGF, they then dimerize and activate the MAPK pathway.

DNA (deoxy ribonucleic acid) A long, spiraling molecule made of two strands that wind around one another to create a double helix. The double helix is held together by relatively simple chemicals called DNA bases that pair up in a particular way. The order of the four bases in a DNA strand is called the DNA sequence. DNA is packaged up in our cells in structures called chromosomes.

DNA base Relatively simple (but vital) chemicals that hold together the DNA double helix. There are four subtly different DNA bases called A (adenine), C (cytosine), G (guanine), and T (thymine). A always pairs with T; C always pairs with G. The order of bases in DNA is critical as this carries the information for making proteins and for constructing the entire organism.

DNA polymerase An enzyme that creates DNA from DNA. Used by our cells to create duplicate sets of chromosomes prior to cell division.

Driver mutation A mutation found in a cancer cell that is thought to play an important role in driving the cell's abnormal behavior.

EGF (epidermal growth factor) A growth factor that stimulates cell growth, proliferation, and differentiation of many cell types by binding to its receptor, EGF receptor (EGFR).

EGFR (EGF receptor) A growth factor receptor found on the surface of many different cell types. It responds to the presence of a number of growth factors, the most important one being EGF. When activated by EGF, two EGFRs will pair up and trigger various cell signaling pathways.

EMA (European Medicines Agency) It is responsible for the scientific evaluation, supervision, and safety monitoring of medicines in the EU. Whether the United Kingdom will follow EMA decisions after it leaves the EU is yet to be decided.

Encode A term often used in relation to genes. Each gene encodes (i.e., contains the instructions to manufacture) one or more proteins.

Endothelial cells Specialized cells that line our body's blood and lymph vessels.

Enhancer Enhancer elements are short sequences of DNA to which transcription factors and other proteins can attach and control the activity of genes. Unlike promoters, they can be found a long way away from the genes they help to control.

Enzyme A protein that catalyzes a chemical reaction; examples include proteases, kinases, and methylases.

Epigenetics Describes changes to a cell's DNA that impact on gene activity but that don't involve changes to the sequence of DNA bases. Epigenetics often refers to changes to the backbone of the DNA molecule (e.g., by methylation) or to the histone proteins that DNA is wrapped around (e.g., by acetylation). These changes alter the accessibility of the gene's DNA to transcription factors and hence influence whether the gene is transcribed.

Epithelial cells A very common type of cell in the body. Sheets of epithelial cells line the body's cavities, organs, and glands and cover flat surfaces.

Epithelial to mesenchymal transition (EMT) A process through which epithelial cells change to become more like mesenchymal cells, which are more mobile, independent, and robust. Cancer cells that go through the EMT are more likely to cause metastasis and survive treatment.

Extracellular matrix (ECM) A network of proteins and complicated sugar molecules that surround the cells in our tissues and organs.

FDA (US Food and Drug Administration) It regulates human drugs and medical devices (among other things) in the United States.

Fibroblasts A cell in connective tissue (e.g., bones, cartilage, tendons, ligaments, and fatty tissue), which produces collagen and other fibers. They are the most common type of connective tissue cell in the body.

Fluorescence in situ hybridization (FISH) A laboratory technique used to detect the presence of DNA mutation such as an amplification, translocation, or gene rearrangement.

Fusion protein A protein made from parts taken from two or more different proteins. These are made by cells when the DNA in two genes has broken and been spliced together to create a new, mutated gene. Often caused by translocations.

Gene A stretch of DNA within a chromosome which contains all the information a cell needs to make one or more proteins.

Gene activity Refers to how often a gene's information is accessed by the cell and used to make a particular protein.

Gene activation When a cell "switches on" a gene and starts using the information it contains to make a protein.

Gene expression When a gene's information is being used by a cell to make a protein, that gene is said to be "expressed," "switched-on," or "active."

Generic treatments These treatments are exact copies of an existing treatment.

Genome The complete set of genetic material in a cell, including all the DNA in a cell's chromosomes and the small amount of DNA found in the mitochondria.

Genomic instability A phenomenon seen in cancer cells. Refers to the fact that cancer cells accumulate DNA damage at a faster rate than other cells, largely due to faulty DNA repair proteins and short telomeres.

G-protein coupled receptors A group of over 1,000 receptor proteins found on human cells that respond to stimuli such as light, lipids, sugars, proteins, and peptides. They perform a vast array of different functions.

Growth factor A small protein that binds to specific receptors on target cells called growth factor receptors. Growth factors often promote cell survival and stimulate cell growth and proliferation.

Growth factor receptor Receptor proteins on our cells that respond to the presence of growth factors. There are 58 different growth factor receptors found on the cells in our body. They are also referred to as receptor tyrosine kinases (RTKs).

Hedgehog pathway A signaling pathway active in some cell types including adult and embryonic stem cells and some cancer cells. Involves a receptor called Patched, to which hedgehog proteins can bind.

HER2 Human EGF receptor-2. A member of the EGF receptor family which comprises EGFR, HER2, HER3, and HER4. Also called ErbB2 or Neu.

Heterodimer A dimer made up of two similar but not identical subunits.

HLA See **MHC protein** for a description.

Homodimer A dimer made up of two identical subunits.

Homologous recombination (HR) Our cells' preferred method for repairing double-strand breaks in its DNA. It is an error-free form of DNA repair.

Homologous recombination deficient (HRD) Cells that cannot perform homologous recombination are HRD. They are forced to use error-prone methods to repair double-strand DNA breaks and consequently accumulate DNA mutations rapidly. There is optimism that HRD cancer cells can be killed with treatments called PARP inhibitors.

Hodgkin lymphoma A hematological (blood) cancer driven by faulty mature B cells called Reed Sternberg (RS) cells.

Humanized antibody An antibody that contains mostly human protein, but a small amount of mouse protein remains.

Hypothalamus A region of the brain responsible for making a variety of important hormones.

Immunoglobulins B cell receptors (BCRs) that have been released by B cells into the blood (also known as antibodies).

Immunomodulators A drug that has the ability to affect (modulate) the patient's immune system. Usually used to refer to thalidomide, lenalidomide, and pomalidomide.

Immunotherapy Treatments that activate or restore the ability of the immune system to fight cancer.

Immunohistochemistry (IHC) A laboratory technique that uses antibodies to detect a particular protein of interest in a sample.

Intracellular Within the cell rather than on the cell surface.

Intratumoral heterogenicity Describes the fact that a single tumor (or blood cancer) can contain multiple populations of cancer cells with different properties.

Kinase An enzyme that can attach phosphate to one or more targets. Their targets are often other proteins. The addition of phosphate might activate or inhibit the target, or alter its ability to interact with other proteins. In many cancers, numerous kinases are overactive or present at abnormally high levels. Drugs that act as kinase inhibitors are used to treat various forms of cancer.

Kinase inhibitors Drugs that block the action of one or more kinases.

Ligand A molecule (often a small protein) that can bind to a particular receptor.

Liquid biopsy (fluid biopsy) A sample of a patient's blood from which scientists purify and analyze whole cancer cells or DNA that has leaked out from cancer cells.

Leukocyte A general name for any white blood cell.

Locus The specific position on a chromosome where a gene is located.

Lymphatic spread When a cancer spreads via the lymph vessels.

Lymph node Small bean-shaped organs located throughout the body. Millions of white blood cells live inside them, and fluid from the body's tissues drains into them.

Lymphocytes These include B cells, T cells, and natural killer (NK) cells.

Lymphoid cells There are two main groups of white blood cells: (1) myeloid cells, such as macrophages and dendritic cells, and (2) lymphoid cells, such as B cells and T cells.

Lymphoma A cancer of mature lymphocytes in a lymph node. Can be non-Hodgkin lymphoma or Hodgkin lymphoma. Most are derived from B cells rather than T cells.

Macrophage A type of white blood cell that engulfs and digests cellular debris, foreign substances, microbes, and cancer cells. Also has many other functions such as playing a pivotal role in inflammation and controlling the activity of T cells in our tissues.

Maintenance therapy A treatment that is given to patients following another treatment. It may include treatment with drugs, vaccines, or antibodies that kill cancer cells, and it may be given for a long time.

Malignant disease (malignancy) A disease (cancer) in which abnormal cells multiply out of control and have the potential to invade nearby tissues.

MAPKs Mitogen-activated protein kinases – a family of closely related intracellular protein kinases that includes ERK, JNK, and p38.

MAP kinase pathway (MAPK pathway) A signaling pathway commonly activated when a growth factor such as EGF binds to a growth factor receptor such as EGFR. The term specifically refers to signaling pathways involving ERK or other MAPKs such as JNK and p38. Other components of the pathway include Ras, Raf, and MEK.

Mast cell A type of white blood cell involved in allergic reactions and other immune responses.

Melanoma skin cancer A cancer of melanin-producing cells (melanocytes) in the skin. This is the most aggressive and dangerous form of skin cancer. It is also referred to as malignant melanoma. (Uveal melanoma develops from cells that make melanin in the eye.)

Menarche The age at which a girl gets her first period.

Messenger RNA (mRNA) Similar to DNA but exists as a single strand rather than a double helix. mRNA is manufactured by RNA polymerase, which detects the order of DNA bases in a gene and constructs a corresponding strand of mRNA to match. The mRNA is then transported to ribosomes in the cytoplasm, which use the mRNA to make proteins.

Metastasis A secondary cancer that has developed from breakaway cells from the original tumor that have spread to another part of the body.

MHC protein (major histocompatibility complex protein) MHC proteins (also called human leukocyte antigen – HLA) are found on the surface of all our cells. Our cells use MHC class 1 proteins to display fragments from the proteins they make to white blood cells. Specialized white blood cells such as macrophages and dendritic cells also have MHC class 2 proteins on their surface, which they use to display fragments of proteins they have picked up from their environment.

Microenvironment The immediate small-scale environment of a cell or tumor.

Missense mutation A single nucleotide change in DNA, which alters the amino acid sequence of the encoded protein. A type of point mutation.

Mitochondria These are tiny structures within our cells that create energy for the cell. They take in glucose and fatty acids and convert them into ATP, a high-energy molecule that the cell uses to power its chemical reactions and other functions. Mitochondria also contain some genes (made of DNA), which it uses to create a series of proteins. In addition, when a cell is damaged its mitochondria may release cytochrome C, which triggers apoptosis.

Mitosis The stage in the cell cycle in which the cell finally splits into two to create two daughter cells.

Monoclonal antibody All antibody treatments for cancer are monoclonal. That is, the millions of copies of the antibody in the treatment are identical to one another and have been manufactured using a population of genetically identical cells (a clone).

MRI scan Magnetic resonance imaging. Uses powerful magnets to generate an image of the inside of the body.

MSI – microsatellite instability A phenomenon seen in cancers in which the cancer cells contain faults in a type of DNA repair called mismatch repair. Regions of the cell's chromosomes called microsatellites consequently contain thousands of mutations.

Mutation Any change to the DNA of a cell. Can occur naturally or be caused by exposure to DNA-damaging agents (carcinogens) such as cigarette smoke and UV light.

Myc An important oncogene; a transcription factor.

Myeloid cells There are two main groups of white blood cells: (1) myeloid cells, such as macrophages and dendritic cells, and (2) lymphoid cells, such as B cells and T cells.

Myeloid-derived suppressor cells A group of white blood cells of myeloid origin that are able to suppress other white blood cells, such as T cells.

Multiple myeloma A hematological cancer that develops from faulty plasma cells. Plasma cells are antibody-producing B cells, which are generally found in the bone marrow.

Next generation sequencing A term that refers to various modern techniques to sequence DNA.

NICE The National Institute for Health and Care Excellence – the body that provides national guidance on the treatment of cancer and decides which treatments should be available through the NHS in England.

Natural killer cell Also known as NK cells. These are a type of lymphocyte white blood cell that play a major role in identifying and destroying faulty cells, including cancer cells and cells infected by viruses.

Neuroblastoma A rare cancer affecting children that develops from embryonic cells of the nervous system.

Neutrophil The most abundant type of white blood cell in the human body. A type of myeloid cell. They are short-lived and very mobile and quickly enter sites of infection.

Non-Hodgkin lymphoma A group of hematological cancers caused by faulty, mature lymphocytes (most are caused by faulty B cells). Some are fast growing, such as diffuse large B cell lymphoma; others are slow-growing, such as follicular lymphoma.

Nonsense mutation A point mutation in a gene that creates a stop codon part way through the gene and hence instructs the cell to make a shortened (truncated) version of a protein.

Nucleus The membrane-bound compartment within a cell which contains the cell's DNA in the form of chromosomes.

Estrogen receptor (ER) A receptor often found in breast cancer cells. In the presence of estrogen, these receptors pair up and act as transcription factors that activate transcription of a wide variety of genes.

Oncogene A gene that has the potential to cause cancer. In cancer cells, oncogenes are often mutated in such a way that the protein made from the gene has become overactive or is produced at abnormally high levels. Many oncogenes control cell proliferation and survival.

Oncogene addiction When a cancer cell is completely dependent on an oncogene for its survival.

Oncolytic virus A virus that preferentially infects and kills cancer cells. As the infected cancer cells are destroyed, they release new infectious virus particles that can infect neighboring cells. In addition, as the cancer cells die, they release cell debris into their surroundings that can be picked up by white blood cells and cause an anti-cancer immune response.

Oxygen free radicals (ROS or reactive oxygen species) These are highly active oxygen atoms that cause DNA damage. They are produced naturally in our body during various essential chemical reactions. They are also released by white blood cells and are present in cigarette smoke, air pollutants, and industrial chemicals.

p53 A very important tumor suppressor protein made from the *TP53* gene. It controls the production of DNA repair proteins and triggers cell death if the cell's DNA is badly damaged.

PARP – Poly (ADP-ribose) polymerase Has various functions, one of which is to detect single-strand breaks in DNA and bring in a team of other proteins to perform repair.

PARP inhibitors Treatments that block PARP. These treatments are particularly effective against cancers that have lost the ability to perform error-free DNA repair

through a process called homologous recombination (HR).

Passenger mutation A mutation found in a cancer cell that is adding little or nothing to the cell's abnormal behavior.

Peptide/polypeptide A chain of amino acids not long enough to be called a protein.

Pericytes These are elongated cells that are wrapped around our capillaries (small blood vessels). They can control blood flow and provide structural support and growth factors to the endothelial cells that line the capillaries.

Perineural spread When a cancer spreads by traveling along nerve bundles.

Pharmacodynamics The study of the effects that a drug has on the body.

Pharmacokinetics The study of the movement, absorption, distribution, metabolism, and excretion of a drug from the body.

Philadelphia chromosome An extra-short version of chromosome 22 created by a translocation affecting chromosomes 9 and 22. This translocation forces the cell to make an abnormal protein – a fusion of two proteins called Bcr and Abl. Found in the cancer cells of chronic myeloid leukemia (CML) and occasionally in the cells of acute lymphoblastic leukemia (ALL).

Phosphate A phosphorous atom surround by oxygen atoms.

Phosphorylation When a phosphate group is added to a molecule, such as a protein, sugar, or lipid. The addition of a phosphate group to a protein usually triggers its activity or changes its ability to interact with other proteins.

PI3K/AKT/mTOR pathway A cell signaling pathway important in controlling cell behavior. The target of some cancer treatments.

Pituitary gland A tiny organ, the size of a pea, located at the base of the brain. It produces various hormones.

Point mutation Mutation of a single base pair (nucleotide) in DNA.

Precision medicine An emerging approach in which the characteristics of a patient's cancer are matched with the treatment most likely to be effective for them.

Predictive biomarker A characteristic of cancer cells that can be measured and that tells you whether a particular treatment is likely to be effective or not.

Prognostic biomarker A characteristic of cancer cells that can be measured and that gives an idea of the likely outcome of the patient independently of what treatment they receive. For example, the presence of a particular mutation might be linked to a shortened survival time.

Proliferation Rapid reproduction of cells through cell division.

Promoter A region of DNA found immediately before the start of a gene. It is a place where transcription factors can attach to the gene and recruit RNA polymerase in order to initiate gene transcription.

Protein A big molecule made up of small chemical compounds called amino acids. Hundreds of thousands of proteins are found in our cells and form the basis of body structures such as skin and hair and of substances such as enzymes, cytokines, and antibodies. The instructions for making proteins are found in our genes.

Protein kinase A protein that can add a chemical group called a phosphate group to other proteins, often resulting in a change in their activity.

Proteasome A complicated, cylindrical structure made up of various different proteins. Thousands of them are found in each of our cells, which use them to break down unwanted proteins into their constituent amino acids.

Proto-oncogene A gene involved in normal cell growth. Mutation of a proto-oncogene may cause it to become an oncogene, which can drive the growth of cancer cells. NB. The distinction between proto-oncogenes and oncogenes isn't always adhered to, and the term *proto-oncogene* seems to be falling into disuse.

Prostaglandin A group of tiny, fatty compounds produced by many cells. They are produced at sites of injury or infection and control inflammation, blood flow, and clot formation.

Pseudoprogression When a tumor appears to be growing but will in fact later stabilise or shrink.

PTEN An important tumor suppressor protein that blocks the PI3K/AKT/mTOR pathway and prevents DNA mutations. The gene for PTEN (*PTEN*) is often suppressed or deleted in cancer cells.

Radioimmunotherapy A term used to describe an antibody which has been linked to a radioactive isotope and that is used to deliver radiotherapy to cancer cells.

Radiolabeled antibody Same as radioimmunotherapy.

Radiotherapy A treatment used in cancer involving the use of high-energy radiation to kill tumor cells.

Randomized control trial A clinical trial in which patients are allocated randomly (randomized) into different groups. Each group is given a specific treatment or allocated to be a control group that receives a comparison treatment or a dummy treatment (placebo).

RAS genes An important set of oncogenes that are mutated in many cancers. There are three versions of the gene (*KRAS, NRAS,* and *HRAS*) which encode three main Ras proteins (K-Ras, N-Ras, and H-Ras). Ras proteins are an integral part of the MAPK cascade. They are not kinases and hence cannot be blocked with a kinase inhibitor.

RB (retinoblastoma protein) An important tumor suppressor protein made from the *RB* gene. RB halts the cell cycle unless phosphorylated by CDKs (cyclin-dependent kinases).

Receptor A protein that binds to specific signals from outside the cell, such as growth factors. Many receptors are on the cell surface, such as growth factor receptors. Other receptors, such as some hormone receptors, are found in the cell cytoplasm and nucleus.

Receptor tyrosine kinase A class of receptors found on the surface of our cells. Many of them are growth factor receptors that respond to the presence of growth factors such as EGF.

Recombinant DNA technology Describes techniques used by scientists to create DNA sequences that wouldn't normally exist.

Reed Sternberg (RS) cells Large abnormal cells derived from B cells that drive Hodgkin lymphoma.

Ribosome A large structure made from ribosomal RNA and various proteins. It uses the information in messenger RNA (mRNA) to select and attach together tens, hundreds, or thousands of amino acids to construct a protein. Thousands of ribosomes are found in the cytoplasm of each of our cells.

RNA (ribonucleic acid) A complex molecule similar to DNA. Made from four bases: A, C, G, and U (uracil). Used in the manufacture of proteins.

RNA polymerase An enzyme that creates RNA from DNA. Used by our cells to create mRNA from genes. Ribosomes use the information in mRNAs to make proteins.

Sarcoma A cancer that has developed from bone, cartilage, fat, muscle, tendons, blood vessels, or other connective tissues.

Senescence A dormant state in which the cell is no longer able to divide. It can be triggered by short telomeres and DNA damage.

Signaling pathway/signal transduction cascade A chain reaction of events triggered by a signal (such as the binding of a growth factor to its receptor) at the cell surface, which is then transmitted through the cell and into the nucleus, where it causes a change in the cell's behavior.

Stem cell A cell which can both self-renew, and give rise to other cell types. Various types of stem cells are found in the developing embryo and in healthy adult tissues.

Stromal cells The cells (such as fibroblasts, endothelial cells, pericytes, and adipocytes) that support a tissue or tumor.

Synthetic lethality When a combination of mutations and/or the inhibition of two or more proteins leads to cell death, whereas the mutation/inhibition of only one of these proteins does not.

Targeted treatment/therapy A treatment that has the ability to target a particular protein or faulty process found in cancer cells. Targeted treatments are designed to discriminate between cancer cells and healthy cells better than other treatments such as chemotherapy, but in reality this isn't always achieved.

T cell (T lymphocytes) A type of lymphocyte (white blood cell) that plays a central role in cell-mediated immunity. T cells can be distinguished from other lymphocytes, such as B cells and natural killer cells, by the presence of T cell receptors on the cell surface.

Telomerase An enzyme that lengthens telomeres.

Telomere Stretches of DNA at each end of our chromosomes. They protect our genes and prevent gene breakages and rearrangements. As we get older, our cells' telomeres get shorter.

Toxin A poisonous substance (often a protein) produced by living cells.

Transcoelomic spread When cancer spreads via the fluid circulating in the abdomen.

Transcription The process by which an enzyme called RNA polymerase reads the order of DNA bases in a gene and uses this information to make a copy of that gene in the form of messenger RNA (mRNA).

Transcription factor A protein that can attach to DNA at particular locations (called gene promoters and enhancers) and that helps switch on the transcription of one or more genes. Examples of transcription factors important in cancer cells include p53, Myc, and the estrogen and androgen receptors.

Translation The process by which a ribosome uses a piece of mRNA to make a protein.

Translocation A chromosome abnormality caused by rearrangement of parts of two different chromosomes. A gene fusion may be created when the translocation joins two otherwise separate genes.

Tumor suppressor gene A gene that encodes a protein that helps control and limit cell growth or that is able to trigger cell death. In cancer cells, tumor suppressor genes are often deleted, mutated, or suppressed so that their protective function is lost.

Umbrella trial A type of clinical trial designed to test the impact of multiple drugs on different populations of patients in a single trial. The patients all have the same type of cancer, but are allocated to specific groups based on properties such as the presence of certain mutations.

Vaccine A biological preparation (such as a protein fragment from a virus or other disease-causing microorganism) that, when administered to a person, stimulates their immune system in such a way that it provides long-lasting protection against that organism. Cancer treatment vaccines are used to provoke an immune response against an existing cancer in the patient's body.

Variable region The front-end of an antibody (also called the Fv). This is the part of an antibody that attaches to its target.

Vascular spread When a cancer spreads via the bloodstream.

VEGF Vascular endothelial growth factor. VEGF attaches to VEGF receptors on endothelial cells that line blood vessels. This causes blood vessels to sprout and grow to create new blood vessels, and this is called angiogenesis.

VDJ recombination The process by which T cells and B cells randomly assemble different gene segments – known as variable (V), diversity (D) and joining (J) genes – in order to generate unique receptors (B cell receptor or T cell receptor) that they place on their surface to allow them to recognize invading microbes or cancer cells.

Whole genome sequencing When the DNA is extracted from a single cell or sample of tissue and subjected to DNA sequencing analysis. "Whole genome" refers to the fact that the entire genome is sequenced rather than just the genes, which only take up about 1%–5% of the cell's DNA.

Wild-type The usual, non-mutated version of a gene.

Index

Page locators in **bold** indicate tables. Page locators in *italics* indicate figures.

A Beginner's Guide to Targeted Cancer Treatments, First Edition. Elaine Vickers.
© 2018 John Wiley & Sons Ltd. Published 2018 by John Wiley & Sons Ltd.